Ludwig M. Auer Vera Van Velthoven

Intraoperative Ultrasound Imaging in Neurosurgery

Comparison with CT and MRI

With 466 Figures
in 547 Separate Illustrations

Springer-Verlag Berlin Heidelberg New York
London Paris Tokyo Hong Kong

LUDWIG M. AUER, M. D., Professor of Neurosurgery
Neurosurgical Department, University Hospital Graz, Austria
Neurosurgical Department, Krankenhaus Nordstadt
Haltenhoffstrasse 41, D-3000 Hannover 1

VERA VAN VELTHOVEN, M. D., Assistant Professor of Neurosurgery
Neurosurgical Department, University Hospital
De Pinte Laan, B-9000 Gent

ISBN-13:978-3-642-74047-3 e-ISBN-13:978-3-642-74045-9
DOI: 10.1007/978-3-642-74045-9

Library of Congress Cataloging-in-Publication Data. Auer, Ludwig M., 1948- . Intraoperative ultrasound imaging in neurosurgery : comparison with CT and MRI / Ludwig M. Auer, Vera Van Velthoven. p. cm. Bibliography: p. Includes index. ISBN-13:978-3-642-74047-3 1. Brain-Surgery. 2. Ultrasonic encephalography. 3. Brain-Tomography. 4. Brain-Magnetic resonance imaging. 5. Operative ultrasonography. I. Velthoven, Vera Van, 1953- . II. Title. [DNLM: 1. Brain--pathology. 2. Surgery, Operative. 3. Ultrasonic Diagnosis. WL 141 A917i] RD594.A84 1990 617'.481059-dc19 DNLM/DLC for Library of Congress 89-6052 CIP

Softcover reprint of the hardcover 1st edition 1990

Reproduction of the figures: Gustav Dreher GmbH, D-7000 Stuttgart

2122/3130 - 543210 - Printed on acid-free paper

Preface

Almost a decade has passed since intraoperative real-time ultrasound imaging became available for routine use in daily practice. Our own initial difficulties in the handling of this technique and the interpretation of images stimulated us to put together this introductory atlas based on the cumulative experience from over 500 neurosurgical intraoperative investigations, the first book to appear on this topic. This volume is thus intended primarily as a practical guide to the handling of the instruments, anatomical orientation in the intracranial cavity and the interpretation of pathomorphological changes on ultrasound images. In order to facilitate recognition of well-known image patterns, we have emphasized the comparison of ultrasound with conventional neuroimaging methods such as computerized tomography (CT) and magnetic resonance imaging (MRI).

Not all of the examples shown in this atlas are typical lesions where ultrasound imaging is of practical use for one reason or another; rather, we selected the cases on didactic grounds, to allow the reader first to become accustomed to the appearance of parts of the brain on ultrasound images, and thereafter to recognize a variety of pathomorphological changes which have previously been diagnosed by means of other imaging techniques such as CT or MRI. A separate chapter is then dedicated to those applications where we found intraoperative ultrasound imaging to be of real practical use.

We are indebted to Prof. Dr. E. Vogler, Head of the Department of Radiology of the University of Graz, and his colleagues for kindly allowing us to use the CT and MR images of our patients for this atlas. We also thank the staff of the Department of Neurosurgery of the University of Graz for their cooperation in so many intraoperative ultrasound investigations, and we are especially grateful to Anton Pein for his technical assistance, to Elga Pöschl for preparing all the photographs of CT and MR images and above all to Elfriede Meier for her patient and reliable secretarial assistance in the preparation of the manuscript.

We also want to thank Mr. W. Bergstedt and Mrs. M. Gründler of Springer-Verlag and their team for their generous assistance and marvellous cooperation in the composition of this atlas.

L. M. Auer
V. Van Velthoven

Contents

General Introduction 1

Technical Remarks 3
Generation of Ultrasound Waves 3
Origin of Tissue Echoes 4
Transformation of Ultrasound Waves 4
Importance of Ultrasound Frequency for Imaging in Neurosurgery 6
Artifacts and Limitations in the Interpretation of Images 6
Biological Effects of Ultrasound Imaging 7
Note on the Technical Equipment 7

Practical Handling of the Ultrasound Probe During Investigation 10
Imaging with Dura Closed or Open? 10
Landmarks for Orientation in the Normal Brain and Intracranium 11
Horizontal View 12
Orientation of the Sector Plane in the Intracranial Space: Hand-Eye Coordination 12
Sagittal View 16
Coronal View 18
Orientation in the Posterior Fossa 20

Intracranial Pathomorphology 23
General Remarks 23
Gliomas 24
Meningiomas 47
Metastases 65
Ventricular Tumors 78
Posterior Fossa Lesions 83
Other Tumors 92
Brain Abscesses 97
Hydrocephalus 99
Subarachnoid Hemorrhage, Aneurysms and Arteriovenous Malformations . . 108
Intracerebral Hematomas 122

Practical Application of Intraoperative Imaging 131
Intraoperative Anatomical Orientation 131
Intraoperative Control After Tumor Removal 147
Ultrasound-Guided Stereotaxy 152
Endoscopic Evacuation of Intracerebral Hematomas 156
Endoscopic Biopsy of Cystic Brain Tumors 159
Ultrasound-Guided Biopsy of Brain Tumors 166
Ultrasound-Guided Drainage of Brain Abscesses 169

References 170

Subject Index 172

General Introduction

The primary objective of any technique for morphological imaging of the brain is to detect pathological structures such as tumor or hematoma. It is also important, e.g., before instituting therapy, to ascertain the exact anatomical relations of a lesion with the surrounding brain tissue, as well as the general topographical situation in the cranial cavity.

The imaging procedure should yield information on the histopathology of the lesion in order to enable selection of adequate therapeutic measures at the earliest possible point of management. Recent developments in noninvasive imaging technology such as computerized tomography (CT) and magnetic resonance imaging (MRI) have revolutionized pathomorphological diagnosis in many cases, permitting precise location and delineation of a lesion and clear demonstration of its anatomical relations. However, reliable information on the histopathology of the lesion can not be expected in the majority of circumstances.

Another piece of information important to the operating neurosurgeon, but not given by any of the modern preoperative imaging techniques, is the direct correlation of the pathoanatomical and topographical information with the reality of the operating field, for instance when the surgeon is confronted with a normal-looking cerebral cortex harboring a tumor less than 1 cm in diameter. This gap can now be closed with the aid of intraoperative real-time ultrasound (US) imaging.

The basic knowledge of US physics dates back to theoretical advances made toward the end of the nineteenth century, the applicability of which is linked to the discovery of the piezoelectric effect of certain crystals by J. and P. Curie in 1880 [9]. The first practical application of acoustic echos for object localization took place under water in the search for the wreck of the Titanic in 1912 [48]; there was further rapid development of techniques during both world wars, the aim being the detection of submarines.

Dussik, of Austria, was the first to apply US for medical diagnosis: this also represented the first application of US in the brain for the demonstration of the lateral ventricles [12]. The first use of US by neurosurgeons dates back to 1950, when French et al. [21] tried to obtain echo signals from tumors in autopsy brains. The technique of using the lateral shift of echo signals from midline structures to detect mass lesions such as hematomas, described by Leksell in 1954 [39], found widespread application until it was replaced by CT. The transformation of echo signals into a gray-scale image made US imaging interesting for clinical diagnostic use; since bone is a barrier for US waves modern real-time sector scanners were first applied in pediatric medicine to obtain images of the brain through the open fontanelles. The opening of the skull in the course of neurosurgery obviously represents another opportunity to image the brain by means of US. The first reports on the successful demonstration of intracerebral pathomorphology were published by Rubin and Dohrmann in 1980 [58] and by Masuzawa et al. in 1981 [45].

The rapidly increasing technical excellence of real-time imaging of intracerebral pathomorphology and the improvements in topographical orientation make the method interesting for use in daily neurosurgical routine. The interpretation of US images together with CT and MR images is thus a challenge for the neurosurgeon. Both the initial practical difficulties and the subsequent enthusiasm on increasing experience stimulated the authors to write this introductory atlas, which is designed to help the reader interpret images of the most common pathomorphological processes as well as some of the less frequent findings in operative neurosurgery.

The first part of the book provides the reader with a necessary minimum of technical background to the useful practical application of the method, together with some comments on sources of artifacts and limitations on the interpretation of images.

The second section describes landmarks for anatomical orientation on US images of conventional planes of brain sections, as also used for CT and MRI, and discusses some of the common oblique US sections.

The third part shows a variety of pathological lesions as they typically appear on US images, with the CT and/or MRI appearance for comparison.

The fourth section of the book goes on to describe the practical day-to-day application of the method. Besides providing anatomical orientation, useful during a wide variety of neurosurgical interventions, this section also goes one step further and demonstrates how US imaging can be used in stereotactic surgery for pathfinding from a point on the skull to a target deep in the brain.

Discussion of US in pediatric neurosurgery is limited to the intraoperative applications. Transfontanellar imaging has been described extensively in the literature (e.g., [3, 40, 50, 31]).

It must be emphasized for the benefit of readers inexperienced in the practical application of this method that the images presented in this atlas are single pictures from real-time sequences like single frames from a movie. The real image encountered on the video monitor of the US apparatus can thus be expected to yield a significantly better two-dimensional impression of a lesion. Moreover, manual movement of the US probe gives the surgeon a three-dimensional impression of the spaces and structures within the brain.

Technical Remarks

It cannot be the purpose of this atlas to provide a detailed description of the technical background to US imaging; however, the basic principles will be briefly outlined inasfar as they are required for the adequate application of this method in daily clinical practice.

Sound is a mechanical energy transmitted in wave form by movement of molecules; this movement is induced by a pressure which pushes one molecule against the next in a chain reaction.

Ultrasound waves, like sound waves and other forms of energy transmitted in wave forms, follow certain physical laws such as those of refraction and reflection. The phenomenon of reflection of US waves, termed "echo" like the reflection of sound waves, is exploited for US imaging, which is thus a method of echography. The method as it is used today and as demonstrated in this atlas can be called "real-time ultrasound echotomography"; what "real time" and "tomo" stand for will be briefly outlined in the following.

As a first step let us consider how the US waves are generated and directed, where they are reflected to give an echo signal, and how this echo is received.

Generation of US Waves

The generator of US waves is a special quartz or synthetic ceramic crystal. How can a crystal distribute US waves? Not on its own, but as a result of the so-called piezoelectric effect (Fig. 1). When a crystal is placed into an electric field, the electrons cause a sudden change in the structure of its grid - the crystal grows or shrinks. This sudden structural change causes a sound wave by pushing the molecules surrounding the crystal. Each crystal is induced to distribute waves at one and only one frequency. For US imaging, frequencies between 3 and 10 MHz are used. When the crystal is exposed to alternating current of 5 MHz, it will distribute US waves oscillating at a frequency of 5 MHz. The same crystal has also the ability to transform an US wave of the same frequency back into an electromagnetic wave. This "incoming" US wave can, for example, be the echo of the wave sent out into biological tissue. The electrical current resulting from transformation of the US echo in the crystal is a measure of its amplitude. The time-delay between the sending of the wave and the return of the echo is a measure of the depth of the point in the tissue where the echo was produced.

Primarily, the crystal sends the US waves into all directions. Therefore, an "acoustic lens", functioning like an optic lens, is used to bundle the waves (Fig. 2). The image resolution, i.e. the sharpness of the US image, depends on the difference in depth between the zone of focus and the section imaged.

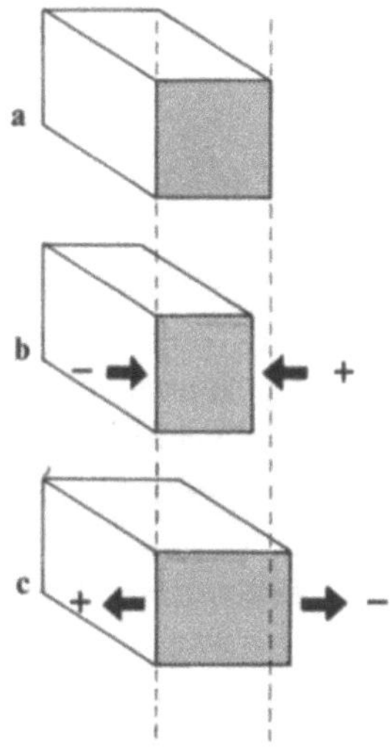

Fig. 1a-c. Piezoelectric effect. Depending on the polarization in an electrical field, the crystal **(a)** will shrink **(b)** or expand **(c)**, emitting mechanical energy in the form of sound waves on rapid fluctuation between the shrunken and expanded states in a field of alternating current

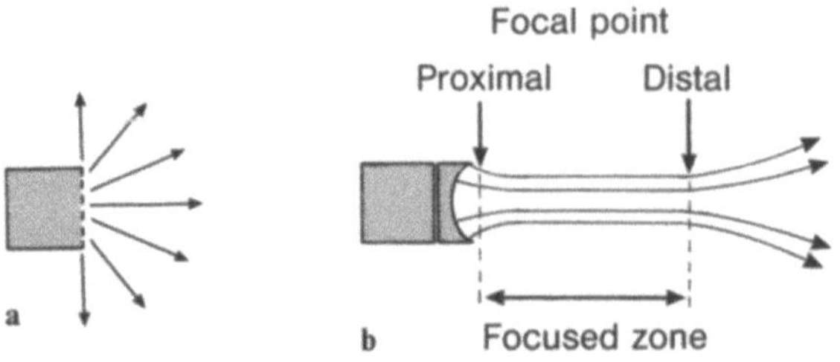

Fig. 2. **a** The crystal emits sound waves in all directions. **b** The acoustic lens in front of the crystal bundles the sound waves to a focal zone (between arrows)

Origin of Tissue Echoes

The US wave energy arriving in biological tissue encounters areas of different density and different mechanical properties - connective tissue, bone, fluids etc. The principle acoustic property of a tissue, its acoustic impedance, is determined by its density and the velocity of US waves through it.

The US wave behaves like other waves, such as light, in that refraction and reflection occur at the interfaces between media of different densities. Thus, it is at the interface between two tissues with different acoustic impedance that the US wave undergoes refraction and reflection; the echo is the part of the wave reflected back toward the crystal. The intensity of the echo depends on the difference in acoustic properties between two adjacent tissue compartments: the greater the difference, the greater the amount of reflected US energy, hence the higher the echo intensity. Therefore, an acoustically homogeneous area such as a CSF space will display a low echo intensity. By contrast, tissues composed of many small compartments of different densities will exhibit a high echo intensity.

At the interface between tissue and air, total reflection occurs. This explains why a layer of air in the field of observations acts as a barrier. Equally, a bubble of air will create a "shadow" where imaging is not possible because no US waves arrive in the area behind the air (Fig. 6). Therefore, it is of great importance to use a perfect layer of gel as a couple between the surface of the crystal (i.e., the surface of the US probe) and the sterile rubber membrane which covers the probe. Moreover, either the rubber membrane must be in direct contact with tissue, such as the dura, or the area in between must be filled with material of similar acoustic impedance, e.g., saline.

The same phenomenon of total reflection of the US wave occurs at the surface of bone. Therefore US imaging can only be performed through bone windows. Bony structures in the US image show up as a hyperechoic barrier with a shadow behind (i.e., a dark area) (Fig. 6).

Transformation of US Waves

We have said that the echo reflected back to the crystal is transformed by the crystal into electrical energy; this again is transformed into a light spot on a television monitor, using a gray scale: low echo signals are depicted as dark spots, high echo signals give a bright or even white spot. Seen in an idealized way, the US waves are sent out along a line (US beam). The point of origin of the echo along this line is calculated by the computer built into the US apparatus from the time delay between the sending of the wave signal and the arrival of the echo back at the crystal.

As long as we hold the US probe in a fixed position, the US image we see on the monitor is produced by automatic movement of the crystal over a plane of tissue or by using a multicrystal detector with electronic guidance (Figs. 3, 4).

Movement of the crystal is achieved either by wobbling (oscillator) or by rotation within the housing of the probe (Fig. 3). Each movement of the crystal over a sector plane gives one image of this plan of tissue, i.e., an echotomogram composed of many echo lines from US beams one next to the other (Fig. 3c, d). This primarily static echotomogram is made into a real-time echotomogram by the motion of the crystal over the sector plane at a frequency of 30-50 movements per second, thus producing 30-50 images per second, which are shown on the monitor like a movie.

As we start to move the US probe by hand over, for example, the dura, the sector plane is changed, and we get a real-time three-dimensional impression of the intracranial space. The left-

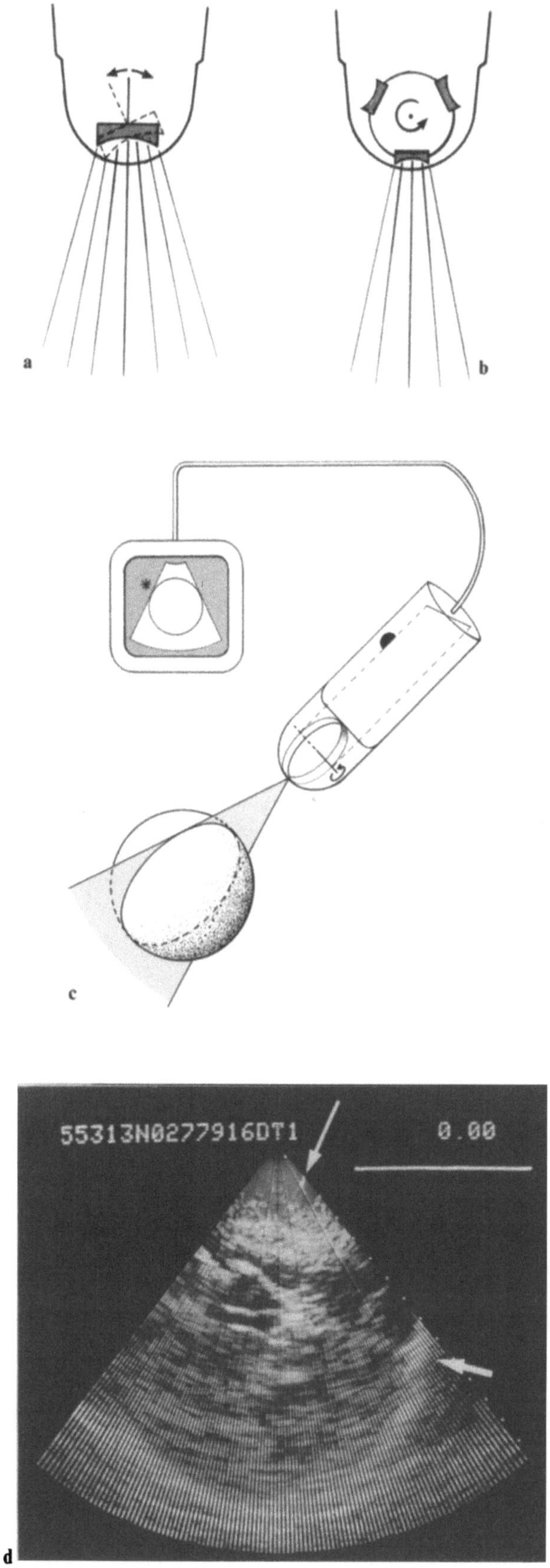

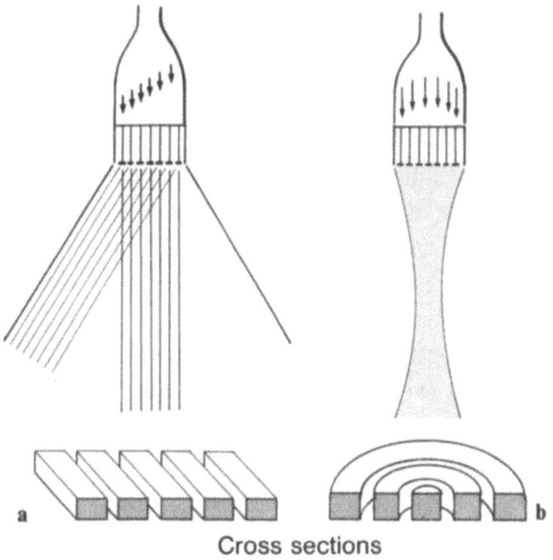

Fig. 4a, b. Multiple-element transducer with juxtaposed or annular elements, electronically activated. **a** Phased array; **b** annular array. The cross sections show the arrangements of the crystals

right and anterior-posterior orientation in space is obtained by observing anatomical landmarks and their movement during manual movement of the US probe (see p. 11 for further explanation). The interpretation of gray values on an image is based on qualitative comparison of the echo intensity with that of normal brain tissue. Thus, an area with lower echo intensity than normal brain wil be called "hypoechoic", while an area with higher echo intensity than normal brain will be termed "hyperechoic".

Fig. 3a–d. Single-element transducer driven by a motor. **a** Production of a sector image of oscillating (wobbling) the crystal. **b** Production of a sector image by rotating the crystal. **c** Production of a sector image by means of rotating the crystal system. The image on the monitor shows the scan of a section through a globe. The black dot on the US probe and the asterisk on the screen correspond to each other and aid left-right orientation. **d** One of the first published real-time US images of the brain, showing the individual echo lines that make up the image (see explanation on p. 1). (From Masuzawa et al. [45] by kind permission of the authors)

Importance of US Frequency for Imaging in Neurosurgery

Principally, there is an inverse relation between the US frequency used and the depth of penetration of the US beam. Employing a low frequency such as 3 MHz, the whole cranial cavity can be reached from a cranial bone window. However, there is also a direct relation between frequency and resolution, i.e., imaging quality: at 3 MHz the image will give only a fairly rough impression of the brain (poor axial resolution), with especially poor demonstration of the area near the US probe (Fig. 5).

By contrast, the use of a high frequency will provide excellent imaging of the immediate surroundings of the US probe (high axial resolution); however, the image reaches only a few centimeters deep. The reason is the high attenuation of high-frequency US waves - so that after the waves have travelled a few centimeters no energy is left for echoing. This is an especially important consideration for intraoperative neurosurgical US, where the lesion may be a few millimeters or over 10 centimeters away from the probe. Even for routine use, therefore, frequencies of 5 MHz and 7.5 MHz or even 10 MHz should be available. With a low-frequency probe only, lesions like a small subcortical metastasis may be missed; if only a high-frequency probe is available, the search for a deep-seated lesion will be unsuccessful.

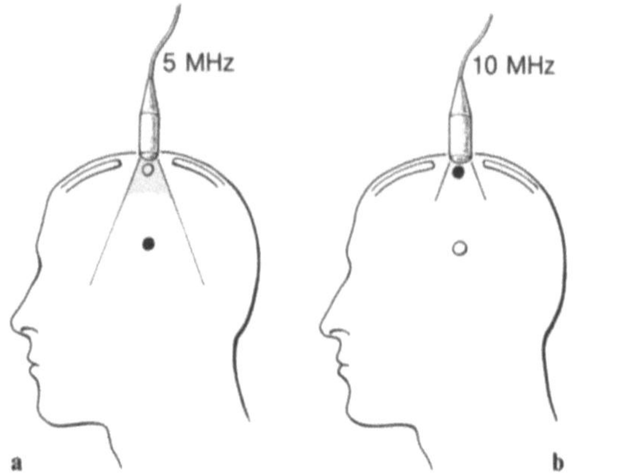

Fig. 5a, b. Use of appropriate frequency. **a** Lower frequency reaches deep but results in a dead zone near the probe. **b** Higher frequency misses more distant lesions

Artifacts and Limitations in the Interpretation of Images

Besides bone and air, metallic objects will cause a shadow in the image, preventing interpretation of tissue behind. Moreover, fresh blood clots and hemostatic material may cause not only an area of high echo intensity, but also a shadow behind this area (Fig. 6).

The exact assessment of the diameter of a lesion is limited by the lateral resolution in a sector plane: outside the focus area of the acoustic lens of the crystal, and object may appear larger than it really is. This error may also be caused by the angular velocity of the US beam in the periphery

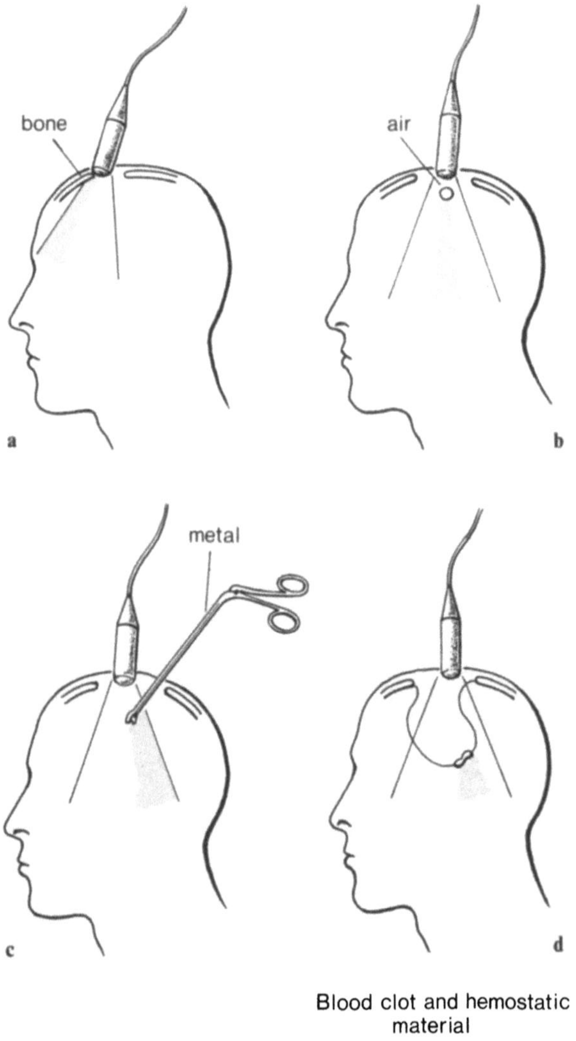

Fig. 6. Shadow artifacts caused by **a** bone, **b** air, **c** metal, **d** fresh blood clot together with hemostatic material

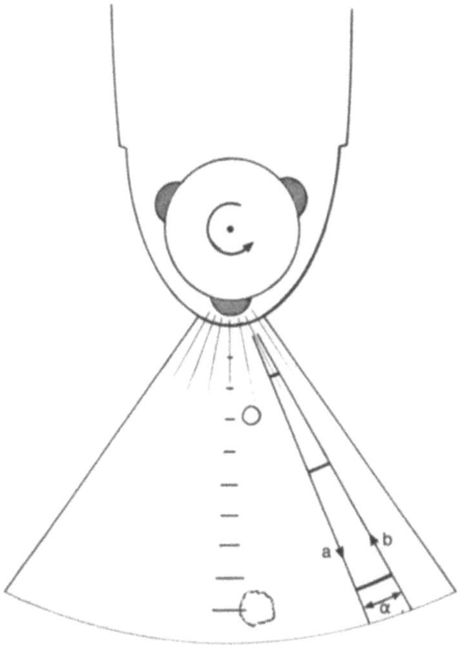

Fig. 7. Lateral resolution. Objects are imaged at their actual size near the transducer but appear larger than they really are in the periphery. Between emission of the US waves and arrival of the echo, the crystal has rotated through the angle α. The distance between arrays *a* and *b* increases with the distance from the transducer, leading to the apparent size difference

of the sector image, where the crystal travels a longer distance between sending US waves and receiving echoes (Fig. 7).

Newer multicrystal probes with complicated phasing of crystal activation allow electronic focusing and electronic change of focus according to individual circumstances. These procedures increase both axial and lateral resolution and reduce the need to use special frequencies for deep-seated lesions and for lesions near the surface (Figs. 4, 8) [36, 64].

Biological Effects of US Imaging

In principle both very high and very low sound frequencies can cause destruction. US wave energy is absorbed in the form of heat energy. Direct transfer of the mechanical energy of sound waves into tissue can cause cavitation and vibration. All these phenomena are highly dependent on the time of application of the sound energy. During US imaging in medicine, the energies used are very low (maximally 50 mw/cm^2), and the time of application is extremely short: during 0.1% of its time of activity, the crystal is in its phase of emitting energy. During the remaining 99.9% of the time it is in the phase of receiving echoes, "listening". The single phases of emission are in the microsecond range.

In experimental and in clinical work, no adverse effects of US have been shown; the effect of multiple repeated investigations is considered less certain. One must bear in mind, however, that the risks entailed by X-ray investigations are much greater [2, 41, 42, 44].

Note on the Technical Equipment

In the legends of all US-images on the following pages, abbreviations describe the technical equipment. The corresponding US-instruments and probes are shown in Fig. 8, pp. 8/9.

Diasonics, type **DRF 100**

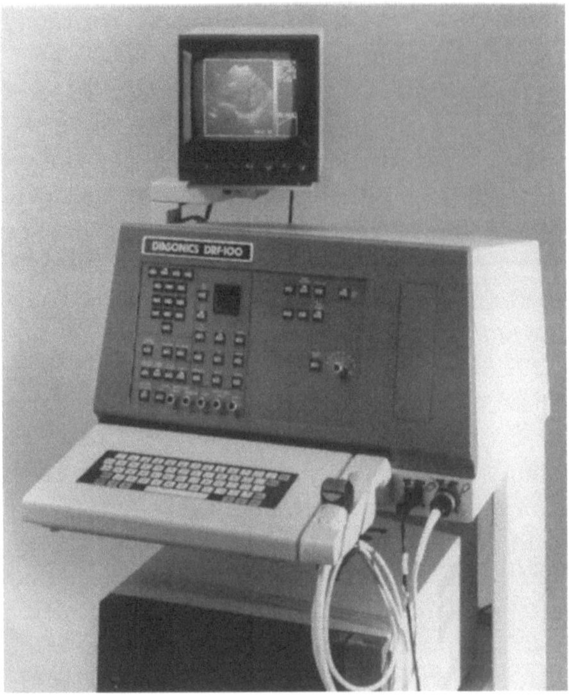

a

Diasonics, type **SPA 1000**

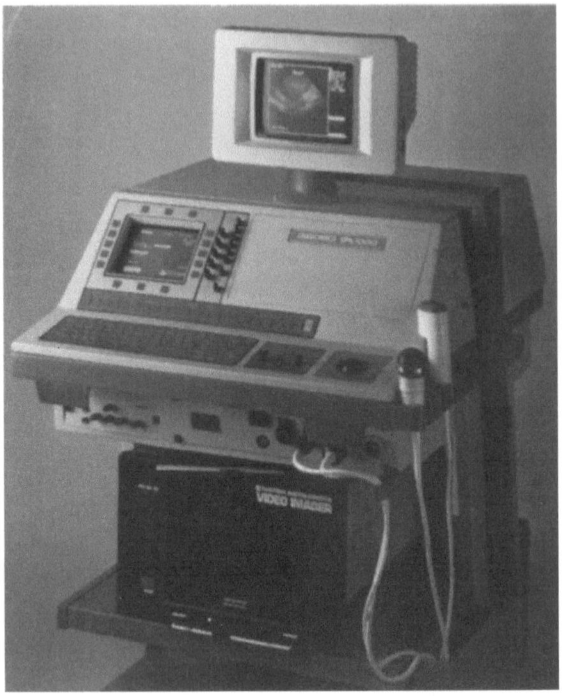

c

Fig. 8. a, c, e, g Various imaging instruments from different companies

Oscillating (wobbling) probe
IOP probe, 5 MHz, 1 cm Ø (Diasonics)

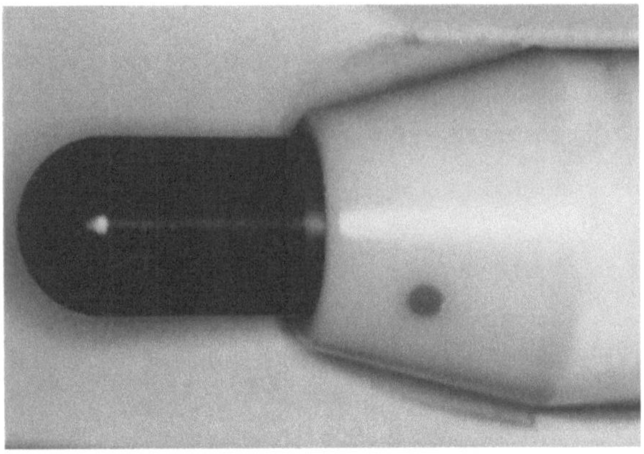

b

b Wobbling crystal, housed in a 5-MHz intraoperative probe with diameter of 1 cm

Oscillating (wobbling) probe
GPS probe, 5 MHz, 3 cm Ø (Diasonics)

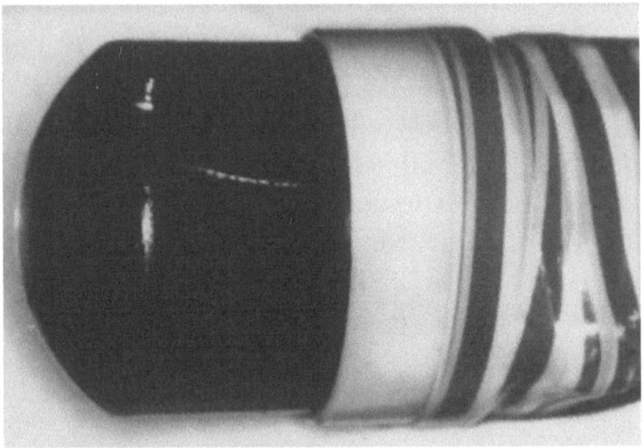

d

d Wobbling crystal, housed in a 5-MHz probe, diameter 3 cm

ATL, type **Ultramark 8** UM 8 (left), and
type **Ultramark 4** UM 4 (right)

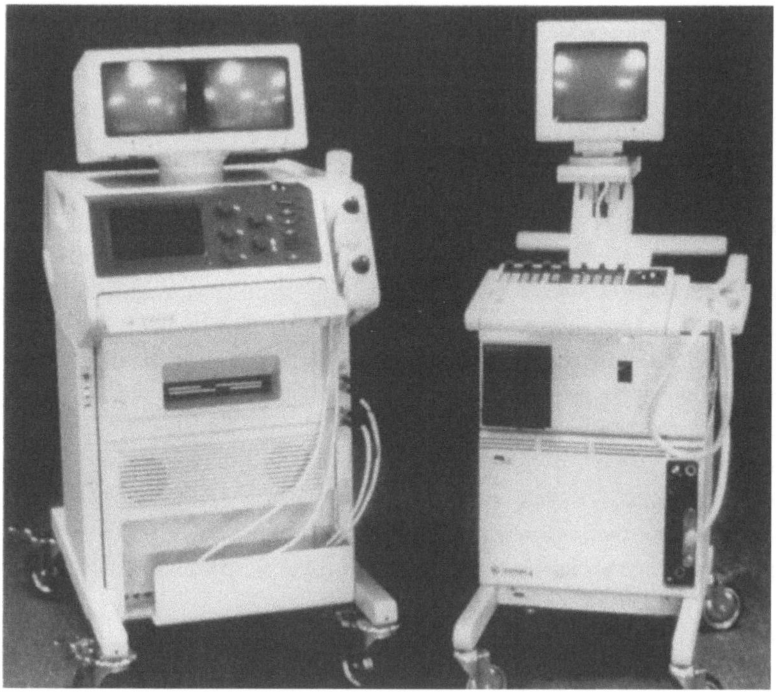

e

Toshiba, type **Sonolayer**
SSA-100A

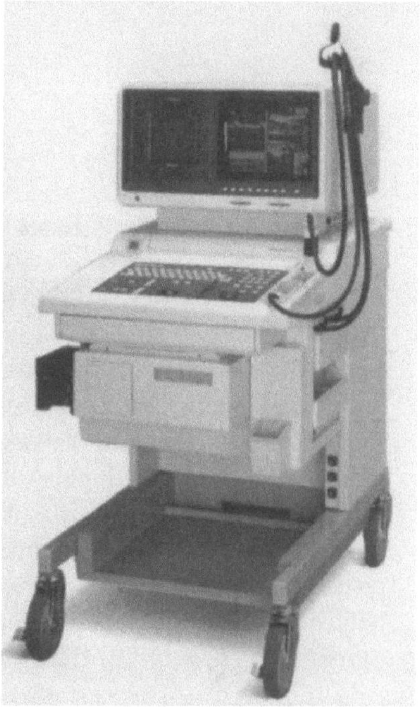

g

Rotating probe
Annular array 3 cm ∅ 3–10 MHz (ATL)

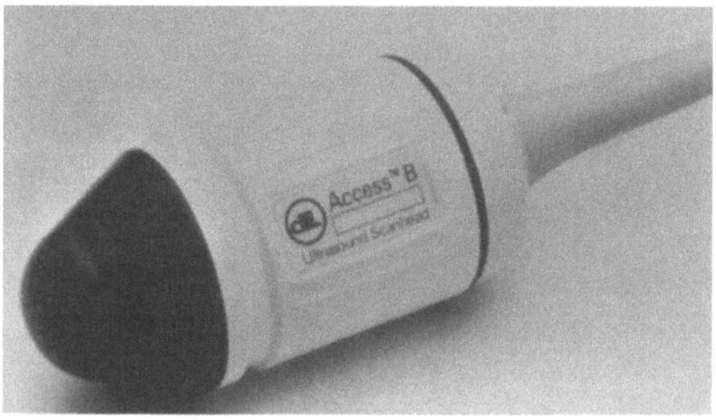

f

f Annular array probe, rotating crystals for 3.5, 5, 7.5, 10-MHz in a 3 cm ∅ housing

Electronic probe
1,5 cm ∅ 5 MHz (Toshiba)

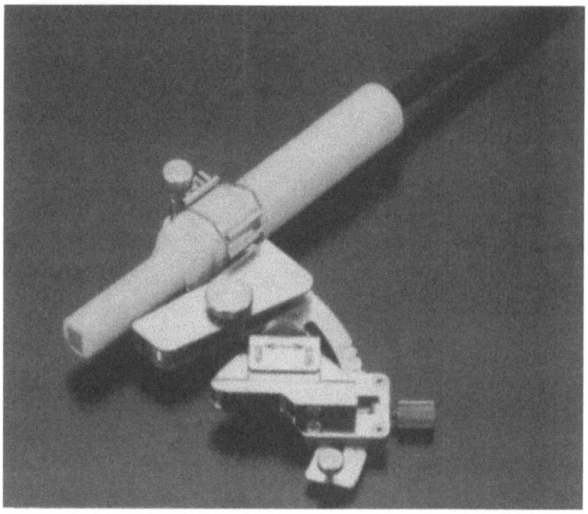

h

h Several immobile crystals mounted in series (juxta-position) in a 5-MHz probe

NF-probe (not shown) = Diasonics Near-Field 10 MHz-probe
NS (not shown) = ATL-Neurosector

Practical Handling of the US Probe During Investigation

Imaging with Dura Closed or Open?

At first glance, it may appear logical to assume that the quality of images will increase if the barrier of the dura mater is removed; indeed, the example of a tumor in the left occipital lobe reaching into the trigonum shows that the echo intensity is generally higher when the dura is open (Fig. 9) than when it is still closed (Fig. 10). Opening the dura does not, however, increase the space resolution, nor does it change the echogenicity of any tissue compartment compared with others. Imaging with the dura closed thus has no basic disadvantages; on the contrary, it has the advantage of applying less circumscribed pressure to the underlying brain tissue and allowing the investigator to move the transducer freely over the dural surface. Movement of the US probe is much more difficult and would sometimes even be traumatizing with the dura open.

As a rule, therefore, initial intraoperative US imaging should be performed with the dura closed. One obvious exception to this rule is US imaging during stereotactic procedures (see also [32]).

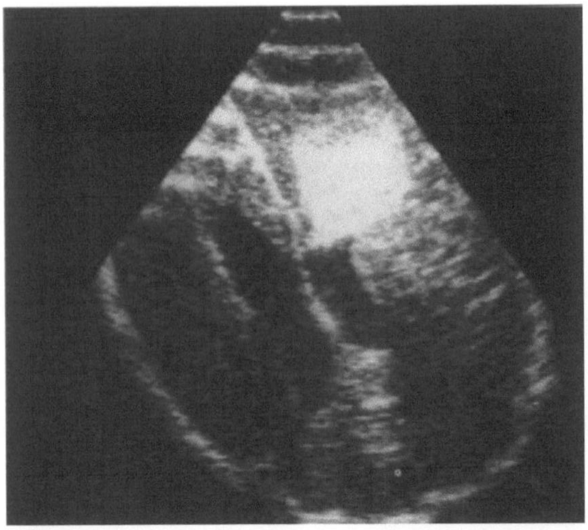

Fig. 9. Dura open. Horizontal US, DRF 100, GPS probe, 5 MHz

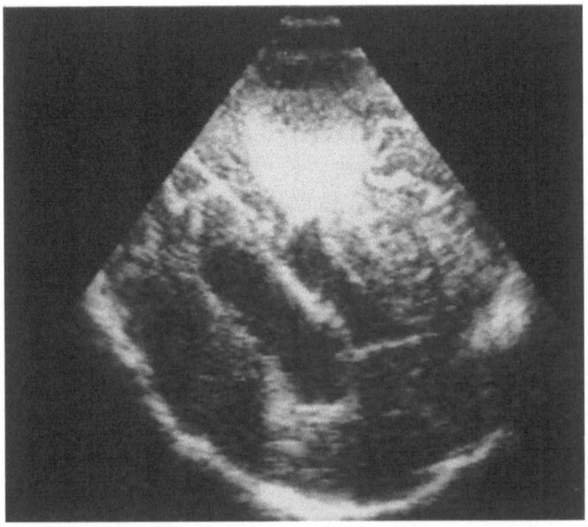

Fig. 10. Dura closed. Horizontal US, DRF 100, GPS probe, 5 MHz

Landmarks for Orientation in the Normal Brain and Intracranium

At first glance, many of the following images will appear unclear and blurred; the longer you look at an image, however, the more well-known anatomical details will appear. The majority of them can not be identified here for fear of obliterating the images with labels.
Initial anatomical orientation is easiest using one or more of the classical planes for brain imaging - horizontal, sagittal and coronal. These three planes will therefore be demonstrated first.

In daily neurosurgical practice, however, it will often not be possible to obtain one of these standard images for orientation, and diagonal and oblique tomograms will have to suffice. For this reason, some of the more common nonstandard planes will also be shown.

On some occasions, for instance in the search for a small subcortical lesion, complete anatomical orientation will not be necessary.

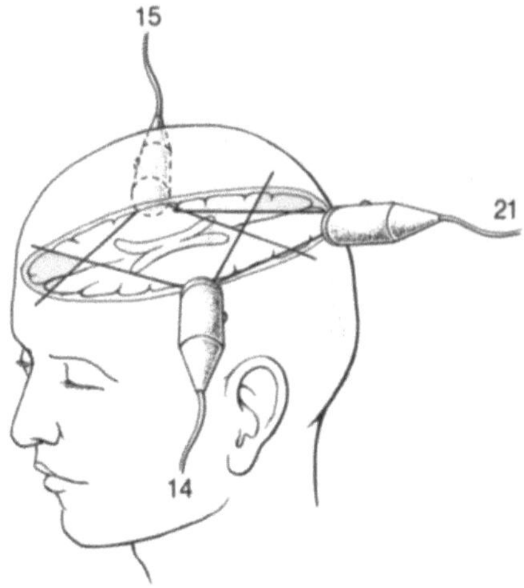

Fig. 11. Horizontal US images from left temporal (probe turned occipitally; see also Fig. 14), right temporal (probe turned frontally; see also Fig. 15) and occipital (see also Fig. 21)

Horizontal View

Horizontal sections of the brain can be obtained via a craniotomy (usually temporal, sometimes frontal or occipital) or via a temporal or occipital burrhole; a frontal burrhole will permit only diagonal images.

The first prominent features in a horizontal image of the supratentorial space from the temporal region (Figs. 14, 15, 18, 19) are the contralateral skull bone and the falx, seen as bright structures (hyperechoic), and the dark spaces of the lateral ventricles (hypoechoic or anechoic) (Figs. 14, 15). Turning the probe somewhat toward the base of the skull yields a lower and slightly diagonal horizontal view in which the bright hyperechoic structures of the choroid plexus appear within the ventricles (Figs. 18, 19).

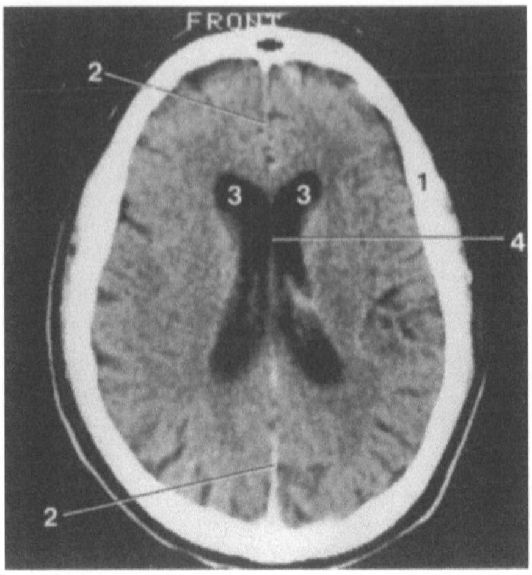

Fig. 12. Horizontal CT

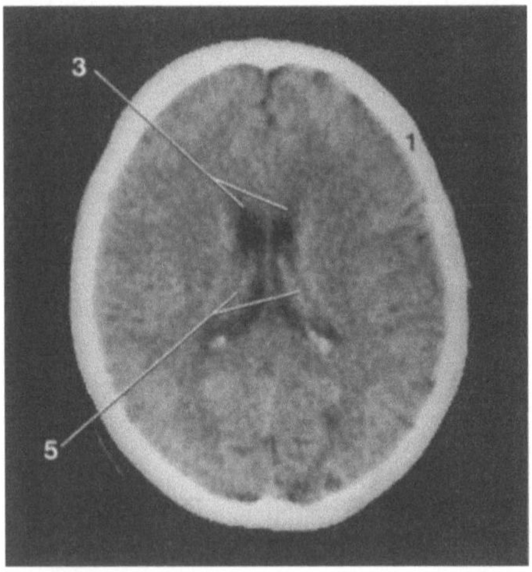

Fig. 16. Horizontal CT (layer below scan shown in Fig. 12)

1 Contralateral skull bone
2 Interhemispheric space and falx
3 Frontal horns of lateral ventricles
4 Septum pellucidum
5 Choroid plexus
6 Occipital horn
P Position of probe

Orientation of the Sector Plane in the Intracranial Space: Hand-Eye Coordination. You must now decide whether you want to look at this horizontal plane from above or from below. In order not to become confused about the location of left and right, frontal and occipital on the image, keep the probe in the chosen plane and turn it so that it points more frontally, at the same time observing how the image changes on the monitor. Decide first what you consider to be the frontal horns of the lateral ventricles and ascertain during movement of the probe whether you indeed look more frontally with your sector plane or whether you move in the wrong direction; in the latter case the probe must be turned through 180 °C. Figures 15 and 19 show images after moving the probe frontally compared with Figs. 14 and 18: the frontal horns move backward, and more of the frontal bone and of the frontal interhemispheric space is seen. Obviously, the left-right orientation is clear from the position of the probe.

Horizontal images taken via an occipital window (Fig. 21) will first of all show the prominent dark areas of the posterior horns and the very bright choroid plexuses in the trigonal areas of the lateral ventricles. The occipital falx will come into view from medial and eventually cross the midline of the image. The falx will appear as a bright line running approximately parallel to the sector boundary of the side of imaging: when imaging is performed from left occipital, then the falx will run parallel to the left sector boundary. Higher up, the pars centralis of the lateral ventricles and the anterior horns may become visible, as may the septum pellucidum; the latter will run parallel to the falx. The contralateral frontal and temporal bones can serve as further landmarks.

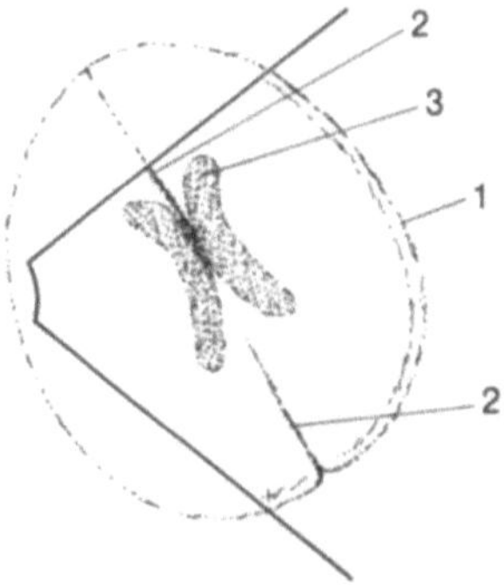

Fig. 13. Landmarks for horizontal image via temporal window

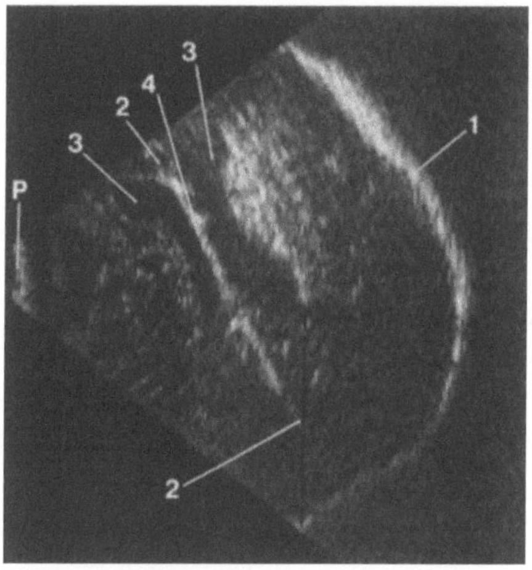

Fig. 14. Horizontal US from left temporal, probe turned occipitally. DRF 100, GPS probe, 5 MHz

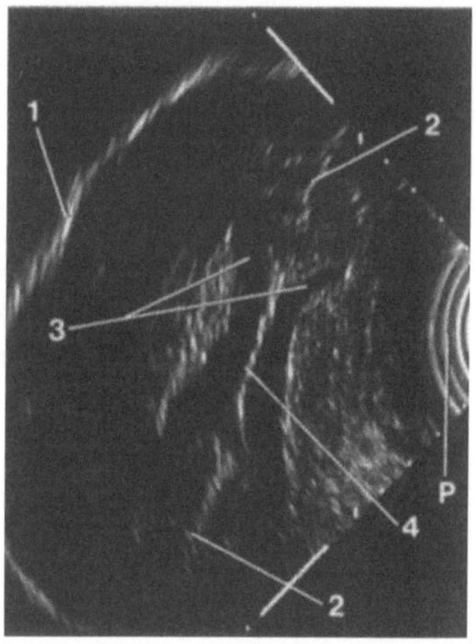

Fig. 15. Horizontal US from right temporal, probe turned frontally. UM 4, annular array probe. 5 MHz

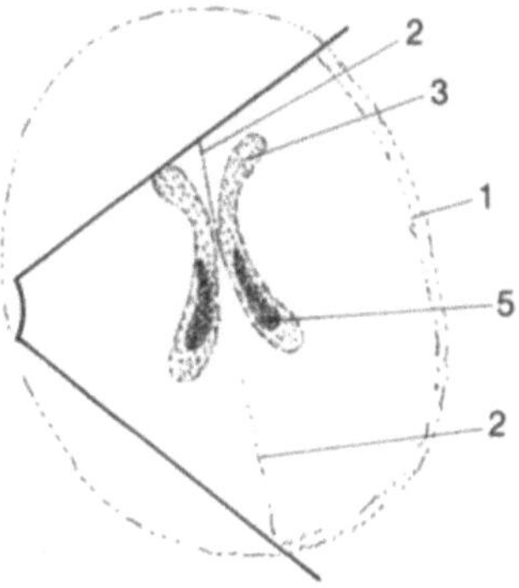

Fig. 17. Landmarks for horizontal image via temporal window

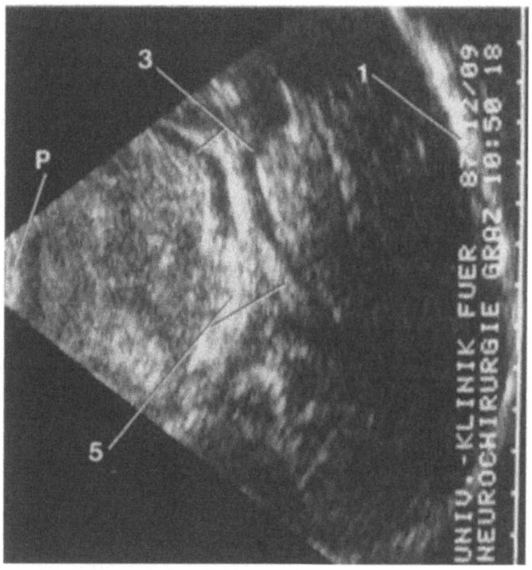

Fig. 18. Horizontal US from left temporal, probe turned occipitally. DRF 100, GPS probe, 5 MHz

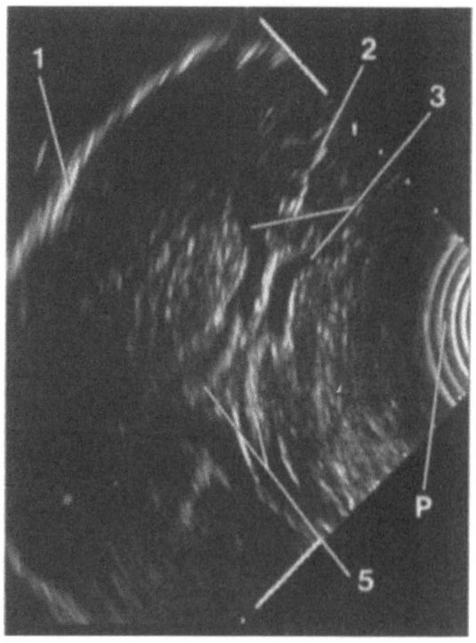

Fig. 19. Horizontal US from right temporal, probe turned frontally. UM 4, annular array probe, 5 MHz

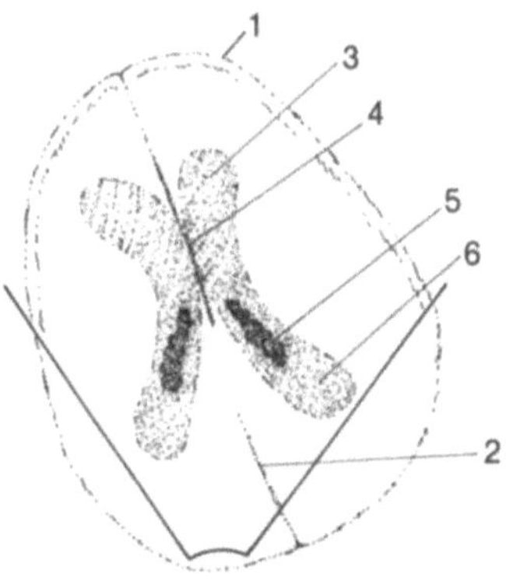

Fig. 20. Landmarks for horizontal image via occipital window

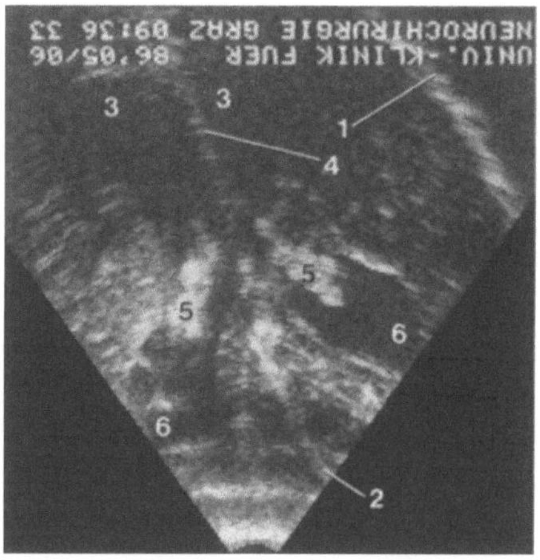

Fig. 21. Horizontal US via an occipital window. DRF 100, GPS probe, 5 MHz

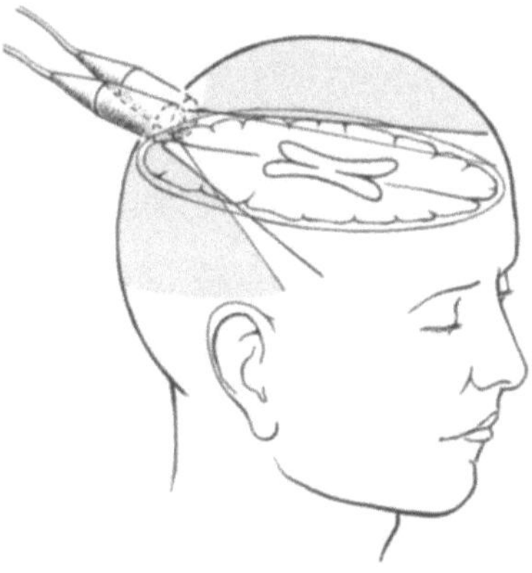

Fig. 22. Landmarks for horizontal image via occipital window

On lower horizontal images, the lateral ventricles are lost as landmarks, and the brainstem appears in the middle of the cranial cavity as a rather dark structure (Figs. 24-26). Behind the brainstem, the upper vermis shows the characteristic lobular structure of the cerebellum. The primary orientation regarding distances is provided by the contralateral skull bone, which should again be observed in the anteroposterior direction (i.e., turn the probe and watch the movement of the skull bone).

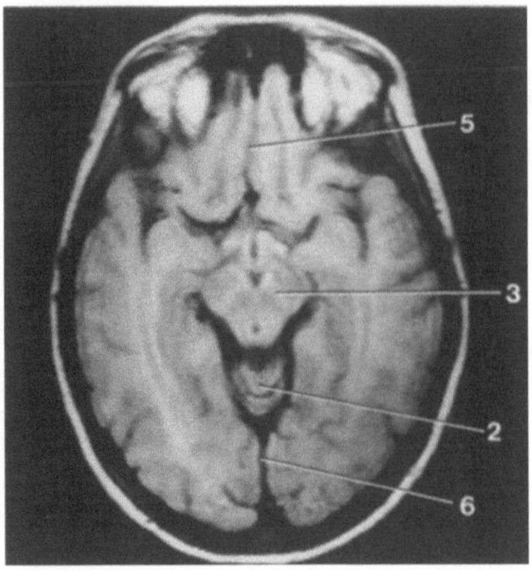

Fig. 23. Horizontal MRI

1 Contralateral skull bone
2 Upper vermis
3 Brainstem (crura cerebri, midbrain, pons)
4 Fourth ventricle
5 Frontal interhemispheric fissure
6 Occipital interhemispheric fissure

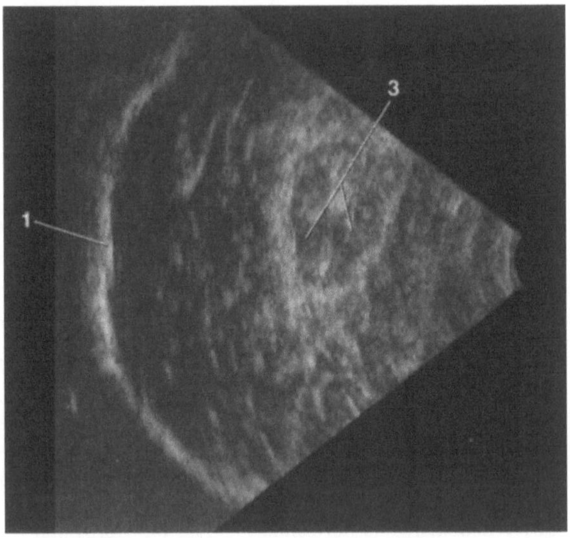

Fig. 24. Lower horizontal US image. DRF 100, GPS probe, 5 MHz

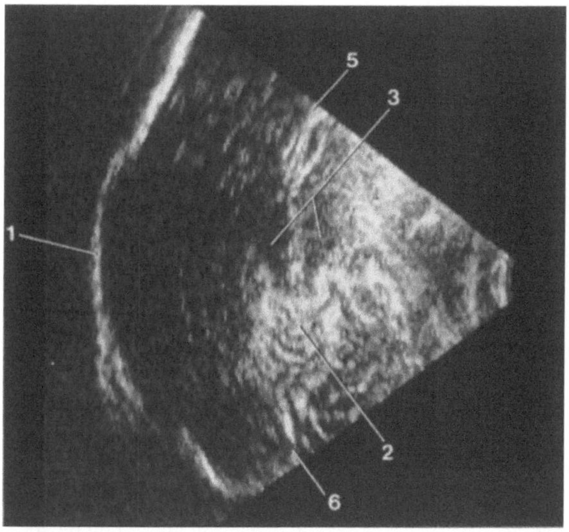

Fig. 25. Lower horizontal US image. DRF 100, GPS probe, 5 MHz

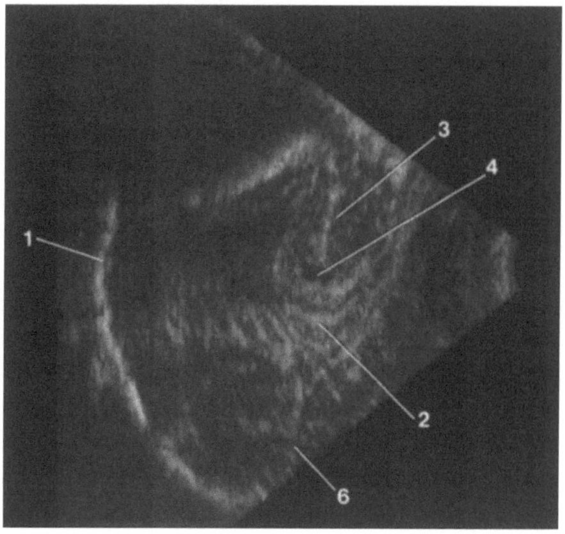

Fig. 26. Lower horizontal US image. DRF 100, GPS probe, 5 MHz

Sagittal View

Sagittal images are, in practice, rarely taken exactly in the median plane. Mostly, parasagittal images cut alongside the ipsilateral ventricle, with its very bright choroid plexus as an obvious landmark. The dominant landmark for all sagittal sections from a frontal or parietal skull window is the frontal skull base, which ends suddenly at the anterior entrance to the sella or the edge of the lesser sphenoid wing.

On midsagittal images, the cingulate gyrus and cingulate sulcus serve as rather clear landmarks, besides a lateral ventricle with a part of its choroid plexus that can be easily visualized by slightly moving the probe to left or right. Again, the anteroposterior orientation is obtained by turning the probe, once toward the front, once toward the occiput, while checking on the monitor to see in which direction the frontal skull base moves.

From an occipital approach, the main landmarks for the midsagittal plane are the clivus, frontal bone and tentorium; the fourth ventricle, cerebellum and corpus callosum (splenium) are also clearly delineated (Figs. 35, 37). On parasagittal views from occipital (Figs. 36, 38), the most prominent structure in the middle of the image is the trigonal choroid plexus. The image of the intracranium is limited by the frontal bone as in the midsagittal section; part of the clivus and the bone structures of the floor of the middle cranial fossa are seen. Depending on the location of the section, different parts of the lateral ventricle can also serve as a reliable landmark.

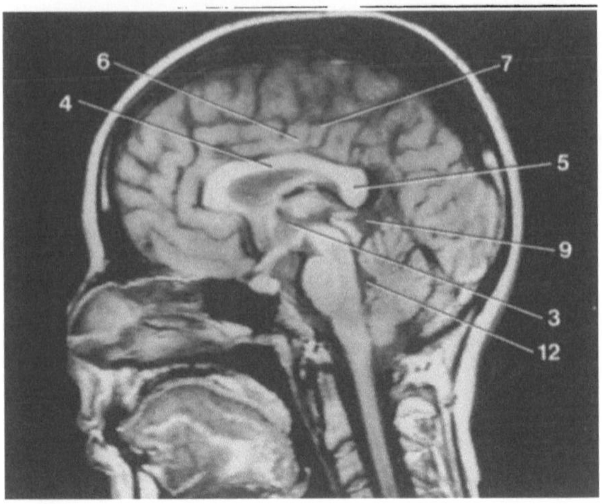

Fig. 27. Sagittal MRI

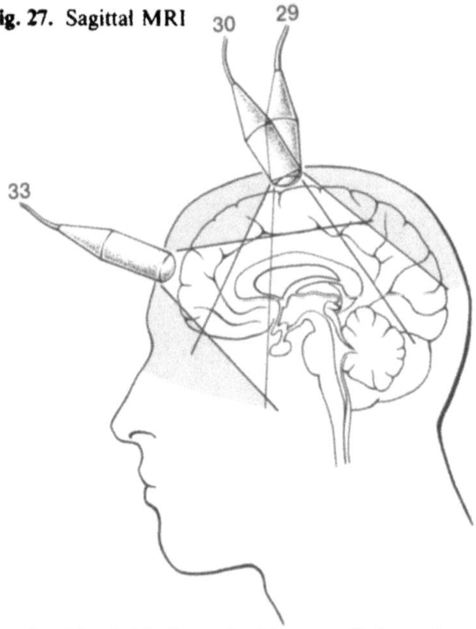

Fig. 31. The field of a sagittal image will depend on the location of the burrhole and the positioning of the US probe. Shown here are the fields for Figs. 29, 30, 33

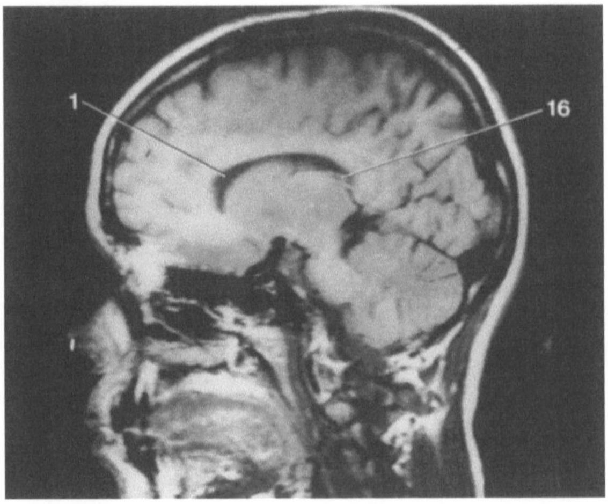

Fig. 34. Sagittal MRI

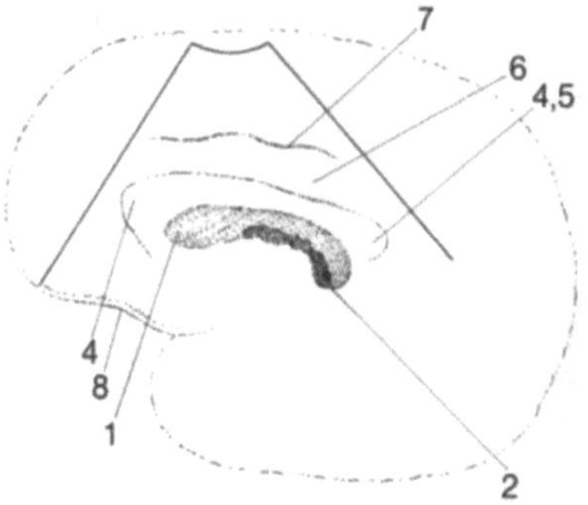

Fig. 28. Landmarks for sagittal images via a frontoparietal window

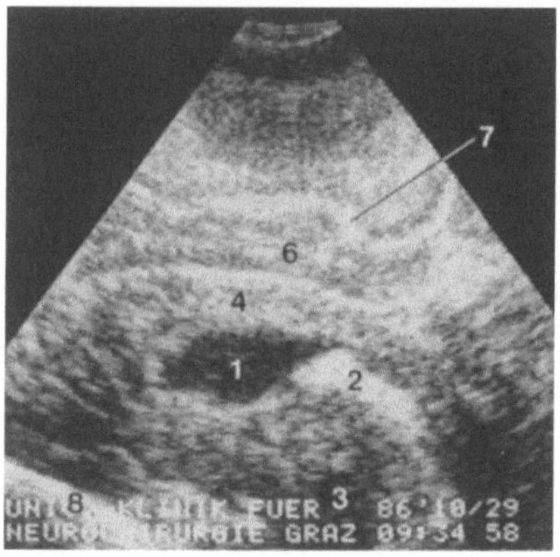

Fig. 29. Sagittal US via frontoparietal window, probe turned frontally. DRF 100, GPS probe, 5 MHz

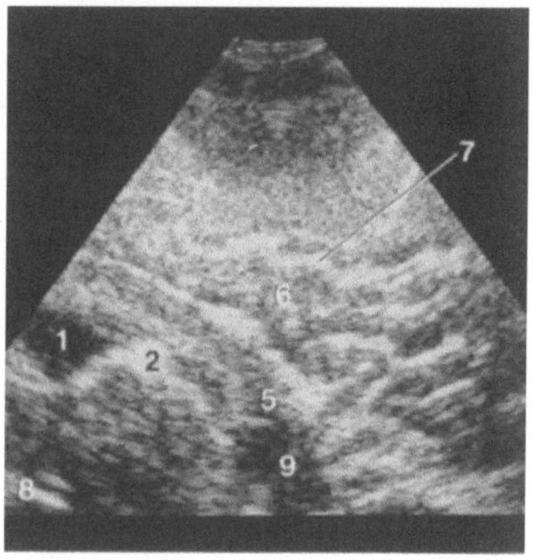

Fig. 30. Sagittal US via frontoparietal window, probe turned occipitally. DRF 100, GPS probe, 5 MHz

1 Frontal horn of lateral ventricle
2 Choroid plexus
3 Third ventricle
4 Corpus callosum
5 Splenium
6 Cingulate gyrus
7 Cingulate sulcus
8 Frontal skull base
9 Quadrigeminal cistern
10 Tentorium
11 Cerebellum
12 Fourth ventricle
13 Clivus
14 Frontal bone
15 Middle cranial fossa
16 Trigonal choroid plexus

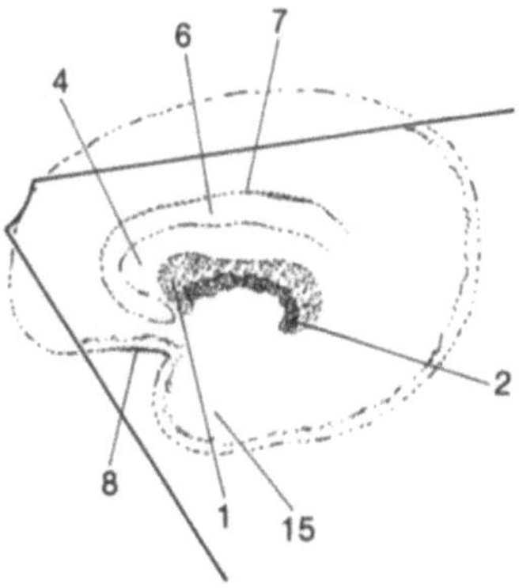

Fig. 32. Landmarks for sagittal images via a frontal window

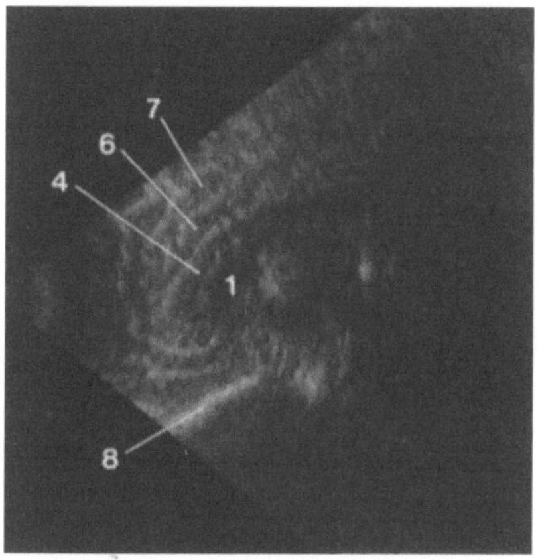

Fig. 33. Sagittal US via frontal window. DRF 100, GPS probe, 5 MHz

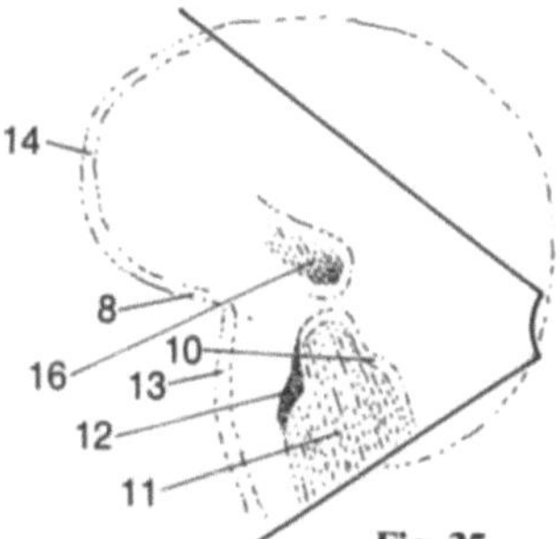

Fig. 35

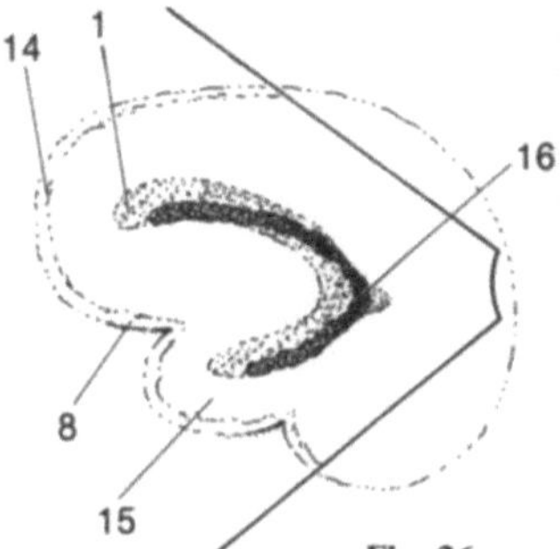

Fig. 36

Figs. 35, 36. Landmarks for sagittal images via an occipital window

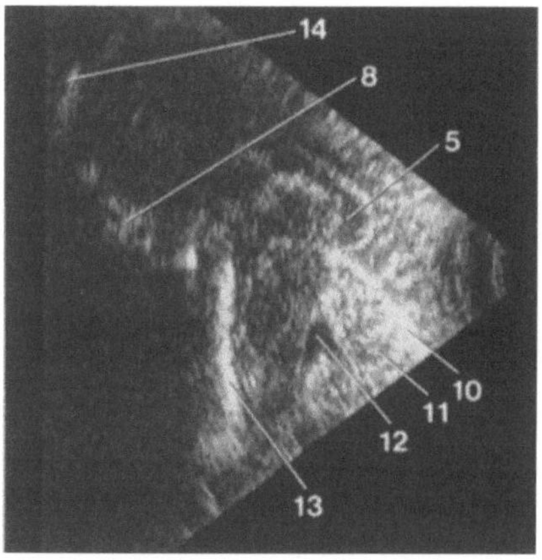

Fig. 37. Sagittal US via occipital window. DRF 100, GPS probe, 5 MHz (see Fig. 35)

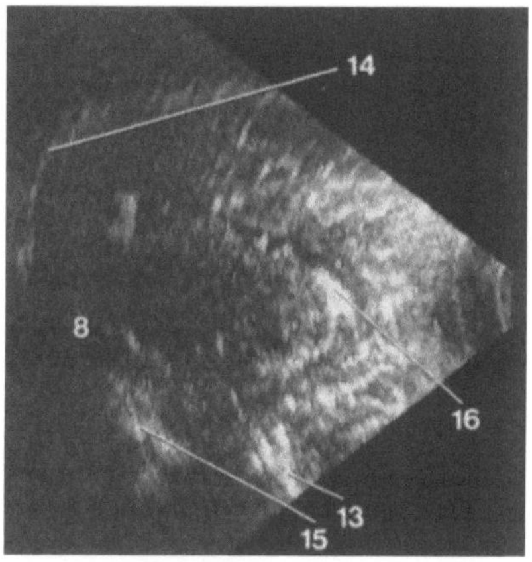

Fig. 38. Sagittal US via occipital window with probe turned laterally. DRF 100, GPS, 5 MHz (see Fig. 36)

Coronal View

Coronal images are mainly obtained via frontal, parietal or temporal approaches. The dominant landmark for coronal sections is the ventricular system: the lateral ventricles are separated by the septum pellucidum. The choroid plexus is either apparent at the bottom of the cross-sectioned lateral ventricles, as bright structures, or leads to the foramina of Monro into the third ventricle. Another clearly visible landmark is the interhemispheric space with the falx. In the case of coronal sections via a temporal window (Fig. 42b), the contralateral skull bone will serve for orientation. When imaging is done through a parietal window (Fig. 41b, c), the floor of the middle fossa and sella region will form a characteristic shape at the lower end of the image. Left-right orientation in this case is obtained by turning the probe to one side and checking whether structures move in the expected direction in the image.

Turning the probe somewhat frontally in the case of imaging through a frontal burrhole, the frontal skull base and the sphenoid wings will be the dominant landmarks. In addition, the middle fossa of either side will be shown more or less symmetrically and lend the image a characteristic pattern (Fig. 41b).

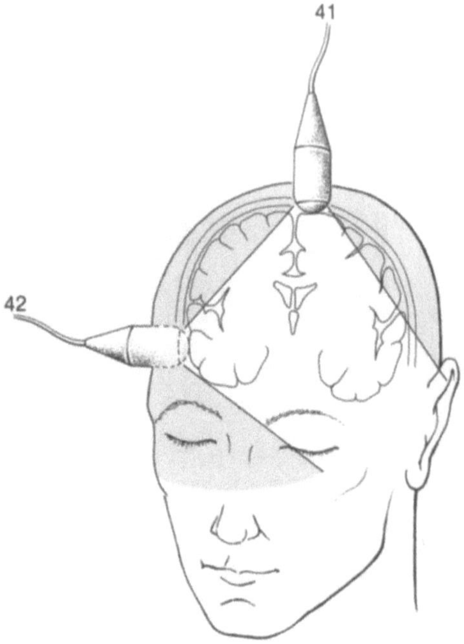

Fig. 39. Coronal images via a parietal window (Fig. 41b, c) or a temporal window (Fig. 42b)

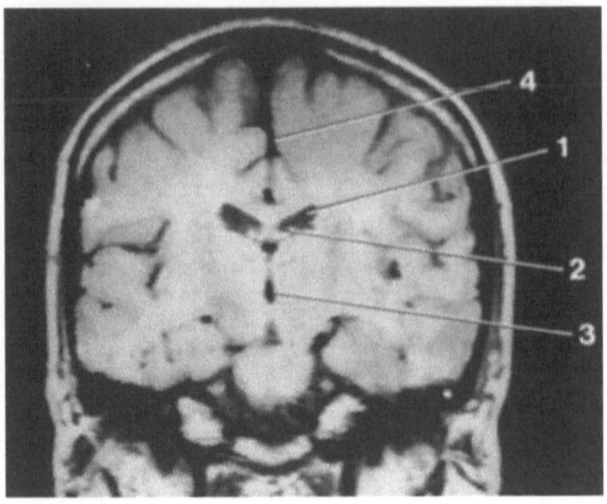

Fig. 40. Coronal MRI

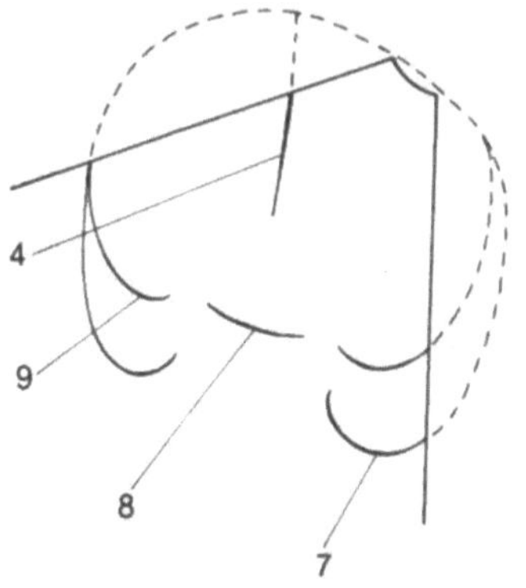

Fig. 41a. Landmarks for coronal images via a parietal window.

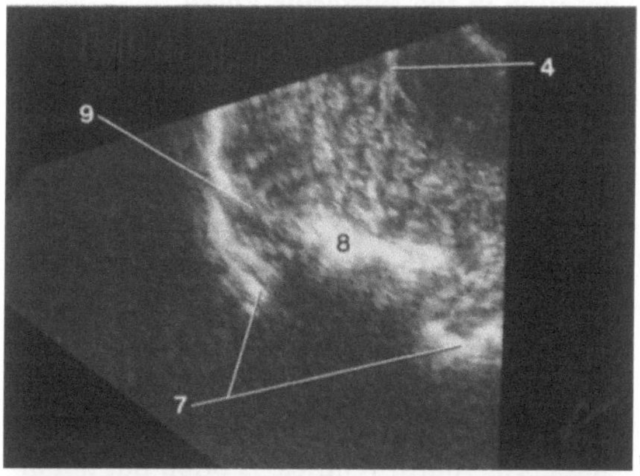

b

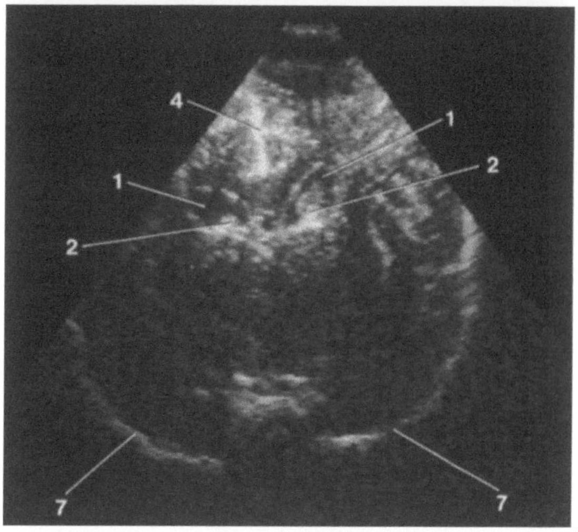

c

Fig. 41b, c. Coronal US via parietal window. DRF 100, GPS probe, 5 MHz

1 Lateral ventricle
2 Choroid plexus
3 Third ventricle
4 Falx and interhemispheric space
5 Septum pellucidum
6 Contralateral skull bone
7 Temporal fossa
8 Frontal skull base
9 Sphenoid wing

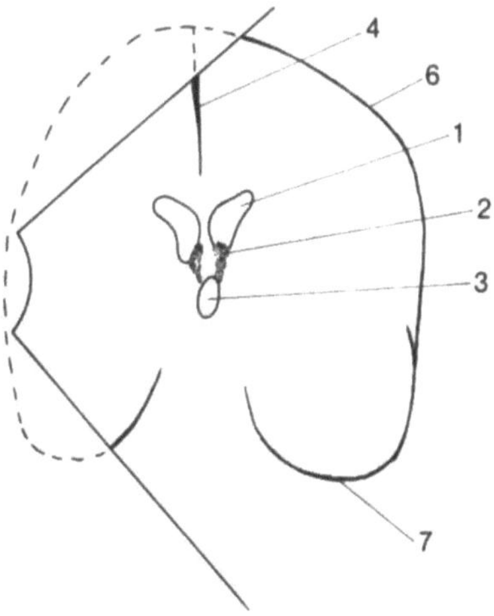

Fig. 42a. Landmarks for coronal images via a temporal window

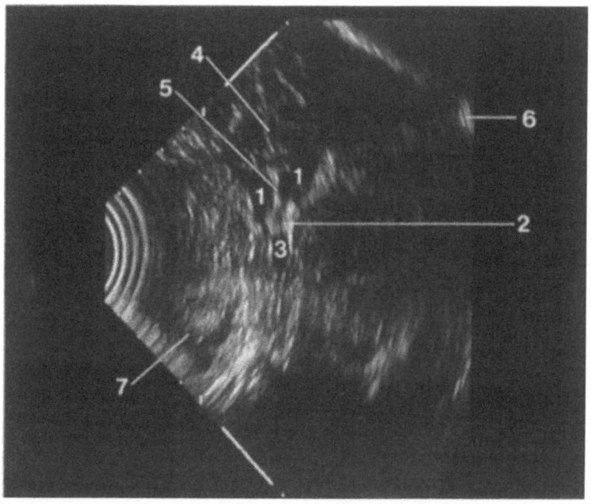

Fig. 42b. Coronal US via temporal window. UM 4, annular array probe, 5 MHz

Orientation in the Posterior Fossa

On sagittal views from an occipital or a suboccipital window (Figs. 44, 45), the arbor vitae of the cerebellum can clearly be recognized. The main landmarks, however, will be the clivus and the tentorium/petrous bone, two structures which almost run in parallel with the fourth ventricle between them.

On coronal/horizontal sections (Figs. 48, 49, 52), a trapezoid or blunt pyramid is formed between the clivus in front and the petrous bones at the sides. The fourth ventricle is often but not always recognized.

As the probe is moved upward, the plane goes over the petrous bones through the tentorium to the supratentorial space. When the supratentorial space is reached, the posterior horns and the trigonal ventricular structures with their extensive and bright choroid plexus are dominant in the image and serve as reliable landmarks.

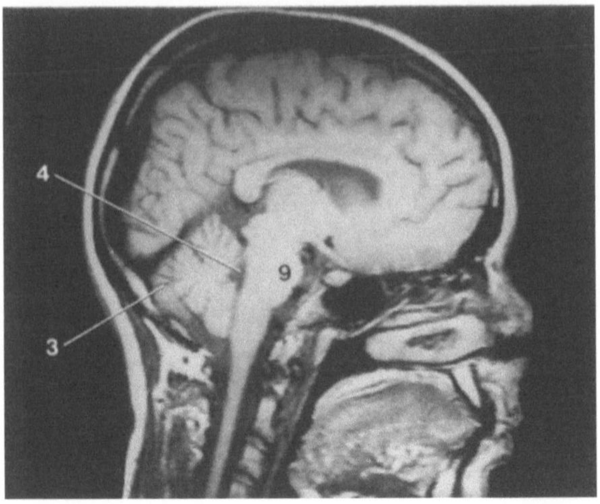

Fig. 43. Sagittal MRI

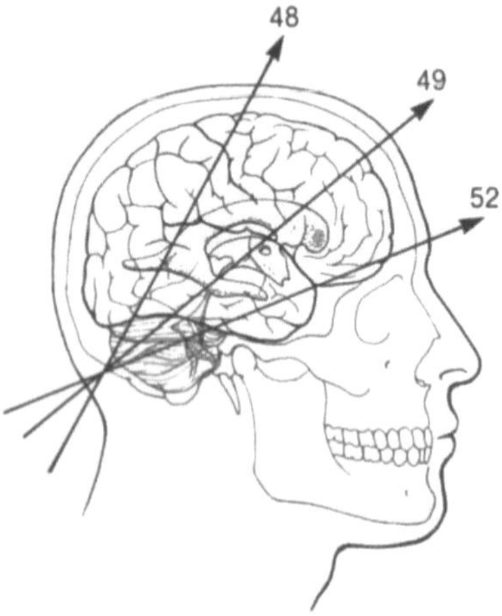

Fig. 46. Coronal/horizontal images via a suboccipital/occipital window (Figs. 48, 49, 52).

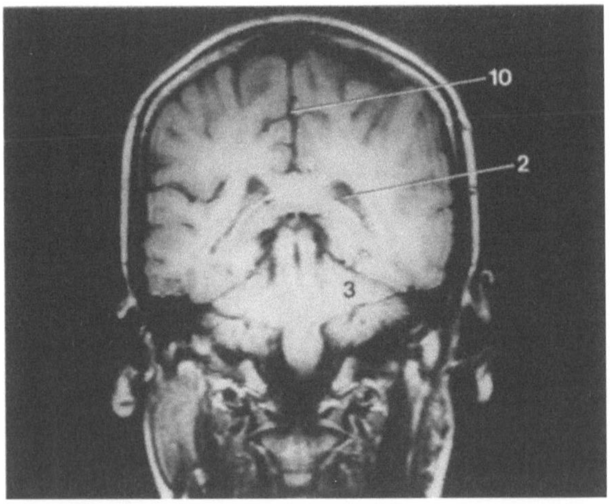

Fig. 47. Coronal MRI

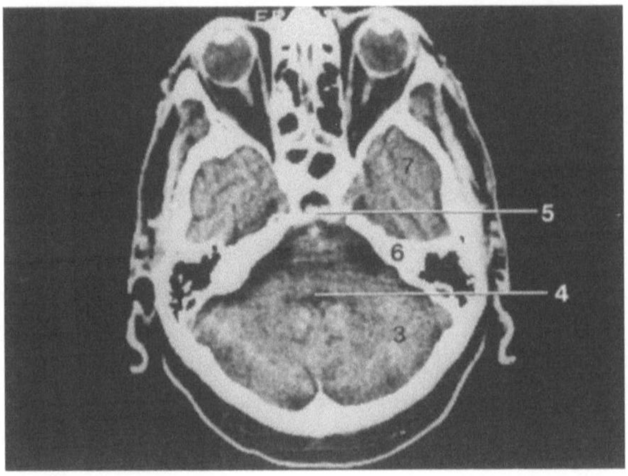

Fig. 50. Horizontal CT

1 Tentorium
2 Lateral ventricle with choroid plexus (trigonum)
3 Cerebellum
4 Fourth ventricle
5 Clivus
6 Petrous bone
7 Temporal lobe with hippocampus
8 Temporal bone
9 Pons
10 Falx

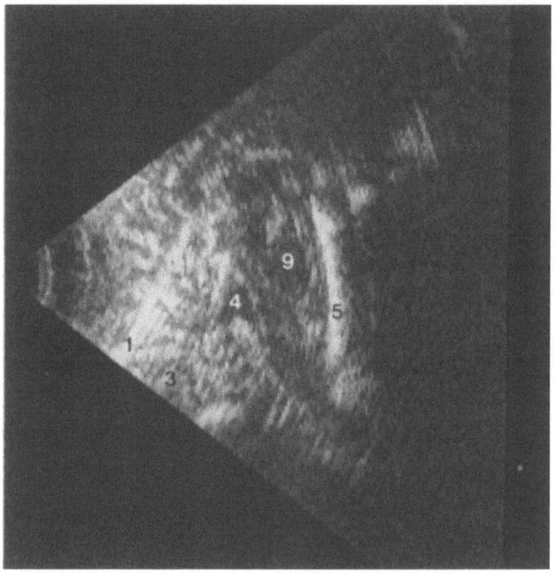

Fig. 44. Sagittal US. DRF 100, GPS probe, 5 MHz

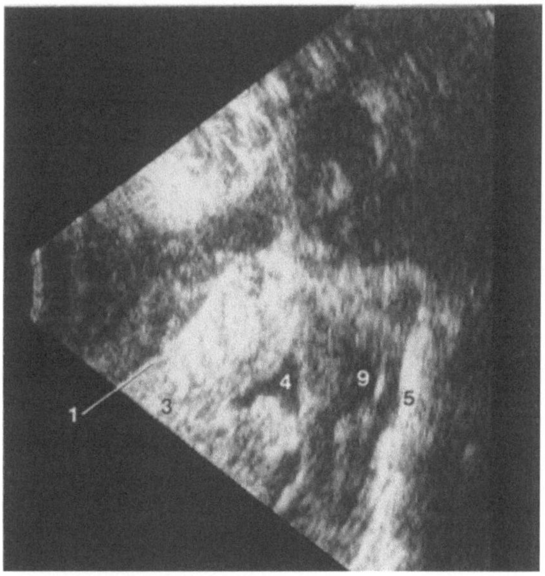

Fig. 45. Sagittal US. DRF 100, GPS probe, 5 MHz

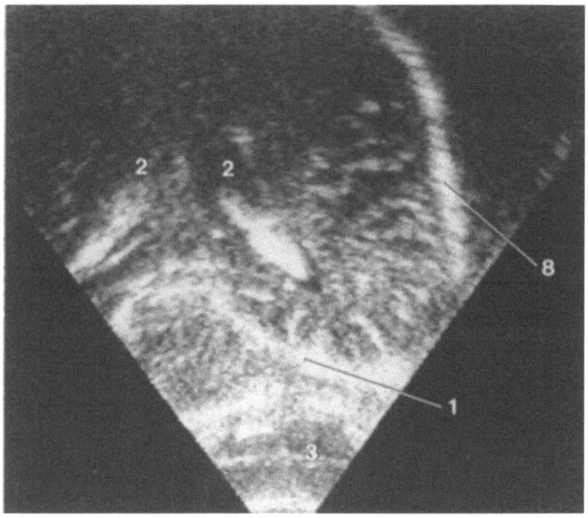

Fig. 48. Coronal or horizontal US via posterior fossa (see schema). DRF 100, GPS probe, 5 MHz

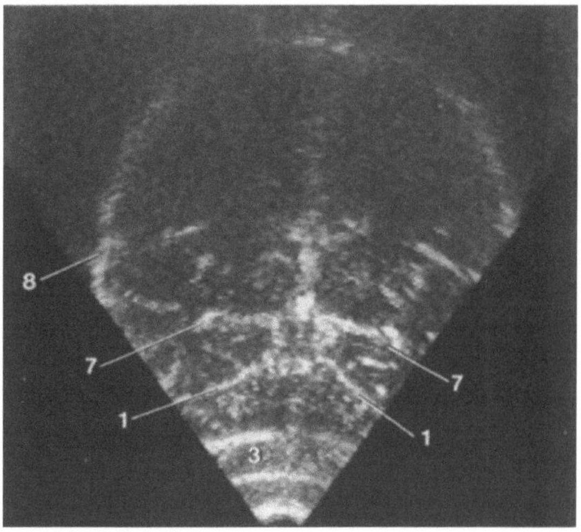

Fig. 49. Coronal or horizontal US via posterior fossa (see schema). DRF 100, GPS probe, 5 MHz

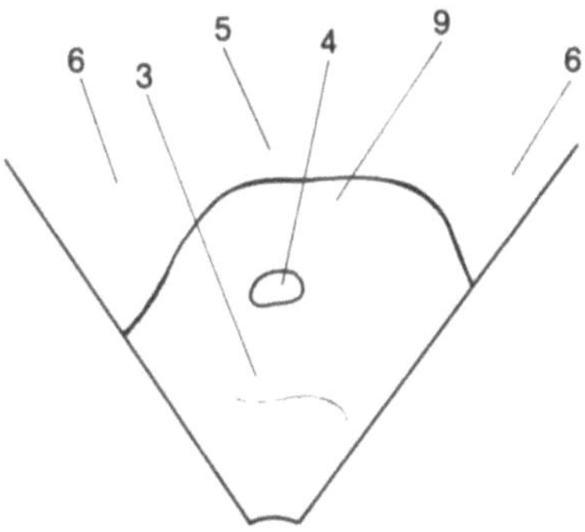

Fig. 51. Landmarks for horizontal images via a suboccipital window

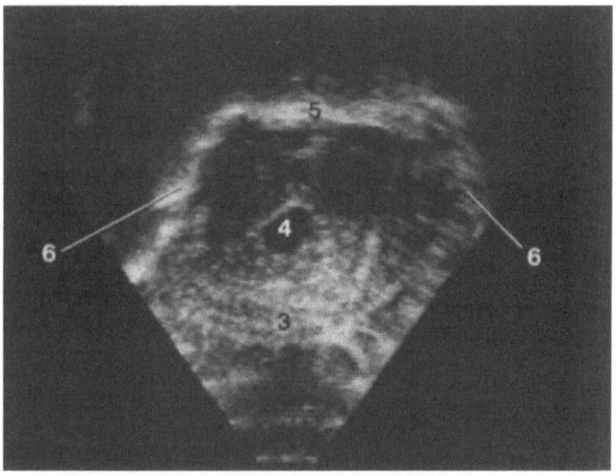

Fig. 52. Coronal or horizontal US via posterior fossa (see schema). DRF 100, GPS probe, 5 MHz

Intracranial Pathomorphology

General Remarks

Comparing pathological intracranial structures on US and CT or MRI, a good correlation of size and shape will generally be found. The few exceptions will be described. The vast majority of lesions will at least partly appear as hyperechoic, i.e., bright structures in the expected area. The only exception to this are arachnoid cysts.

It will become apparent that US is generally more accurate than CT or MRI in showing details of the interior of lesions, while the borders and immediate surroundings are sometimes delineated less clearly by US than by the other modalities. The reason for this is frequently perifocal edema, which is mostly hyperechoic on US, while it shows up, for example, as a hypodense area on CT. The only exception are meningiomas, which seem either to produce a different type of edema or to cause atrophy of the surrounding brain, which appears as hypoechoic (again hypodense on CT).

Differentiation between cyst and necrosis, sometimes difficult on CT, which shows a misleadingly hypodense zone, is generally rather easy with US, because necrosis will be seen as isoechoic or even slightly hyperechoic, while cysts have at least compartments which are clearly hypoechoic.

Finally, it will become clear from the following examples that the structural details depicted clearly on US cannot serve for reliable histopathological correlation.

For further reading see also reference [25] (cited by [38/47]), reference [53], and the references listed in "Practical Applications of Intraoperative Imaging" (p. 131).

Gliomas

One of the major problems in the surgical treatment of many gliomas is the definition of the border between the tumor and the surrounding edema. One of the major hopes placed in intraoperative US, therefore, was that the surgeon would be guided along the tumor surface deep in the brain and that, toward the end of the operation, the US image would reveal any residual tumor that might have been left behind.

This hope initially seemed justified, because some of the morphological peculiarities of gliomas are indeed depicted with more accuracy on US than on CT or MRI. However, a peculiarity of US is that it shows edematous brain tissue around gliomas as a hyperechoic area, whereas edema gives a lower density than normal brain on CT and low-signal areas on T_1-weighted MRI. Gliomas mostly also give high echo densities, i.e., they are either entirely hyperechoic or show a mixture of hyperechoic and hypoechoic (cyst) compartments. At the border between solid tumor and surrounding edema, therefore, two hyperechoics zones meet, and the border zone is less, rather than more, clear than with other imaging techniques. In some cases, the unclear US image is closer to reality than the misleadingly clear tumor border on CT.

Intraoperative US imaging thus does not really improve the surgeon's ability to define the line of dissection for radical removal with preservation of viable surrounding tissue. Especially toward the end of the operation, when the surgeon would like to make sure that the procedure has indeed been radical, US is of little help; not only for the reason given above, but also because even minor blood clots on the surface of the tumor bed shadow the tissue behind, thus making the image even more blurred and unclear (see Figs. 6, 404, 406, 408, 410, 411, 416).

US can, however, be very helpful in the detection of a subcortical low-grade astrocytoma which has been difficult to identify on CT and MRI, or is hard to detect simply by observation of the cortical surface. US will help to clarify the exact location of the tumor and enable the surgeon to chose the least traumatic transcortical aproach. The echo density of gliomas does not seem to correlate with their biological behavior, i.e., benignity is not clearly linked to lower echo density. Intratumoral details are shown with higher accuracy than with other imaging techniques, as are tissue bridges and trabeculae within them. Especially when using high imaging frequencies, it may be easier with US than with other methods to differentiate between cystic and necrotic compartments of a glioma. Central necrosis mostly gives isoechoic or even slightly hyperechoic signals, while CT, for example, shows a marked central hypodensity which might be mistaken for a cyst [27, 25]. Even in the absence of macroscopically visible necrosis or cysts, the interior of a glioma appears heterogeneous in the vast majority of cases. Hyperechoic compartments thus show a variety of gray values, possibly due to multiple microscopically small cysts beyond the spatial resolution of the method. Hypoechoic cysts often vary in echo signal due to sedimentation of proteins and cellular detritus. Only few cysts are homogeneously hypoechoic. As mentioned before, surrounding edema is slightly hyperechoic; the difference is rather clear cut in two-thirds of cases, but in the remaining one-third tumor and edema cannot be differentiated.

For further reading see references [20, 27, 57, 53, 25, 59, 17, 15, 52, 16].

CASE 1 (Figs. 53, 54)

Temporoparietal *pilocytic astrocytoma* in a 25-year-old man, operated upon via left parieto-temporo occipital craniotomy.

The tumor does not appear as well demarcated on US as on contrast-enhanced CT. However, the tumor was found to be larger during operation, and the US image finally turned out to be more precise in its depiction of the tumor border, whereas the CT scan was rather misleading. Both US and CT show that the tumor was filled with small cysts; in addition, the US image shows the larger cysts on the temporal surface that were encountered during operation. The echoicity of the tumor is rather inhomogeneous and slightly higher than that of normal brain tissue. The brain edema surrounding the tumor in the depth, hypodense on CT, appears hyperechoic on US. Note that the CT densities of surrounding brain edema and the larger cysts at the brain surface are very similar; by contrast, their US echogenicities are distinctly different.

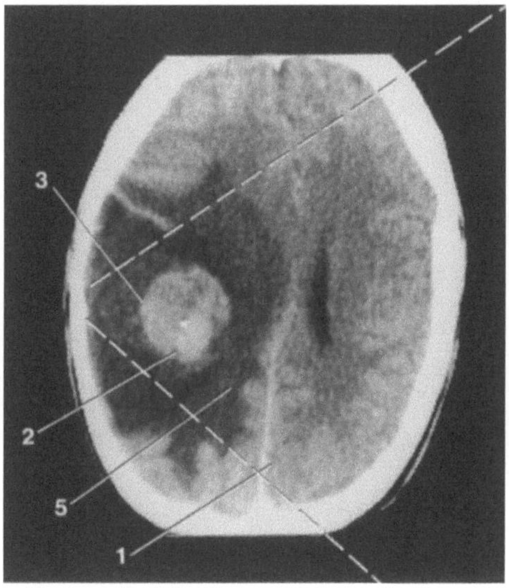

Fig. 53. Horizontal CT

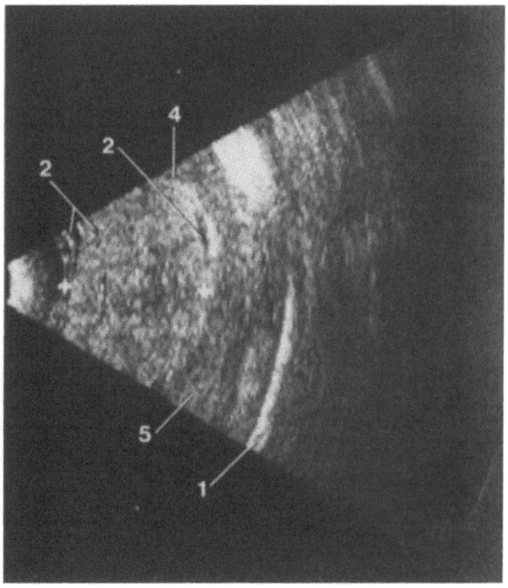

Fig. 54. Horizontal US. DRF 100, IOP probe, 5 MHz

1 Falx
2 Small cysts
3 False impression of tumor surface on CT
4 Tumor surface as seen on US and confirmed during operation
5 Edema

CASE 2 (Figs. 55-63)

Anaplastic oligoastrocytoma grade 2 with central necrosis in the left temporal lobe of a 27-year-old woman operated upon via temporal craniotomy.

The hypoechoic necrotic center is surrounded by a hyperechoic area that decreases in signal intensity with increasing distance from the center. At 5 MHz differentiation between echo intensity of tumor and edema is impossible (Figs. 56-60), but at 7.5 MHz and 10 MHz (Figs. 61-63) the higher signal of the tumor is more or less clearly seen; nevertheless, the border of the tumor remains rather unclear. The gray matter of the parahippocampal gyrus (Fig. 61) adjacent to the horizontally sectioned collateral fissure gives a lower signal than the apparently edematous white matter. Moreover, the necrotic center of the tumor (especially in Fig. 62) turns out to show a higher signal intensity than at 5 MHz. Note that the gray matter of the inferior temporal gyrus in which the tumor is embedded has a slightly higher echoicity than the parahippocampal gyrus.

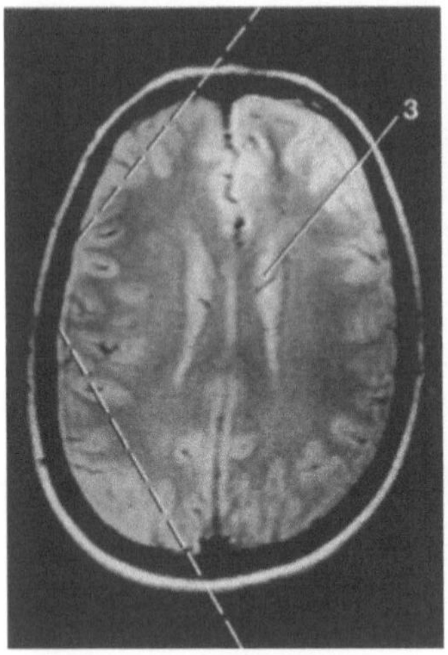

Fig. 55. Horizontal MRI

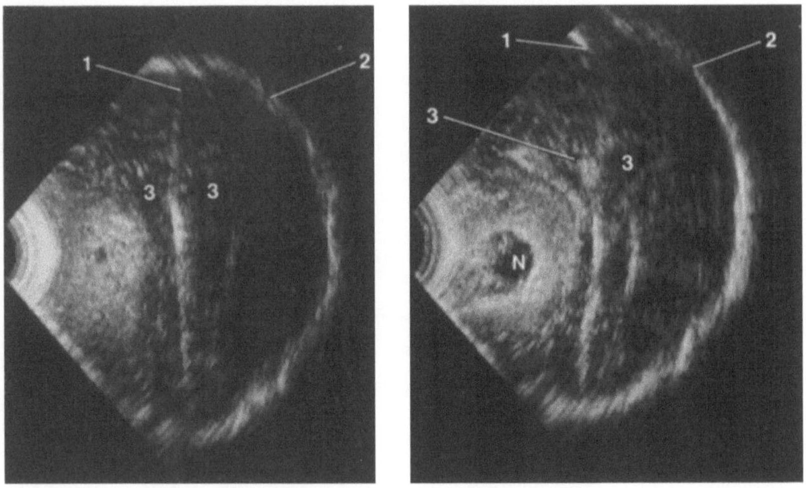

Figs. 56, 57. Horizontal US. UM 8, annular array probe, 5 MHz

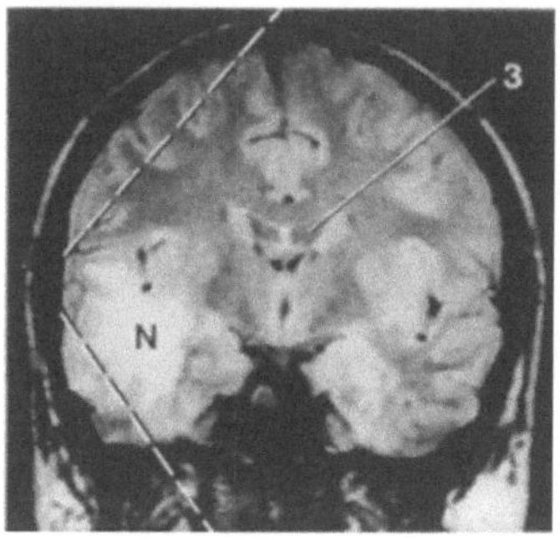

Fig. 58. Coronal MRI

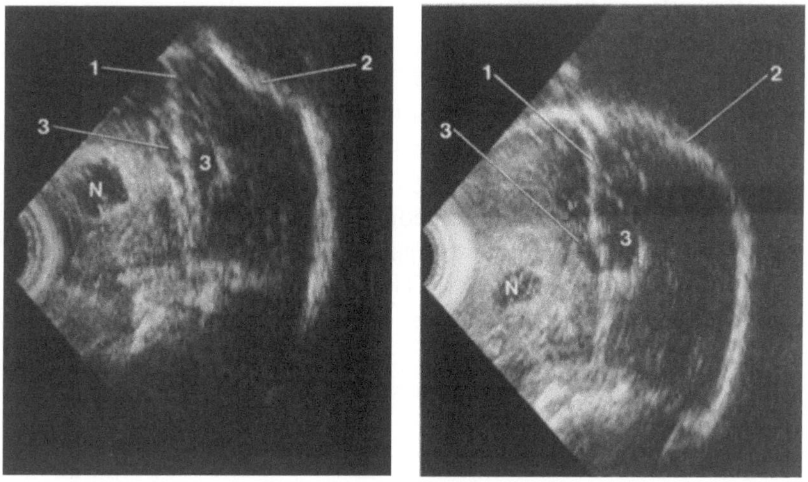

Figs. 59, 60. Coronal US. UM 8, annular array probe, 5 MHz

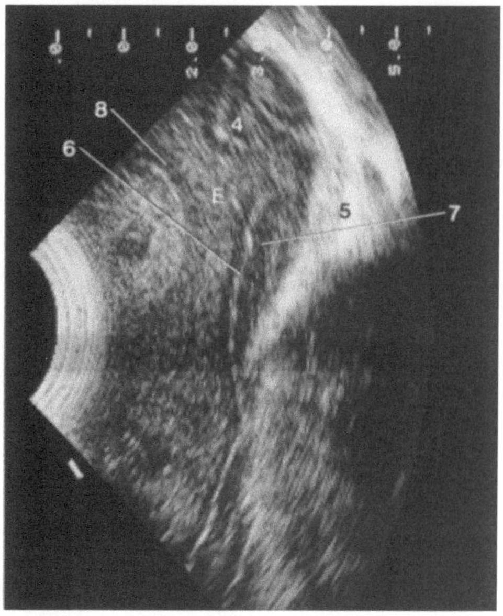

Fig. 61. Horizontal US. UM 8, annular array probe, 7.5 MHz

1 Falx
2 Contralateral skull bone
3 Lateral ventricles
4 Temporal lobe
5 Cavernous sinus
6 Collateral fissure
7 Parahippocampal gyrus
8 Inferior temporal gyrus
E Collateral white matter edema
N Necrotic center of tumor

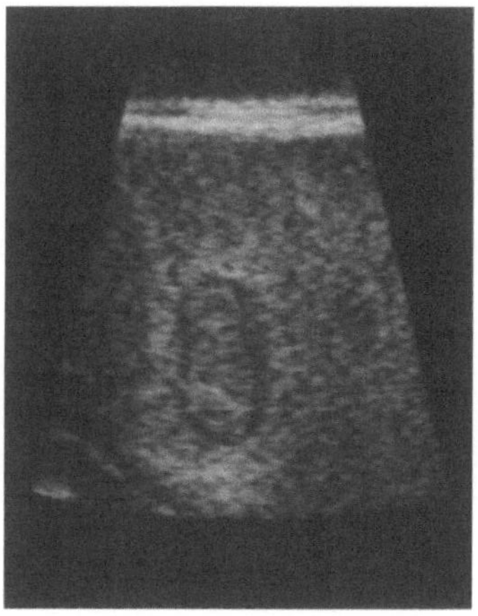

Fig. 62. US at 10 MHz. DRF 100

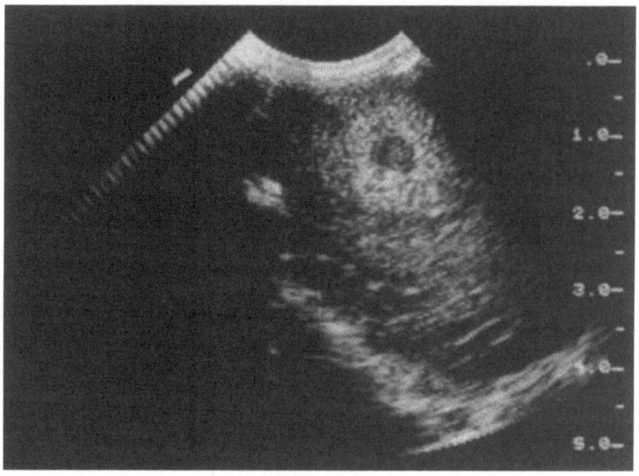

Fig. 63. US at 10 MHz. UM 8

CASE 3 (Figs. 64–68)

Astrocytoma grade 2 in a 26-year-old woman operated upon via a left pterional as well as subtemporal approach.

The tumor is rather homogeneous and markedly hyperechoic, filling the sylvian, suprasellar and interpeduncular cisterns. The ipsilateral cerebral peduncle is compressed by the tumor.

1 Frontal horns with septum pellucidum, foramina of Monro and choroid plexus
2 Third ventricle
3 Insula
4 Superior temporal gyrus
5 Sylvian cistern filled with tumor
6 Uncus
7 Interhemispheric space
8 Contralateral skull bone
9 Ipsilateral gyrus rectus
10 Left crus cerebri compressed by tumor
11 Tentorium
12 Cerebellum
T Hyperechoic tumor filling suprasellar and interpeduncular cisterns

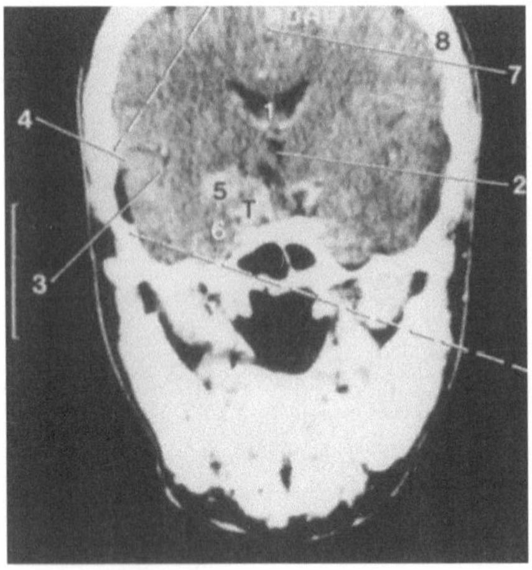

Fig. 64. Coronal CT

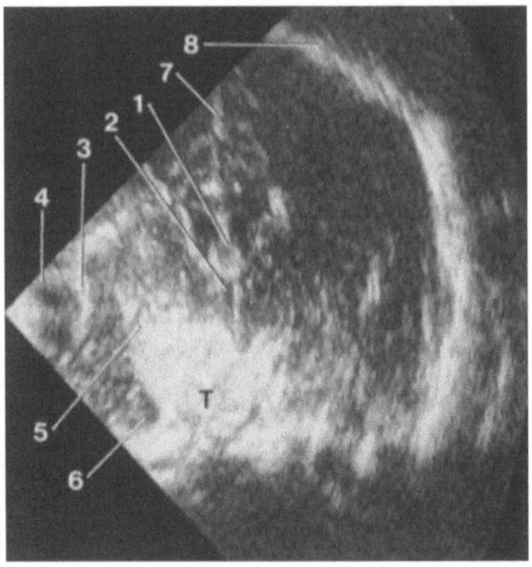

Fig. 65. Coronal US. SSA 100A, 5 MHz

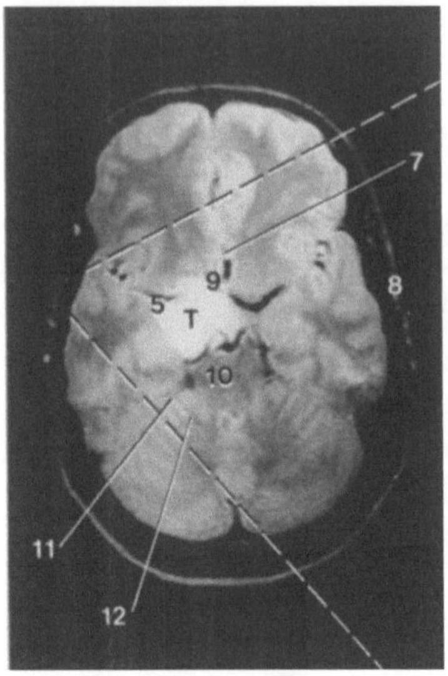

Fig. 66. Horizontal MRI

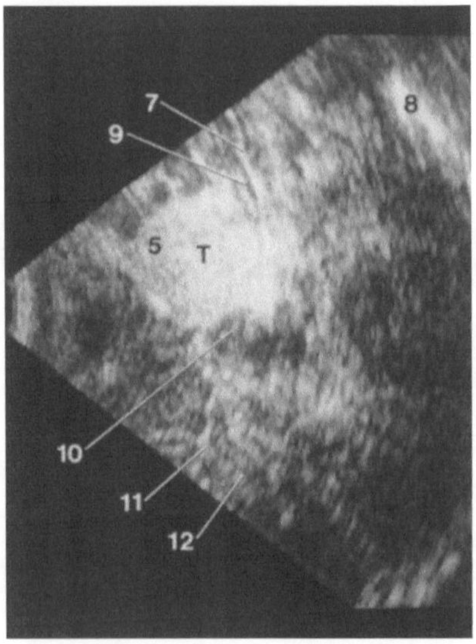

Fig. 67. Horizontal US. DRF 100, GPS probe, 5 MHz

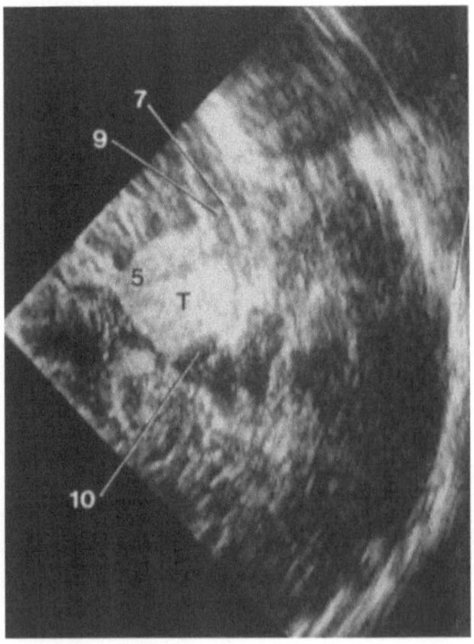

Fig. 68. Horizontal US. SSA 100A, 5 MHz

CASE 4 (Figs. 69, 70)

Anaplastic astrocytoma in a 35-year-old man operated upon via right temporooccipital craniotomy.

Despite contrast enhancement, the tumor is hypodense on CT. On US, the homogeneous tumor is hyperechoic; moreover, it is very ill defined because of the equally hyperechoic edema surrounding the tumor.

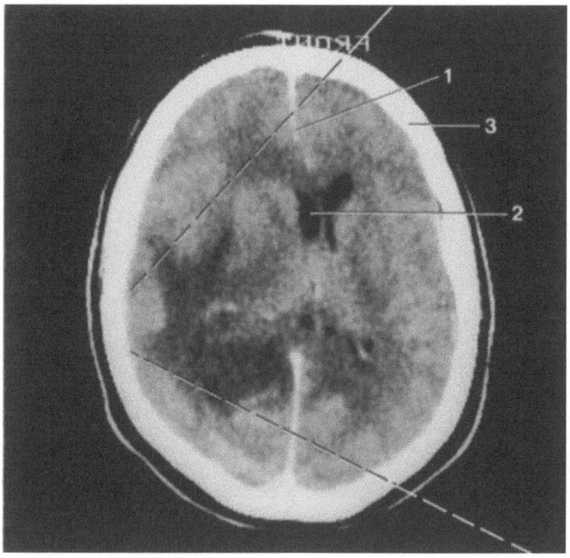

Fig. 69. Horizontal CT

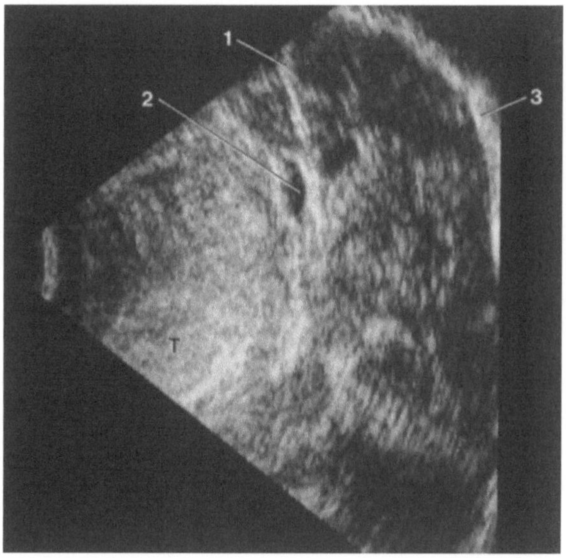

Fig. 70. Horizontal US. DRF 100, GPS probe, 5 MHz

1 Falx
2 Shifted ipsilateral frontal horn
3 Contralateral skull bone
T Hyperechoic tumor with ill-defined border

CASE 5 (Figs. 71–74)

Polycystic low-grade astrocytoma in the pineal region of a 41-year-old man operated upon via an occipital supratentorial approach.

The solid center of the tumor and the capsule of the cystic compartments are almost isoechoic with the cerebellum, but hyperechoic compared with the pons and medulla oblongata. The cystic content is markedly hypoechoic.

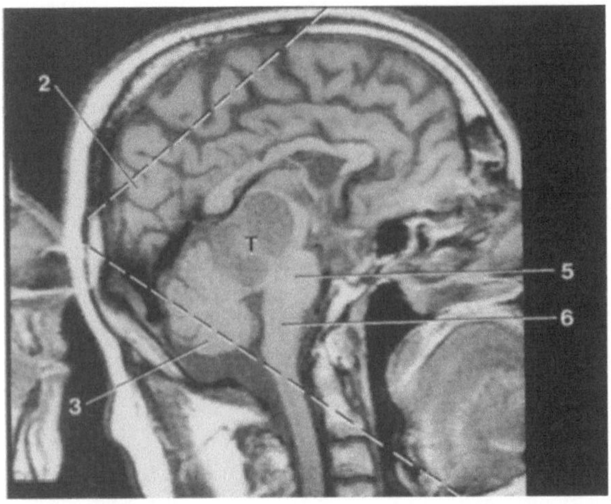

Fig. 71. Sagittal MRI

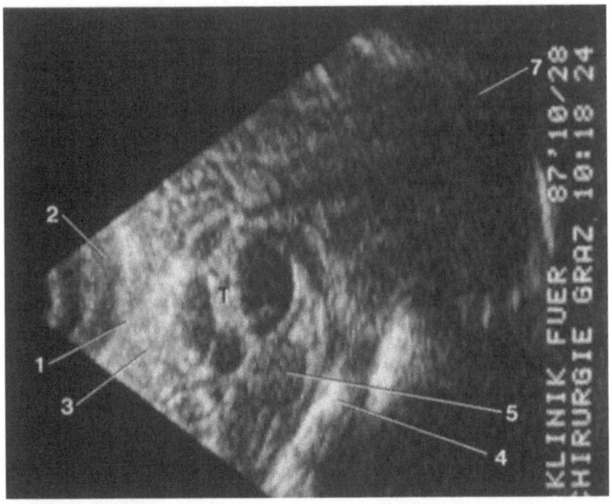

Fig. 72. Sagittal US. DRF 100, GPS probe, 5 MHz

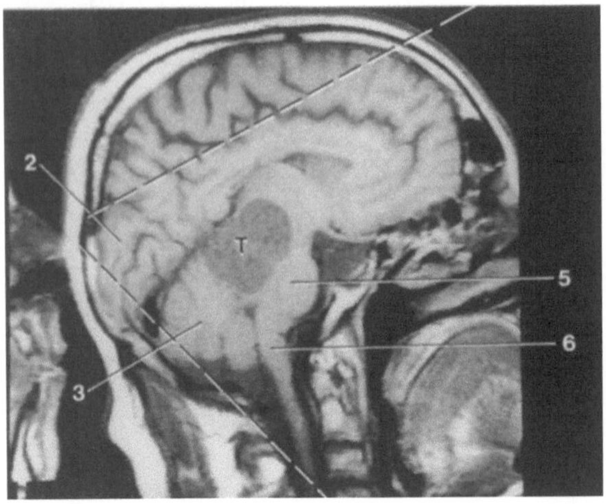

Fig. 73. Sagittal MRI

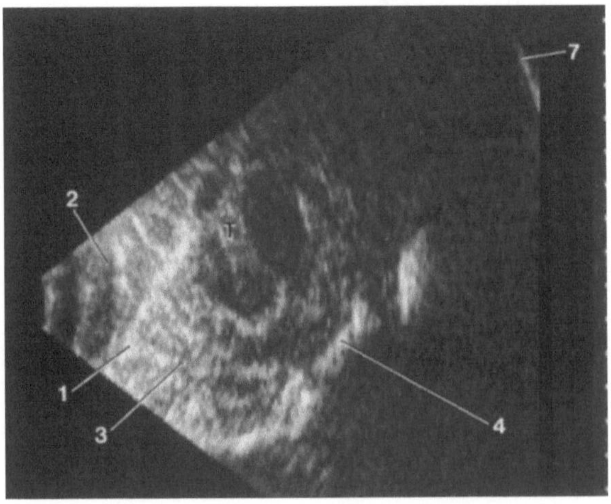

Fig. 74. Sagittal US. DRF 100, GPS probe, 5 MHz

1 Tentorium
2 Occipital lobe
3 Cerebellum
4 Clivus
5 Pons
6 Medulla oblongata
7 Frontal bone
T Tumor

CASE 6 (Figs. 75–77)

Astrocytoma grade 3 in a 52-year-old woman operated upon via left frontal craniotomy.

The tumor appears hyperechoic with a hypoechoic necrotic center. The demarcation of the tumor from its surrounding edematous brain tissue, rather clear on contrast-enhanced CT, is blurred on US, because both tumor and edematous tissue are hyperechoic.

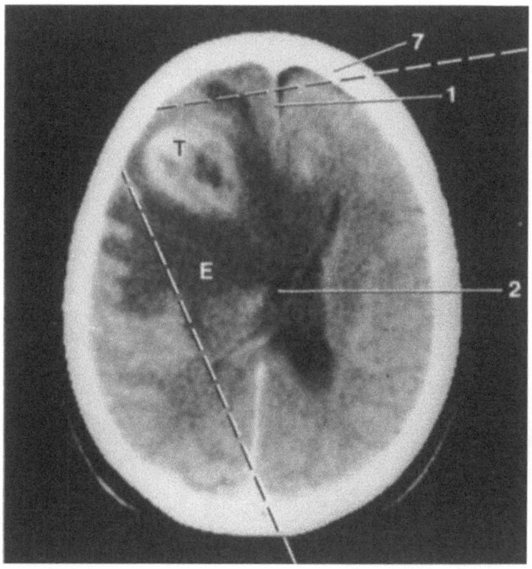

Fig. 75. Horizontal CT

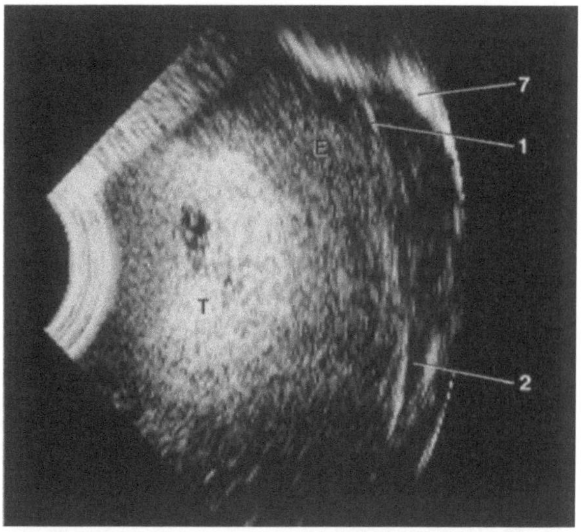

Fig. 76. Horizontal US. UM 8, 5 MHz

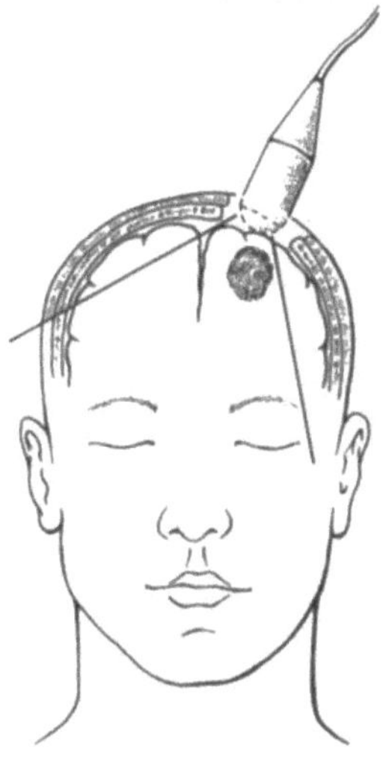

For Fig. 77
(see also Fig. 41 b, c)

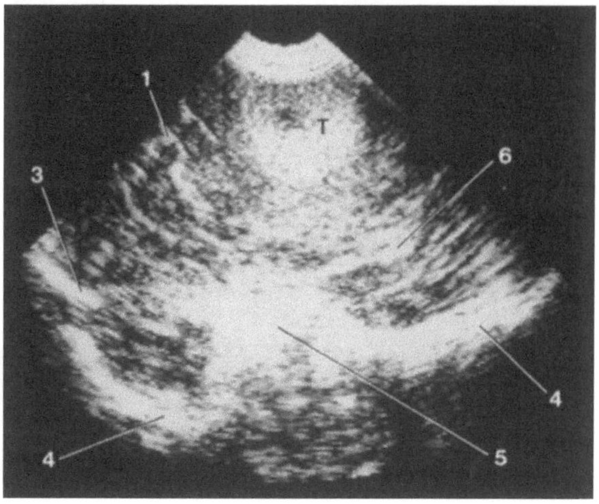

Fig. 77. Coronal US. UM 8, 5 MHz

1 Falx
2 Left lateral ventricle shifted rightward
3 Lesser sphenoid wing
4 Temporal fossa
5 Sphenoid body
6 Medial part of sphenoid wing
7 Skull bone
E Edema
T Tumor with necrotic center

CASE 7 (Figs. 78–81)

Anaplastic astrocytoma in a 55-year-old man operated upon via left temporoparietal craniotomy.

On CT (especially Fig. 78) the tumor has a markedly hyperdense capsule with contrast enhancement and is surrounded by hypodense, probably edematous, tissue. On US the hyperechoic tumor capsule is surrounded by slightly hyperechoic tissue. The interior of the tumor is isoechoic or even slightly hyperechoic. On CT, by contrast, the interior is markedly hypodense, suggesting a cyst.

On operation the interior of the tumor was found to be necrotic, but there was no cyst.

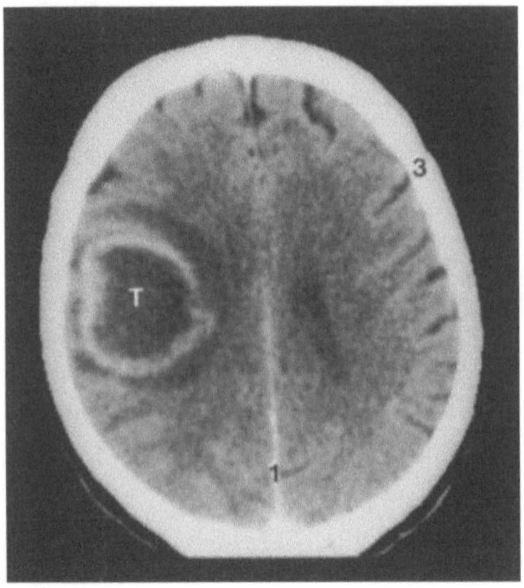

Fig. 78. Horizontal CT

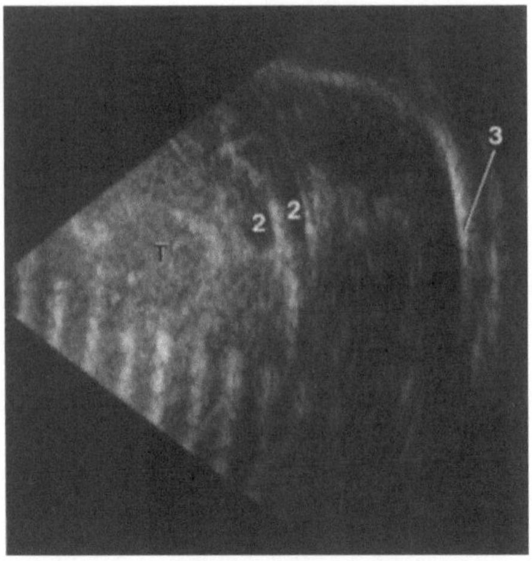

Fig. 79. Horizontal US. DRF 100, GPS probe, 5 MHz

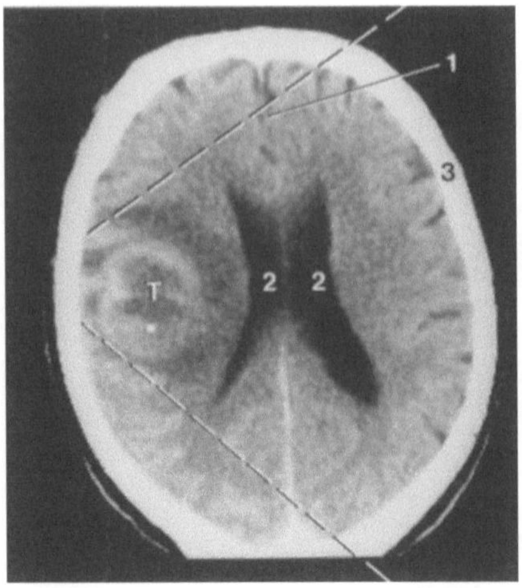

Fig. 80. Horizontal CT

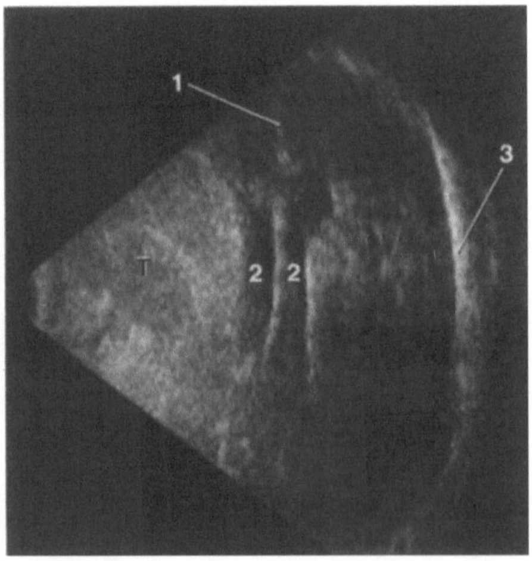

Fig. 81. Horizontal US. DRF 100, GPS probe, 5 MHz

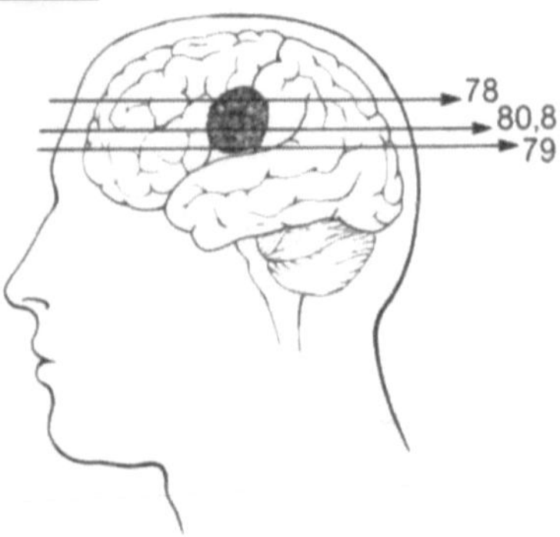

1 Falx
2 Lateral ventricles
3 Right temporoparietal bone
T Tumor

CASE 8 (Figs. 82-84)

Anaplastic astrocytoma in a 33-year-old man operated upon via right occipital craniotomy.

The surrounding edema, characteristically hypodense on CT, is hyperechoic on US; thus, the tumor cysts seem to be surrounded by a thicker rim of solid tumor on US than on CT. US thus blurs rather than clarifies the border between the two. Higher magnification at 5 MHz (Fig. 84) does not make the situation clearer (arrows).

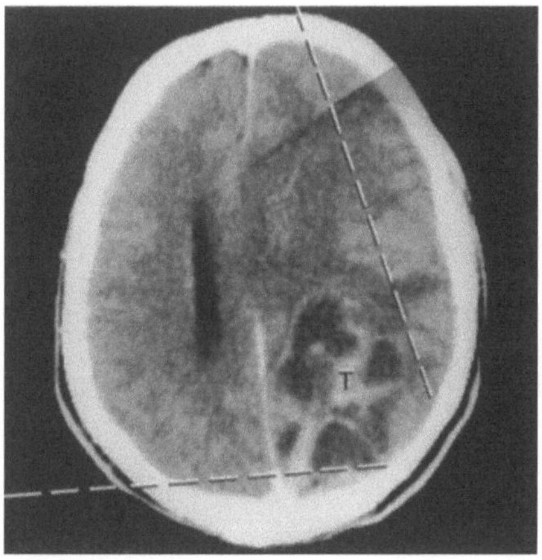

Fig. 82. Horizontal CT

1 Temporal fossa
2 Left sphenoid wing
T Polycystic tumor

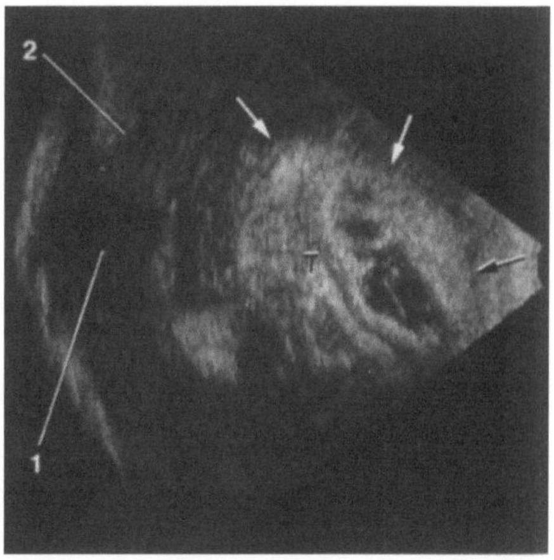

Fig. 83. Horizontal US. DRF 100, GPS probe, 5 MHz

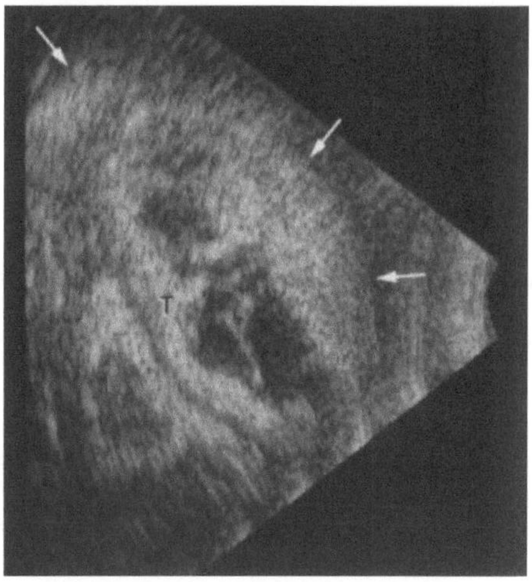

Fig. 84. Higher magnification of Fig. 83

CASE 9 (Figs. 85, 86)

Anaplastic astrocytoma in a 49-year-old man operated upon via temporal craniotomy.

The solid part of the polycystic tumor is hyperechoic. The difference in CT density between cysts and solid tumor is more marked than the difference in US echoicity. The border between the tumor and the surrounding edema is very ill defined on US, as the edema, hypodense on CT, is hyperechoic on US.

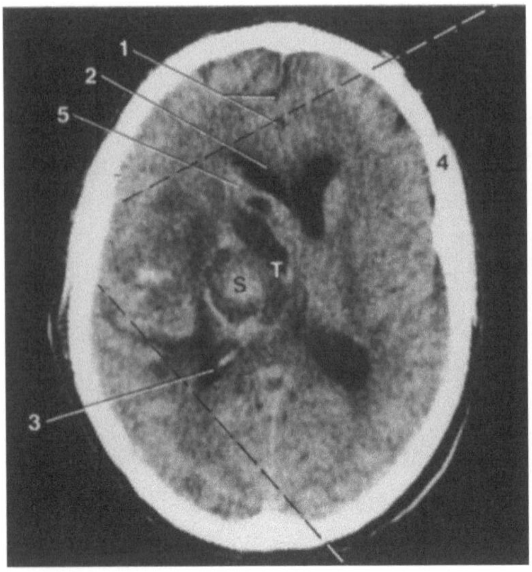

Fig. 85. Horizontal CT

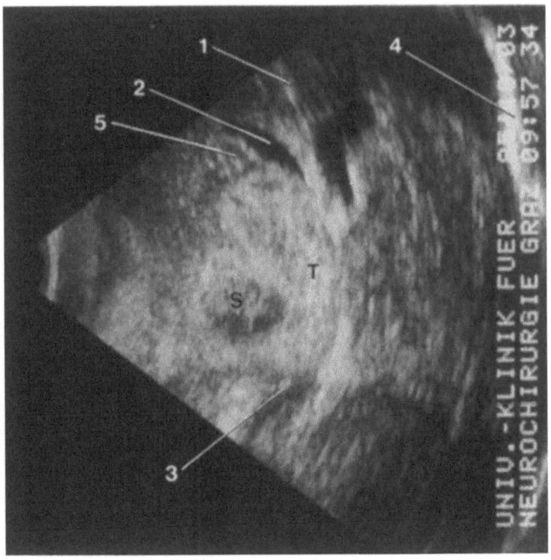

Fig. 86. Horizontal US. DRF 100, GPS probe, 5 MHz

1 Interhemispheric space
2 Displaced left frontal horn
3 Left trigonum with choroid plexus
4 Contralateral skull bone
5 Left caudate nucleus
T Polycystic tumor poorly demarcated from surrounding edema
S Solid nodule within tumor cyst

CASE 10 (Figs. 87-90)

Anaplastic astrocytoma in a 65-year-old man operated upon via occipital craniotomy.

On CT, the tumor is isodense to slightly hyperdense in its periphery and hypodense in the necrotic interior. The hypodense surrounding is interpreted as edema. On US at 5 MHz, the tumor is clearly hyperechoic both on the surface and interiorly; it appears more ill defined, because the surrounding edema is also hyperechoic. On higher magnification at 7.5 MHz (Fig. 89), the US image becomes more similar to the CT picture; the necrotic center is isoechoic, while the periphery is slightly hyperechoic.

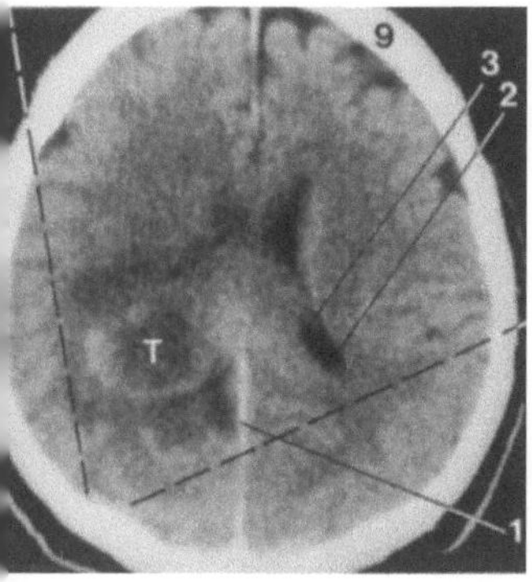

Fig. 87. Horizontal CT

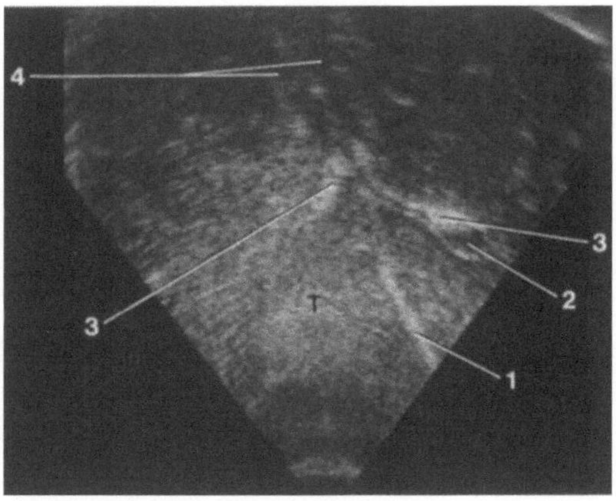

Fig. 88. Horizontal US in plane of CT scan. DRF 100, GPS probe, 5 MHz

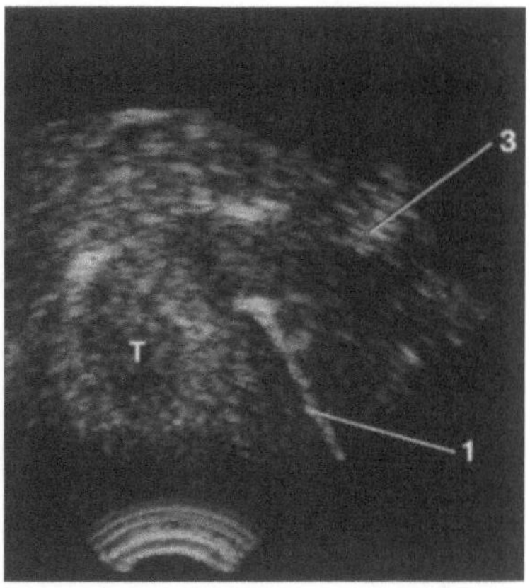

Fig. 89. Horizontal US in plane of CT scan. NS, 7.5 MHz

1 Occipital falx
2 Right posterior horn
3 Choroid plexus (trigonum)
4 Frontal horns
5 Tentorium
6 Cerebellum
9 Frontal bone
10 Occipital bone
11 Choroid plexus in temporal horn
12 Putamen
13 Temporal fossa
14 Sphenoid wing
T Tumor

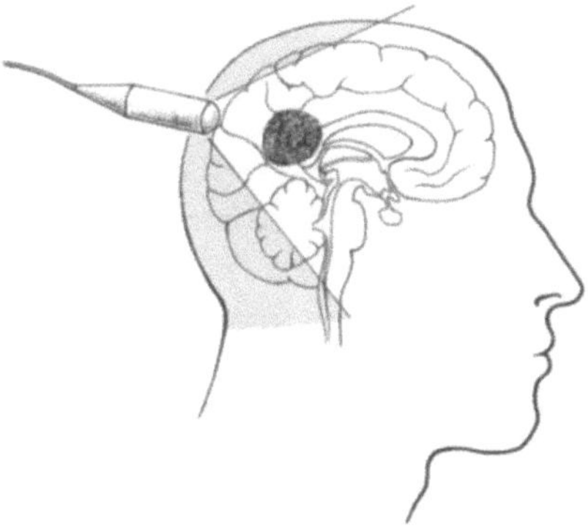

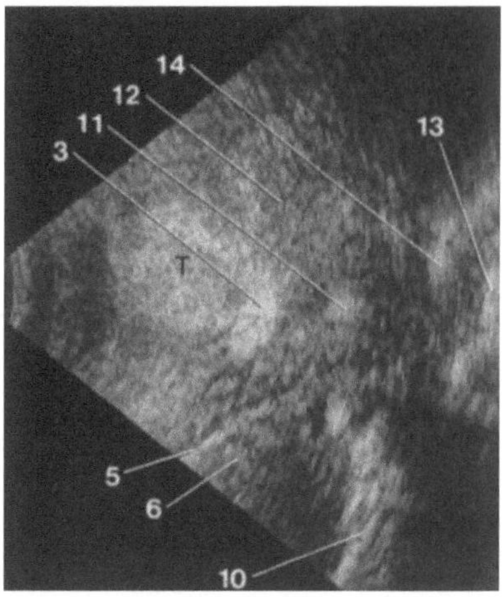

Fig. 90. Sagittal US. DRF 100, GPS probe, 5 MHz

CASE 11 (Figs. 91, 92)

Left temporoparietal *glioblastoma* in a 49-year-old woman operated upon via temporoparietal craniotomy.

The tumor shows a variable density on CT as well as variable echoicity on US. It seems to be rather well defined both on CT and US; the border gets blurred by hyperechoicity only in the area, where CT shows hypodensity (*).

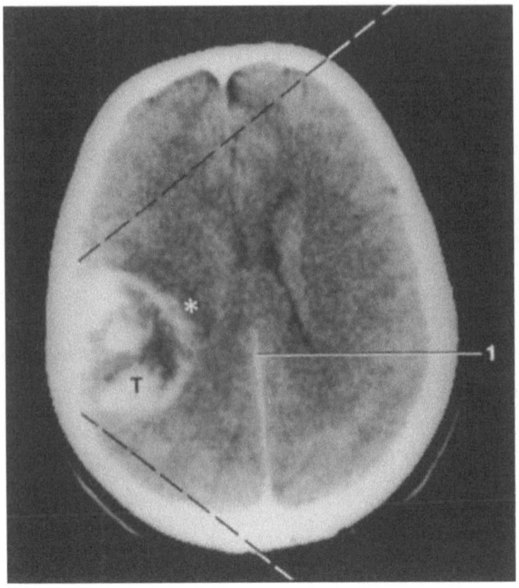

Fig. 91. Horizontal CT

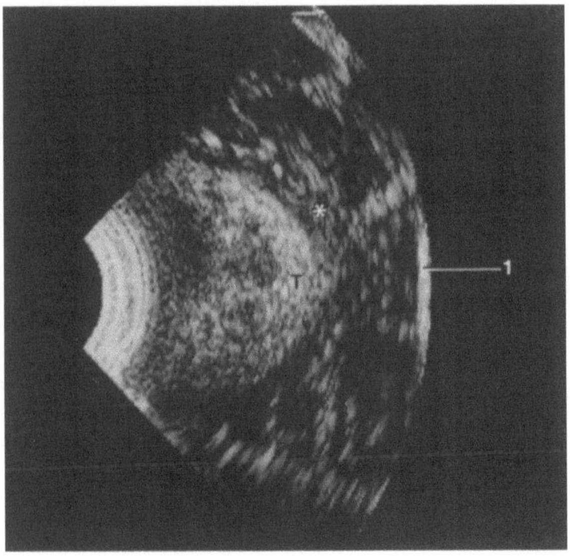

Fig. 92. Horizontal US.NS, 5 MHz

1 Falx
T Tumor

CASE 12 (Figs. 93-95)

Left frontocentral *glioblastoma* in a 26-year-old man operated upon via frontal craniotomy.

At first glance at lower magnification (Fig. 94), one gets the false impression of a well-defined, almost isoechoic tumor with hyperechoic rim (arrows). At higher magnification, the image shows a diffuse variety of signal intensities and the border of the tumor is less clear than on CT.

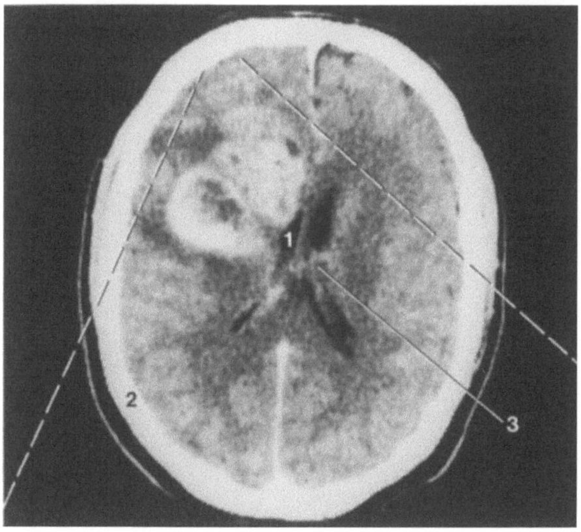

Fig. 93. Horizontal CT

1 Displaced left frontal horn
2 Left occipital bone
3 Choroid plexus in right lateral ventricle

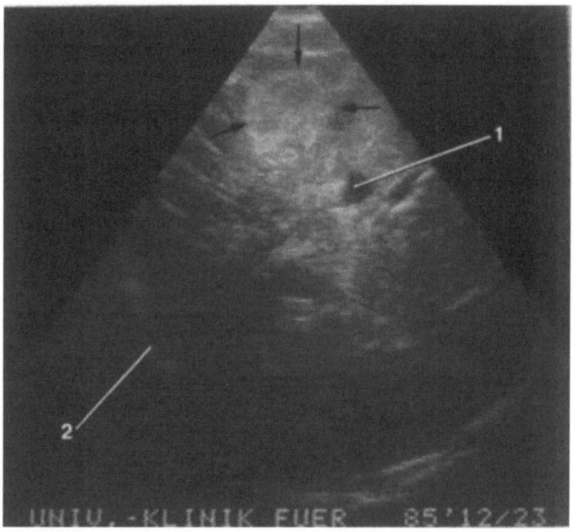

Fig. 94. Horizontal US. DRF 100, GPS probe, 5 MHz

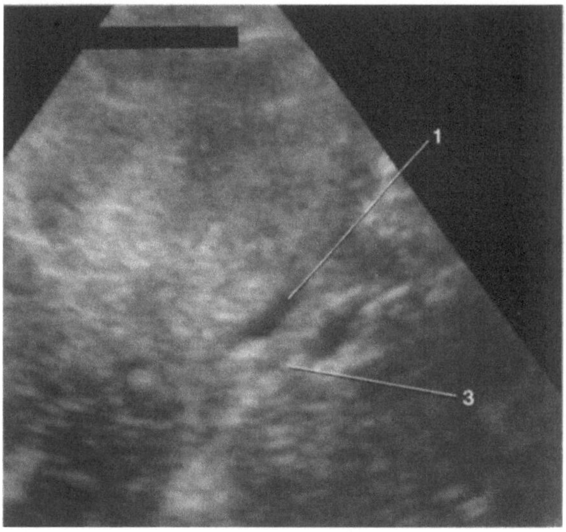

Fig. 95. Higher magnification of Fig. 94. DRF 100, GPS probe, 5 MHz

CASE 13 (Figs. 96, 97)

Left temporofrontal *glioblastoma* in a 54-year-old woman.

CT shows a seemingly well-defined, hyperdense solid tumor which contains several hypodense cysts. US shows a markedly hyperechoic lesion with hypoechoic cysts; however, the hypodense zone around the solid tumor on CT is hyperechoic on US (*).

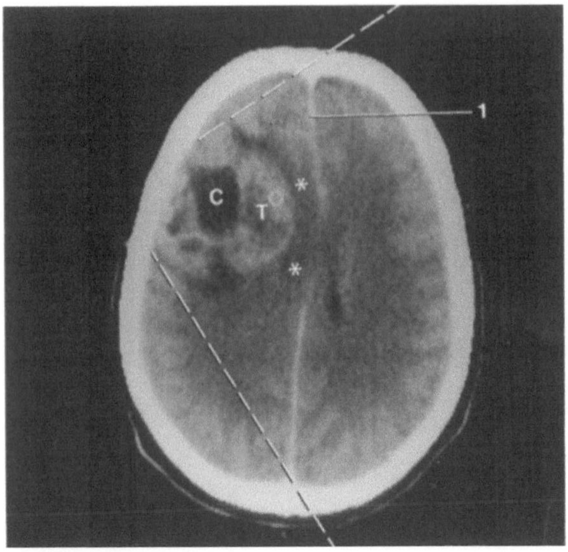

Fig. 96. Horizontal CT

1 Falx
C Cystic tumor
T Solid tumor

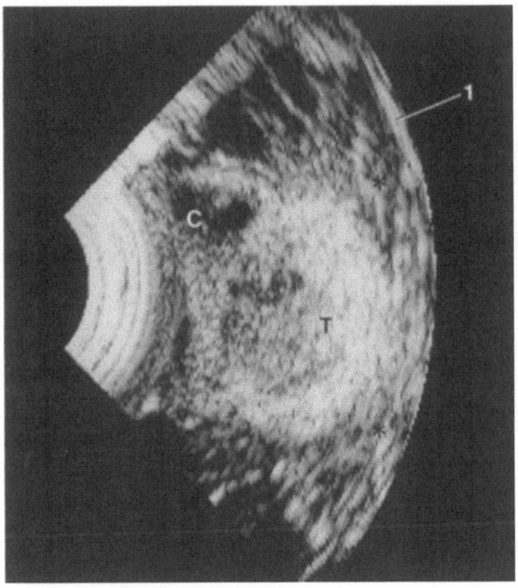

Fig. 97. Horizontal US. NS, 5 MHz

CASE 14 (Figs. 98, 99)

Glioblastoma in a 49-year-old man operated upon via left occipital craniotomy.

The center of the tumor is hypodense on contrast-enhanced CT, but markedly hyperechoic (except for a small area) on US. The tumor seems to be clearly demarcated on both CT and US.

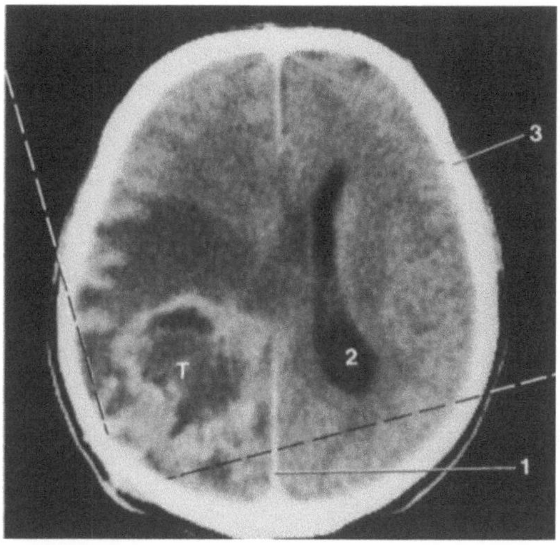

Fig. 98. Horizontal CT

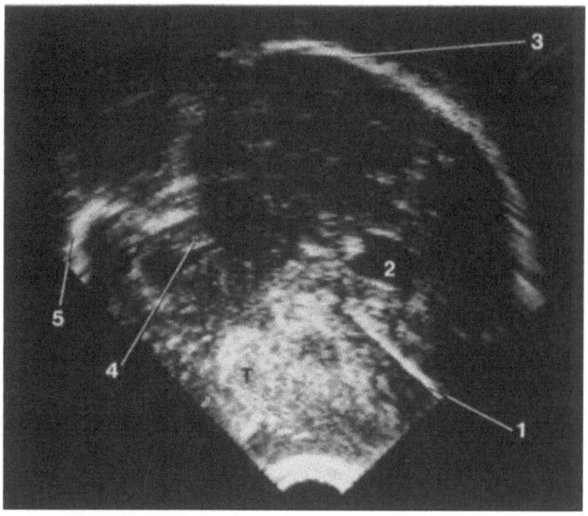

Fig. 99. Diagonal horizontal US. NS, 5 MHz

1 Falx
2 Right posterior horn
3 Right frontotemporal bone
4 Left sphenoid wing
5 Left temporal fossa
T Tumor

CASE 15 (Figs. 100–103)

Right temporocentral *glioblastoma* in a 40-year-old man operated upon via temporal craniotomy. The solid part of the tumor creates a diffuse hyperechoicity in the temporocentral region; thus, US does not differentiate between the CT hyperdense and hypodense areas (the latter of which might be edema). The cystic part of the tumor appears dark with both imaging techniques, hypodense on CT and hypoechoic on US.

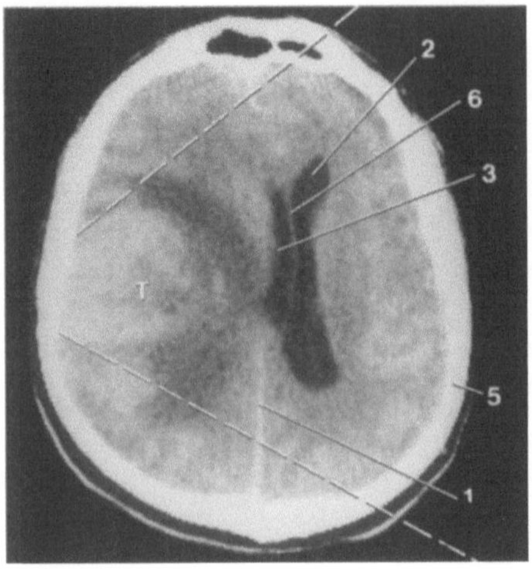

Fig. 100. Horizontal CT

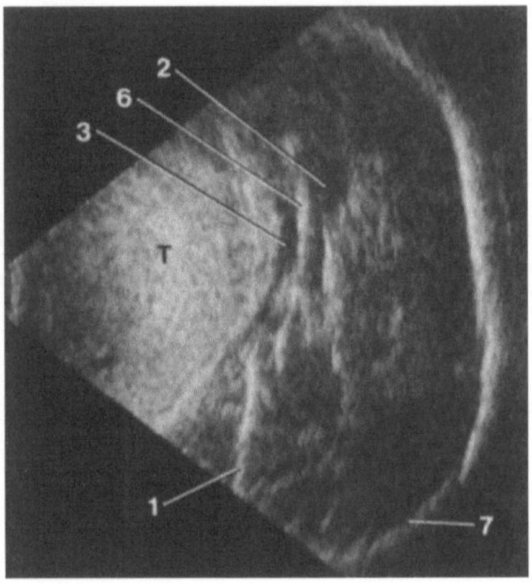

Fig. 101. Horizontal US seen from below. DRF 100, GPS probe, 5 MHz

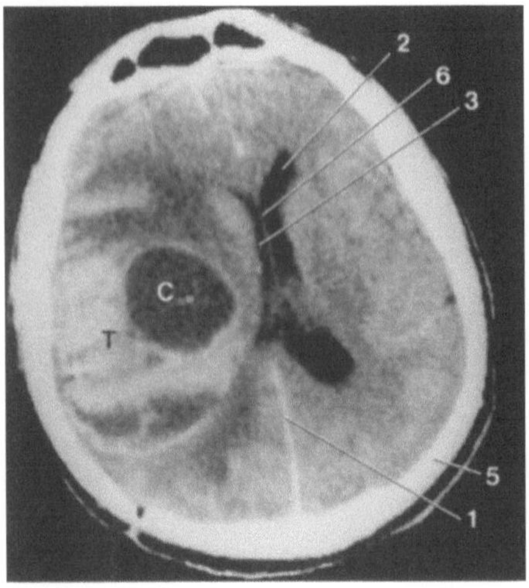

Fig. 102. Horizontal CT

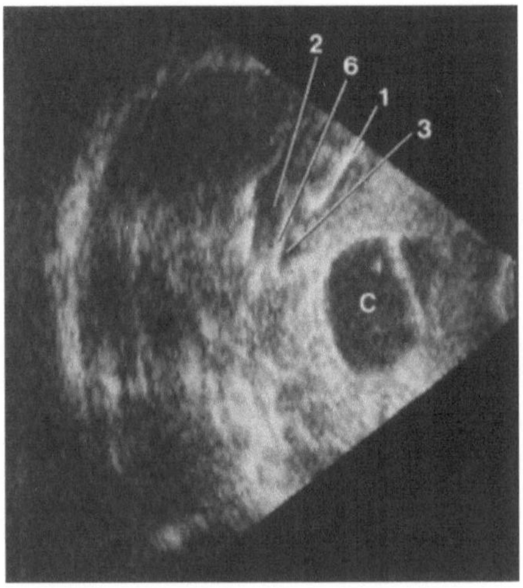

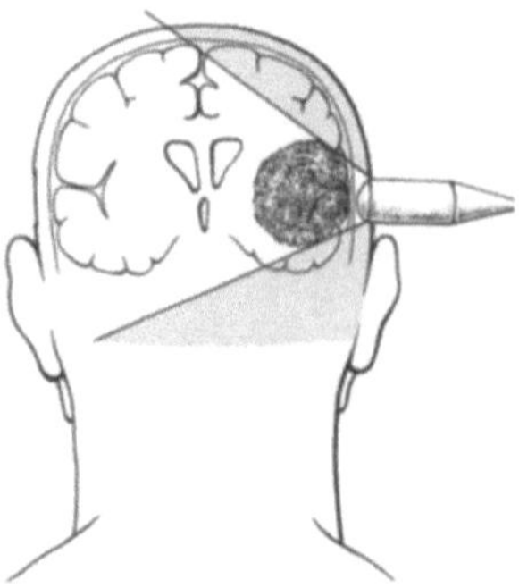

Fig. 103. Coronal US. DRF 100, GPS probe, 5 MHz (see schema)

1 Falx
2 Left lateral ventricle
3 Displaced right pars centralis
5 Left occipital bone
6 Septum pellucidum
7 Occipital bone
C Cystic tumor
T Solid tumor

CASE 16 (Figs. 104-108)

Left parietal *glioblastoma* in a 75-year-old woman operated upon via parietal craniotomy.

Images at 7.5 MHz (Figs. 105, 106) show the partly solid, partly cystic tumor with a variety of different signal intensities. The peripheral aspect of the tumor shows moderate hyperechoicity of homogeneous character, probably edema, that cannot be differentiated from the tumor itself (U). Imaging at 10 MHz shows more detail of the tumor's interior, especially the cysts; however, the border of the tumor does not become more clearly apparent.

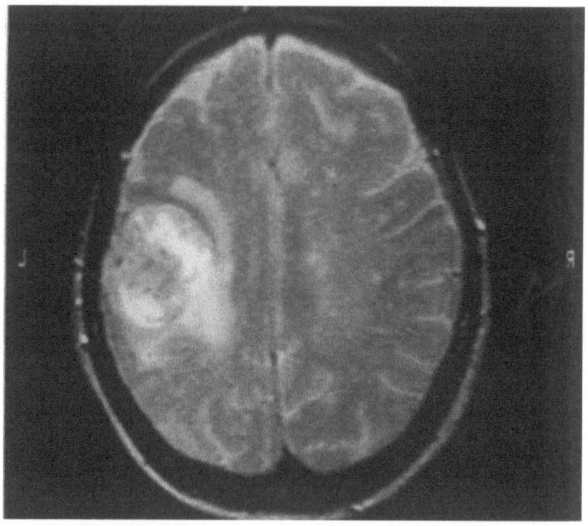

Fig. 104. Horizontal MRI

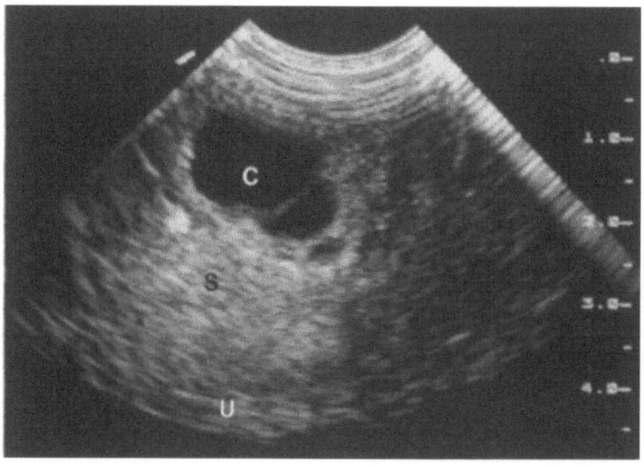

Fig. 105. Diagonal magnified view. US at 7.5 MHz. UM 8, annular array probe

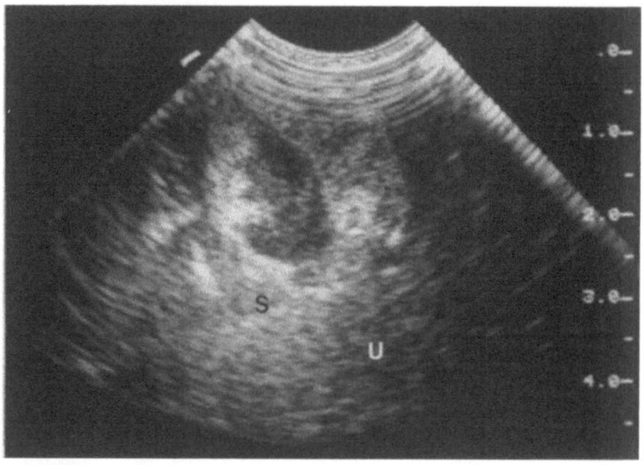

Fig. 106. Diagonal magnified view. US at 7.5 MHz. UM 8, annular array probe

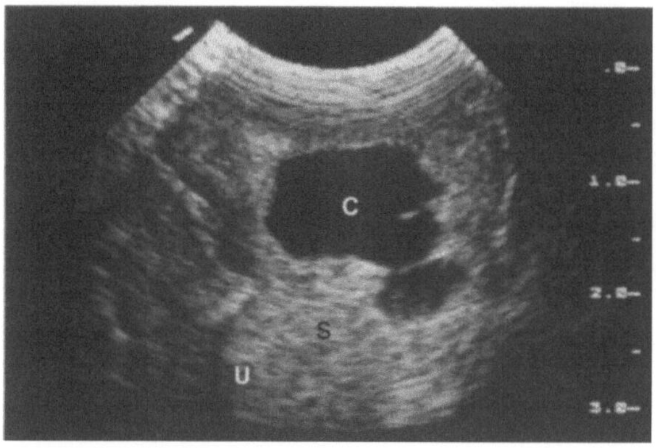

Fig. 107. Diagonal magnified view. US at 10 MHz. UM 8, annular array probe

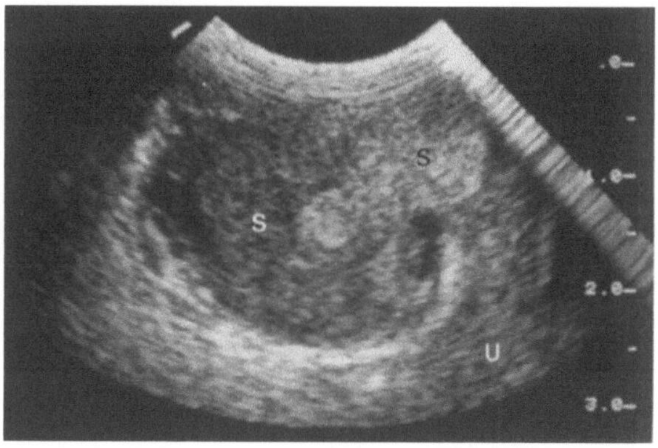

Fig. 108. Diagonal magnified view. US at 10 MHz. UM 8, annular array probe

C Cystic tumor
S Solid tumor
U Uncertain border zone

CASE 17 (Figs. 109-114)

Cystic oligodendroglioma in a 53-year-old man operated upon via right frontal craniotomy.

On US and during surgery, the tumor turned out to consist of two compartments. At the frontal skull base intradurally, a small calcified nodule of bone-like appearance is seen (S in Figs. 111-114); from there, a cyst reaches upward into the right frontal horn (Fig. 114). A tumor capsule of this cyst cannot be identified on US.

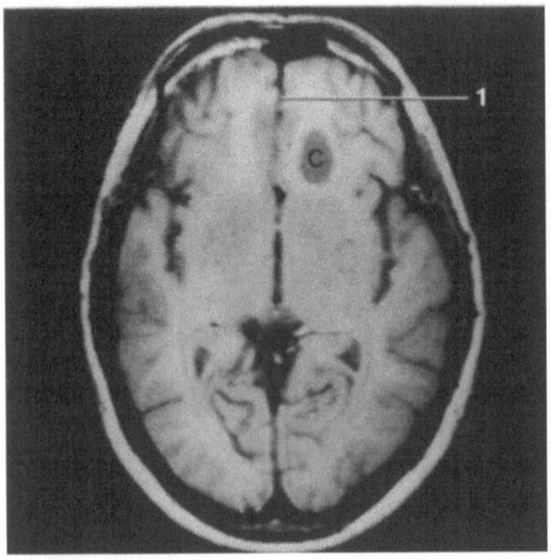

Fig. 109. Horizontal MRI

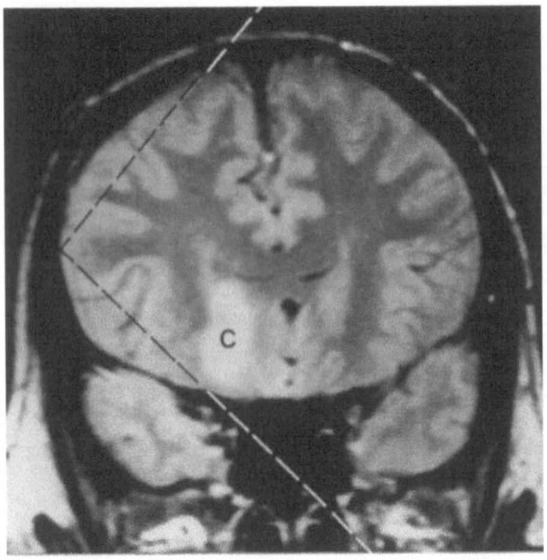

Fig. 110. Coronal MRI

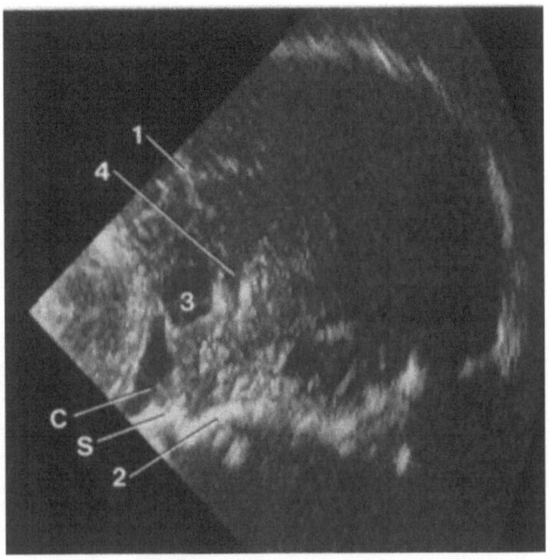

Fig. 111. Coronal US. SSA 100A, 5 MHz

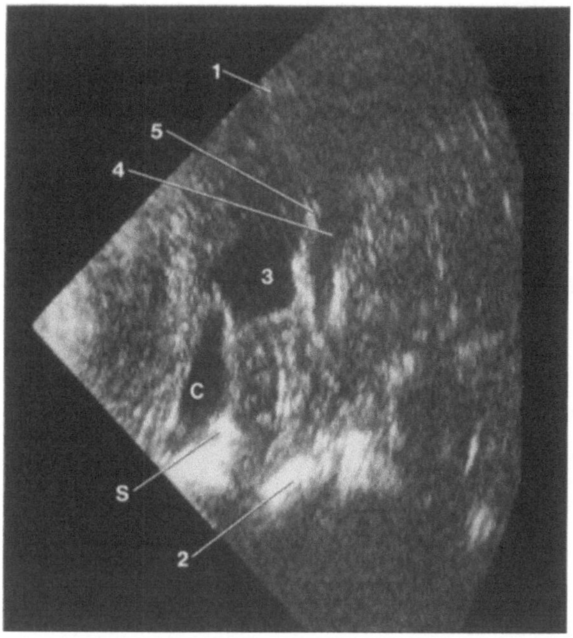

Fig. 112. Slightly diagonal coronal US. SSA 100A, 5 MHz

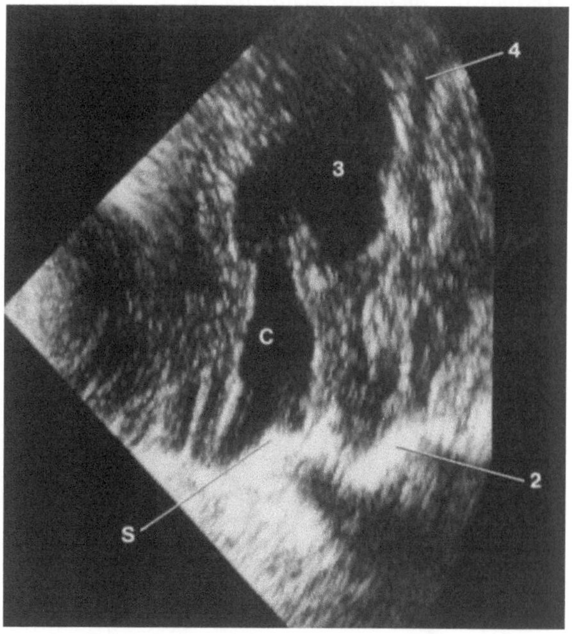

Fig. 113. Slightly diagonal coronal US. SSA 100A, 5 MHz

1 Interhemispheric space
2 Bony floor of anterior fossa
3 Right frontal horn
4 Left frontal horn
5 Septum pellucidum
C Cystic part of tumor bulging into right frontal horn
S Solid nodule of calcified tumor at skull base

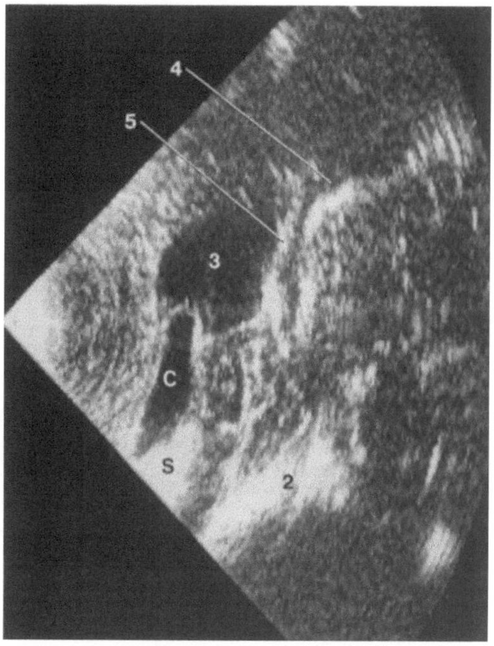

Fig. 114. Slightly diagonal coronal US. SSA 100A, 5 MHz

CASE 18 (Figs. 115-119)

Anaplastic oligodendroglioma in a 27-year-old woman operated upon via right parietooccipital craniotomy.

The tumor is variable in echoicity, mostly hyperechoic toward its border. The latter seems to be clearly defined in the parietomedial area, whereas it is rather ill defined toward the basal circumference (Fig. 116) and toward the internal capsule (Fig. 117).

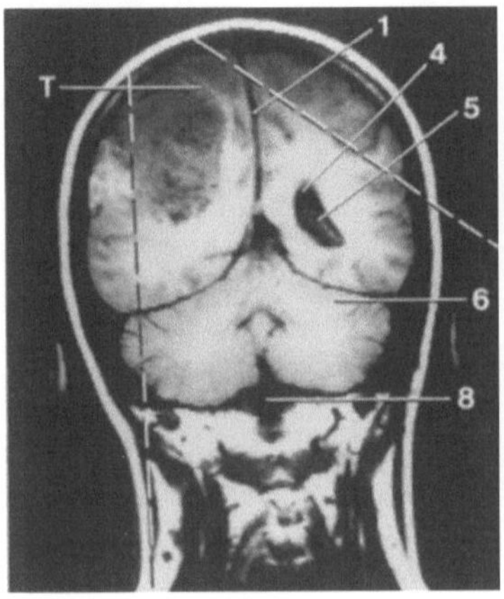

Fig. 115. Coronal MRI

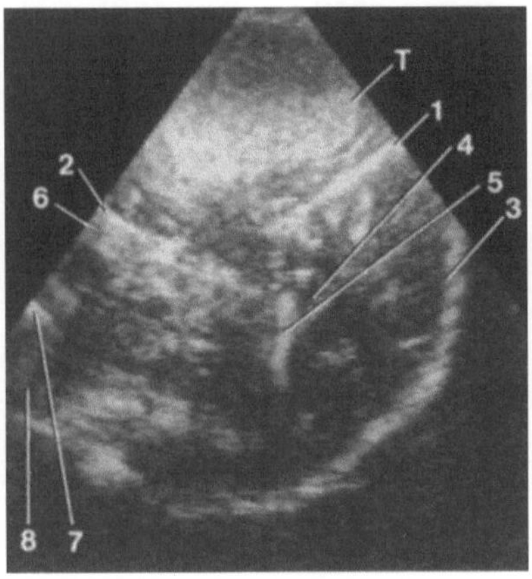

Fig. 116. Coronal US through center of tumor. DRF 100, GPS probe, 5 MHz

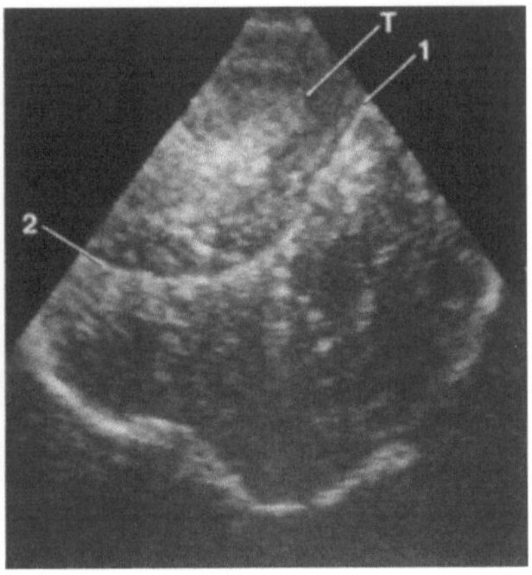

Fig. 117. Coronal US through posterior part of tumor. DRF 100, GPS probe, 5 MHz

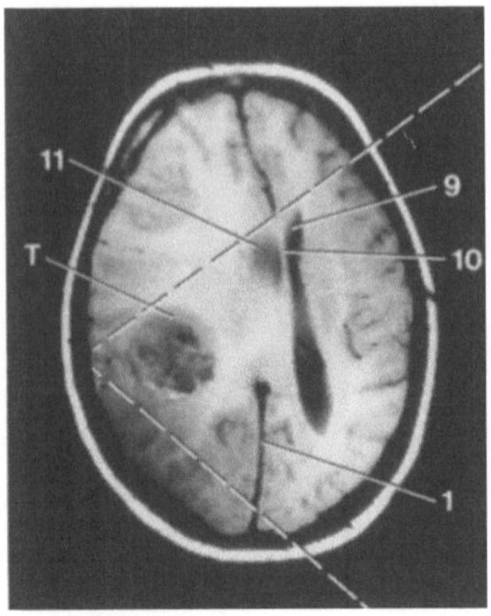

Fig. 118. Horizontal MRI

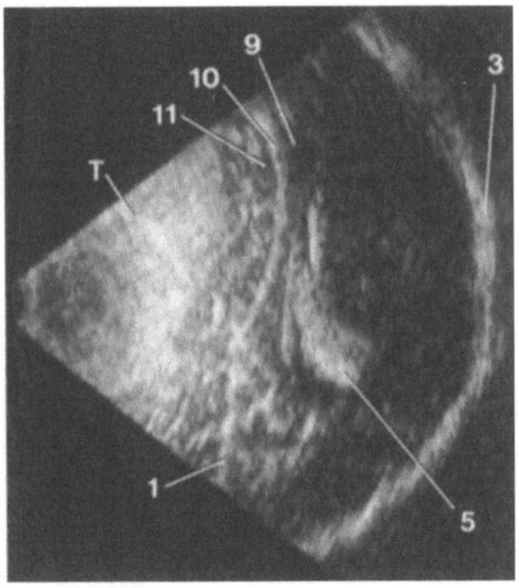

Fig. 119. Horizontal US. DRF 100, GPS probe, 5 MHz

1 Falx
2 Ipsilateral tentorium
3 Contralateral parietal bone
4 Trigonum of contralateral ventricle
5 Choroid plexus
6 Cerebellar cortex
7 Edge of foramen magnum
8 Cisterna magna
9 Contralateral anterior horn
10 Septum pellucidum
11 Ipsilateral anterior horn
T Border of tumor

CASE 19 (Figs. 120, 121)

Ependymoma in a 1-year-old child with a very minor neurological deficit, operated upon via left temporal craniotomy.

The solid parts of the tumor are markedly hyperechoic. The cysts, clearly hypodense on CT, appear rather isoechoic on US. The border of the tumor in the occipital region, where it is visible on the US image, seems well defined.

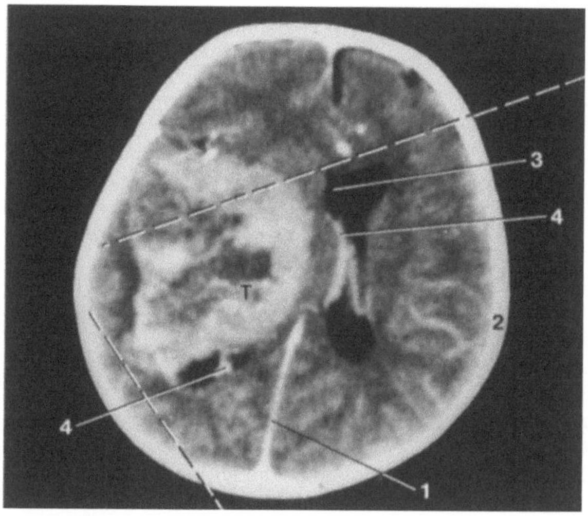

Fig. 120. Horizontal CT

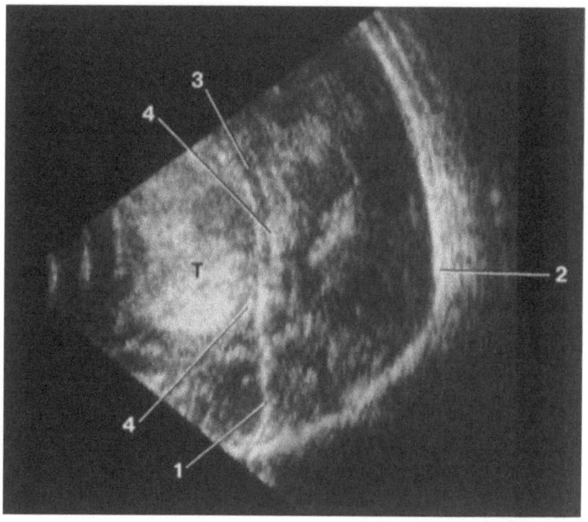

Fig. 121. Horizontal US. DRF 100, GPS probe, 5 MHz

1 Falx
2 Contralateral skull bone
3 Displaced ipsilateral lateral ventricle
4 Choroid plexus
T Tumor

CASE 20 (Figs. 122–124)

Ganglioglioma in a 23-year-old man operated upon via temporoparietal craniotomy.

The markedly hypoechoic cystic compartment seems to have a very thin hyperechoic wall. However, the surrounding white matter is hyperechoic either because of edema or because the tumor continues or both. Subcortically, the solid part of the tumor, which is slightly hyperechoic and apparently better defined at its border, contains several hypoechoic cysts, as shown at higher magnification and higher frequency (10 MHz).

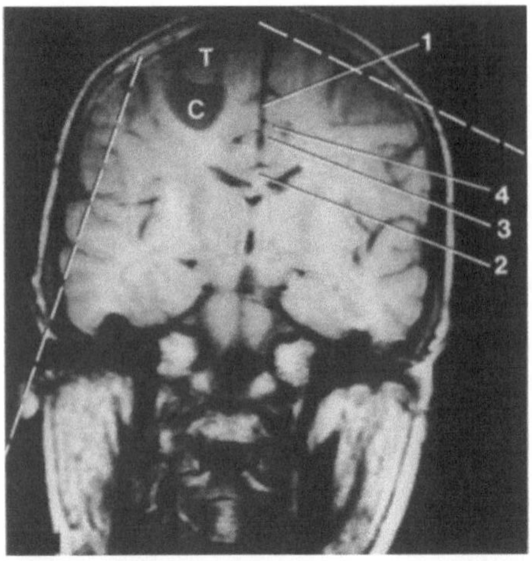

Fig. 122. Coronal MRI

1 Interhemispheric space
2 Corpus callosum
3 Cingulate gyrus
4 Cingulate sulcus
C Large cyst
T Polycystic (→) solid tumor

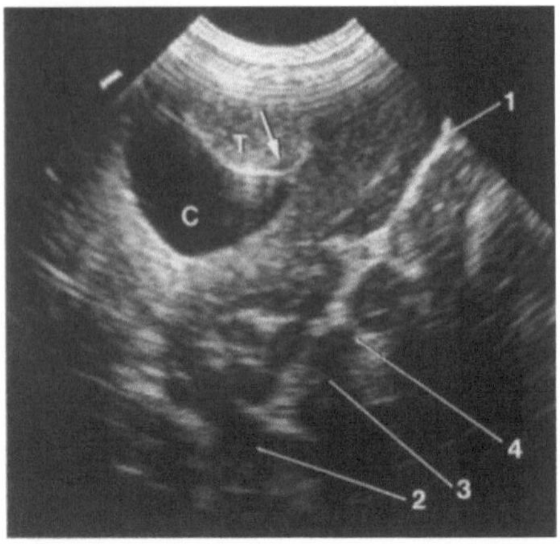

Fig. 123. Coronal US. UM 8, annular array probe, 7.5 MHz

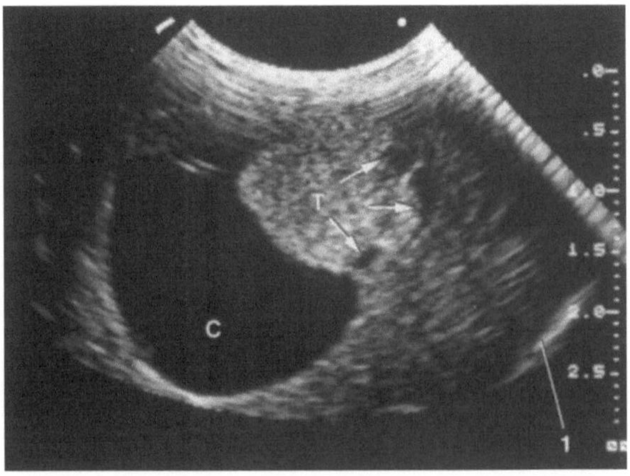

Fig. 124. Coronal US, higher magnification. UM 8, annular array probe, 10 MHz

Meningiomas

Most meningiomas display homogeneously high echo intensity (see also ref. [52]); thus they usually appear on US images as clearly demarcated white areas surrounded by the dark-gray structure of brain tissue. Usually the capsule is even more hyperechoic, which underlines the clear delineation. In some cases, parts of the tumor are isoechoic or even hypoechoic; when this is due to tissue necrosis, good agreement is found with CT and MRI images. In other instances, however, CT and MRI fail to show such intratumoral areas, or density differences on CT are very minor, while US shows markedly hyperechoic areas next to markedly hypoechoic zones. In this latter case, differences of echo intensity correlate well with the consistency of tumor tissue encountered during operation, i.e., soft nonnecrotic tumor tissue of mostly younger age is hypoechoic, while harder tissue is hyperechoic.

Small meningiomas in particular can be surrounded by significant amounts of edema. This edema appears hypoechoic on US and hypodense on CT (see also ref. 59). Interestingly, edema on US is not always hypoechoic: perifocal edema is hyperechoic around gliomas and metastases, while it is hypodense on CT under all circumstances.

CASE 21 (Figs. 125–133)

A temporoparietal *convexity meningioma* in a 62-year-old man operated upon via a left temporoparietal craniotomy.

The tumor, ill-defined and isodense on native CT, enhanced markedly with contrast to show up as a well-defined hyperdense lesion which causes no midline shift and no brain edema (Fig. 125). External carotid angiography (Fig. 128) shows no tumor vessels but a hypovascularized area in the capillary phase. Horizontal views from left parietal (Figs. 126, 129) show both lateral ventricles and both choroid plexuses. A hyperechoic tumor border appears. The major part of the tumor appears misleadingly as hypoechoic, because it is in the dead zone, the near field of the 5-MHz probe. The tumor is surrounded by a hypoechoic zone which is not readily seen on CT. At higher magnification (Fig. 130) the tumor appears homogeneous and isoechoic, hyperechoic only at its border. Demarcation from the surrounding brain tissue is clear, but differentiation between the surrounding brain tissue and the CSF space is difficult.

The 10-MHz probe (Figs. 131–133) shows a clearly hyperechoic, very well demarcated tumor with hypoechoic areas (cysts). It now seems possible to differentiate between the tumor capsule, the surrounding brain tissue and the intervening subarachnoid space (arrows).

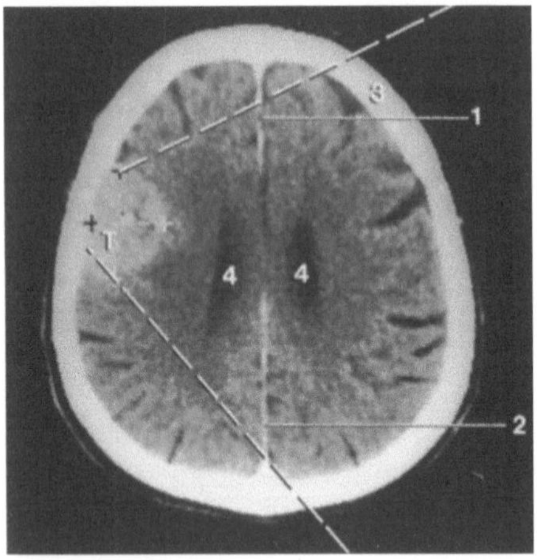

Fig. 125. Horizontal CT

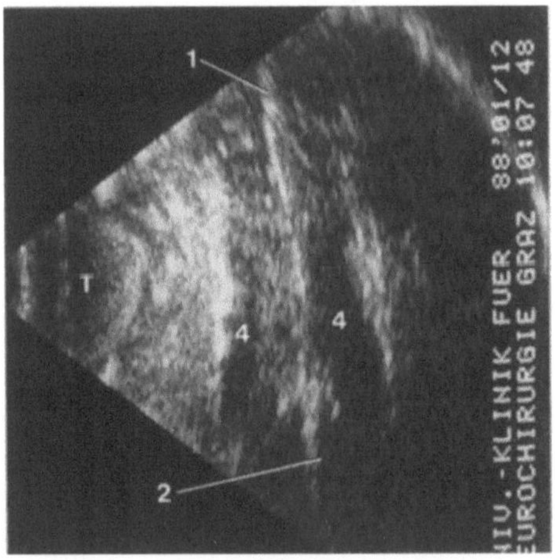

1 Frontal falx
2 Occipital falx
3 Right frontal bone
4 Pars centralis
5 Frontal horns
6 Caudate nucleus
7 Septum pellucidum
8 Choroid plexus
T Tumor
→ (black) Tumor capsule
→ (white) Brain surface of tumor bed
* Intratumoral cyst
• Peritumoral CSF space

Fig. 126. Horizontal US. DRF 100, GPS probe, 5 MHz

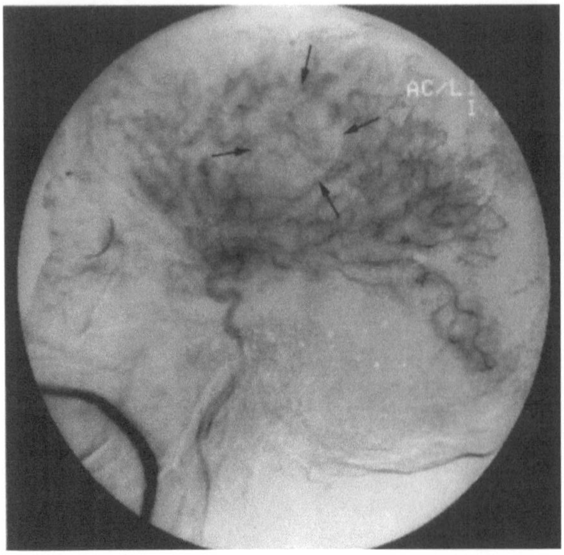

Fig. 127. Left lateral internal carotid angiography

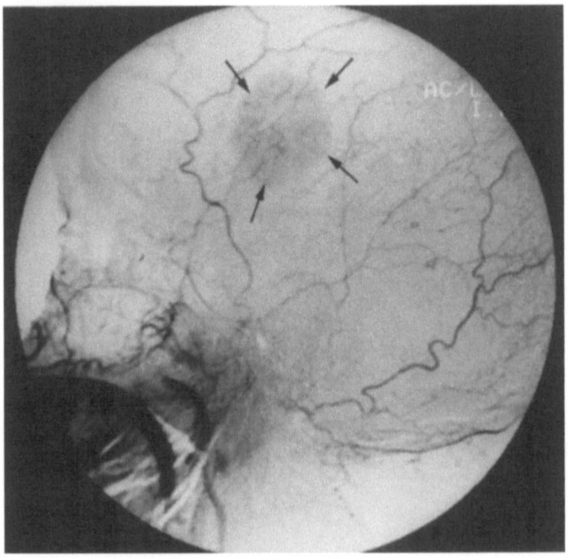

Fig. 128. Left lateral external carotid angiography

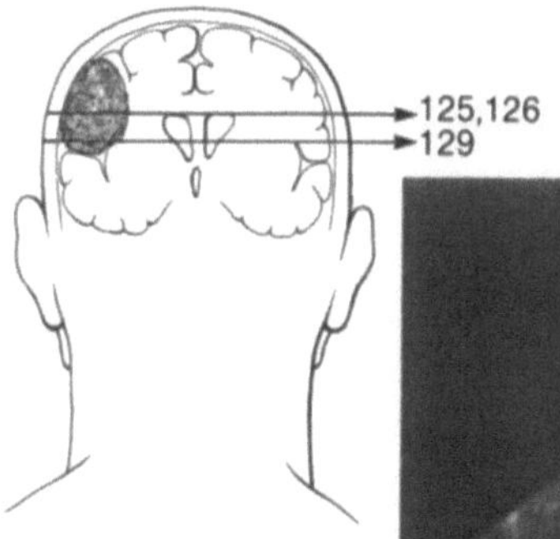

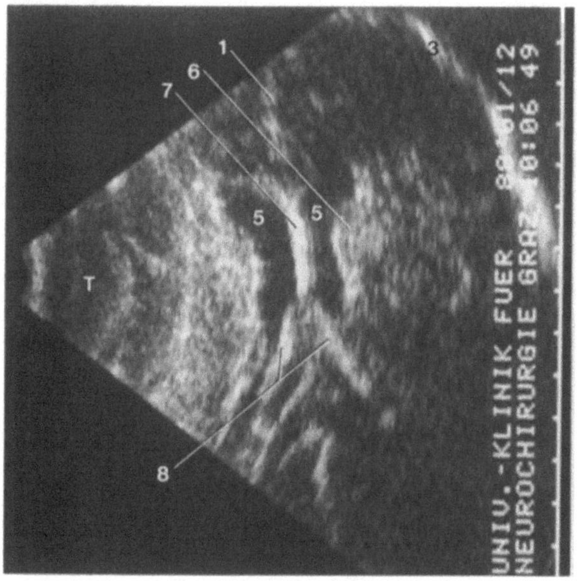

Fig. 129. Horizontal US. DRF 100, GPS probe, 5 MHz

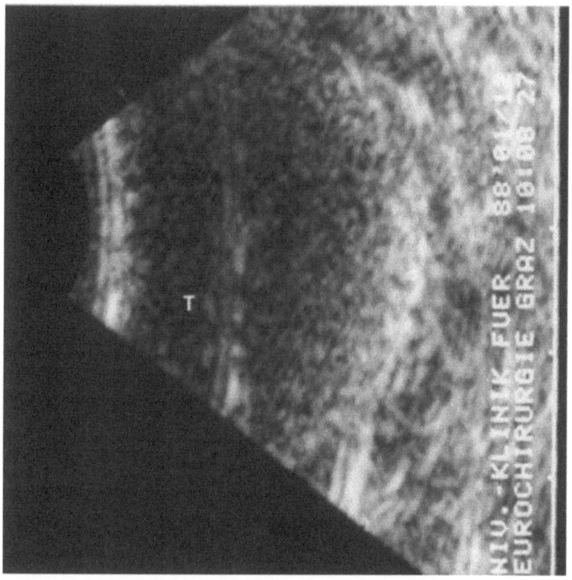

Fig. 130. Horizontal US, higher magnification. DRF 100, GPS probe, 5 MHz

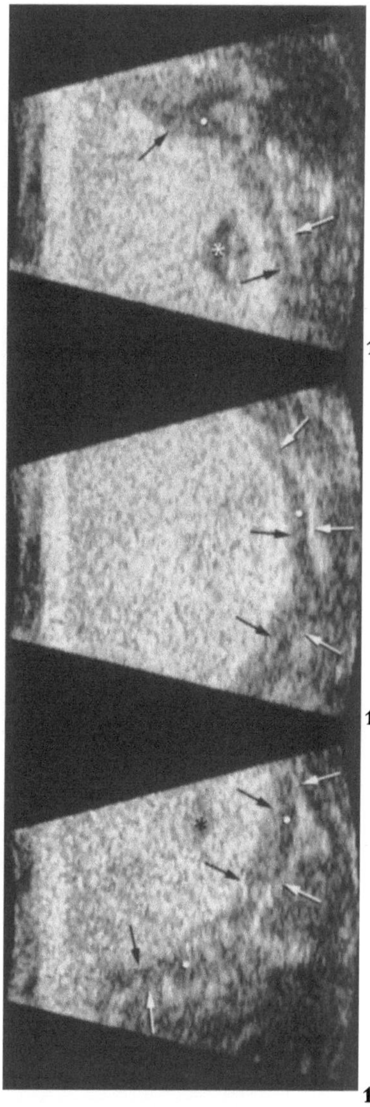

131

132

133

Figs. 131–133. Horizontal US. DRF 100, NF probe, 10 MHz

CASE 22 (Figs. 134–139)

Parasagittal *convexity meningioma* in a 76-year-old woman operated upon via left parietooccipital craniotomy.

The tumor is well demarcated and markedly hyperechoic, although the intratumoral signal intensity is somewhat inhomogeneous. The CSF space surrounding most of the tumor surface on MRI can be clearly distinguished on a 7.5-MHz image (Fig. 139), whereas it is appreciated only with difficulty on 5-MHz images (Fig. 137). The coronal 5-MHz image shows a slightly hyperechoic area in the deep white matter of the left hemisphere (Fig. 138).

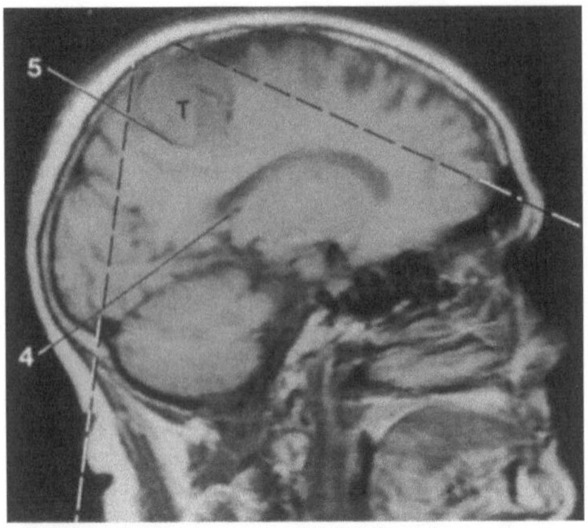

Fig. 134. Sagittal MRI

1 Falx
2 Lateral ventricles
3 Choroid plexus
4 Trigonal choroid plexus
5 CSF space around tumor
E Edema
T Tumor

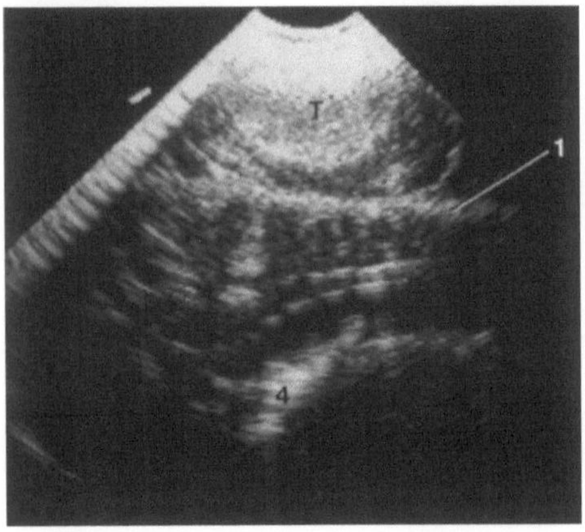

Fig. 135. Diagonal sagittal US. UM 8, annular array probe, 5 MHz

Sector plane for Fig. 135

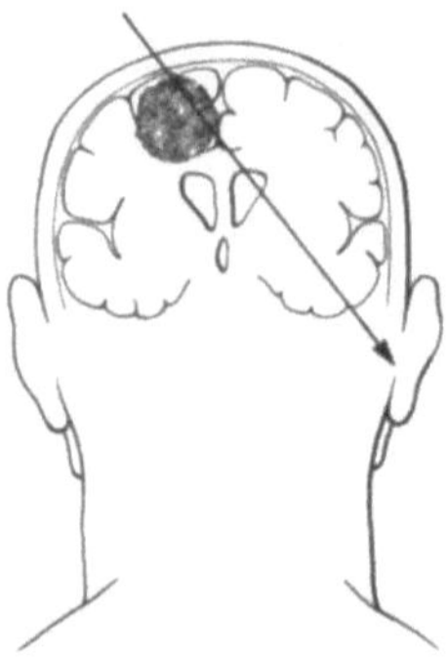

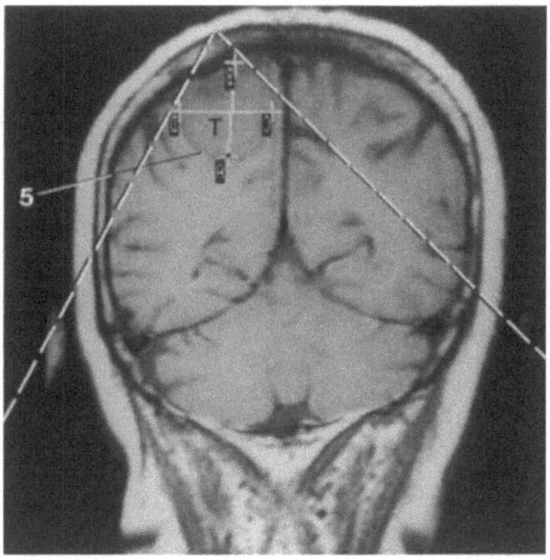

Fig. 136. Coronal MRI

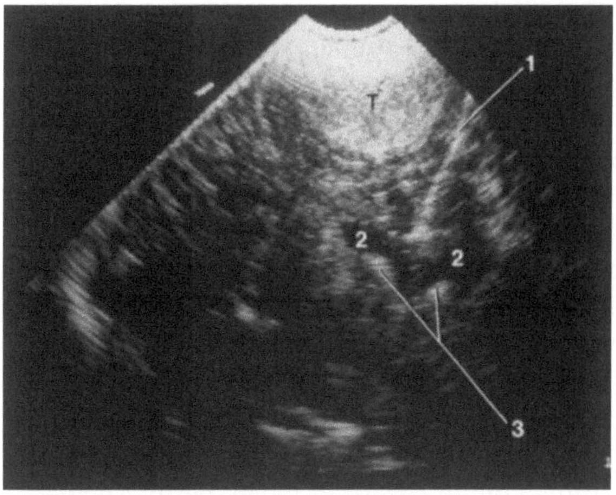

Fig. 137. Diagonal coronal US. UM 8, annular array probe, 5 MHz

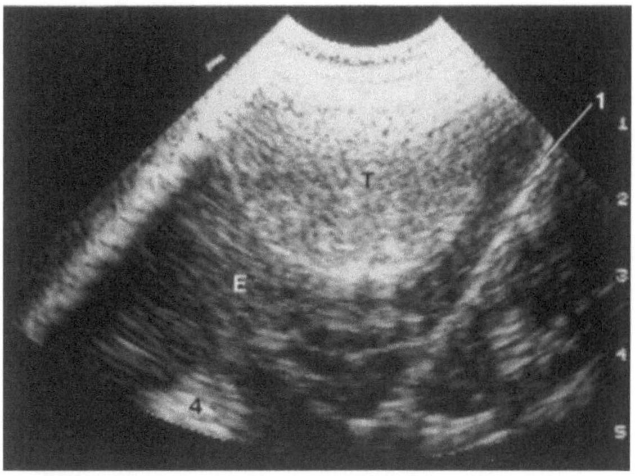

Fig. 138. Coronal US. UM 8, annular array probe, 5 MHz

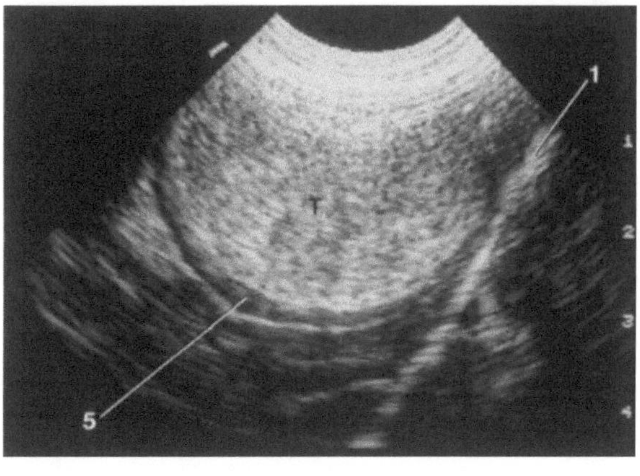

Fig. 139. Coronal US. UM 8, annular array probe, 7.5 MHz

CASE 23 (Figs. 140–145)

Parasagittal *convexity meningioma* in a 53-year-old woman operated upon via right parietal craniotomy.

CT shows that the tumor has two compartments, one hyperdense and located at the parietal convexity (T_I), the other isodense and growing toward the depth of the interhemispheric space (T_{II}), displacing the falx to the right side. Little edema is seen in the depth of the white matter and near the occipital suface of T_{II}. On US, T_I is hyperechoic, T_{II} very slightly hypoechoic. Both are well demarcated, and T_{II} has a clearly hyperechoic capsule. During operation, T_I turned out to consist of tough, partly calcified tissue, whereas the tissue of T_{II} was soft.

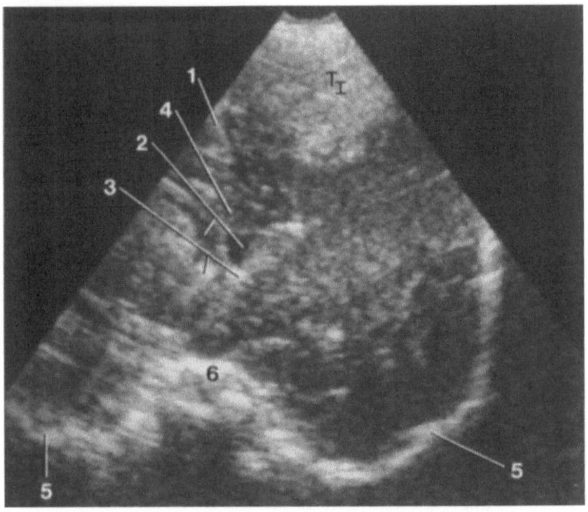

Fig. 141. Coronal US. DRF 100, GPS probe, 5 MHz

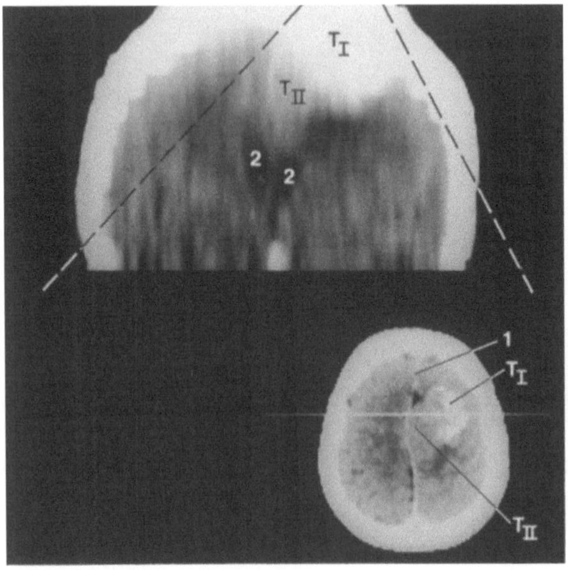

Fig. 140. Coronal and horizontal CT

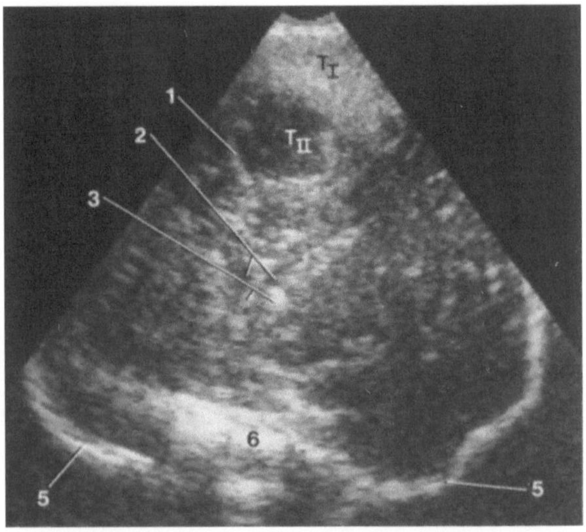

Fig. 142. Coronal US. DRF 100, GPS probe, 5 MHz

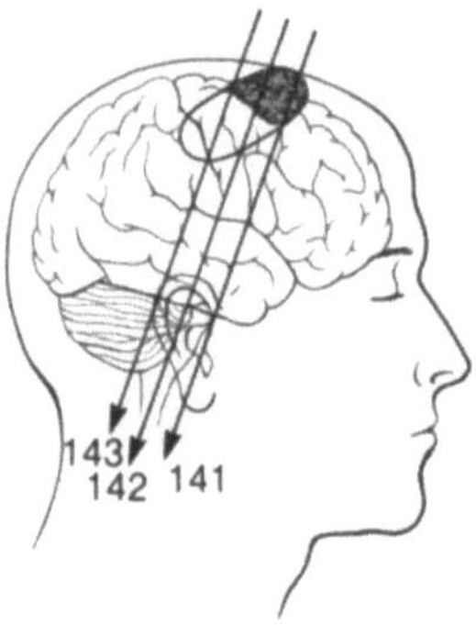

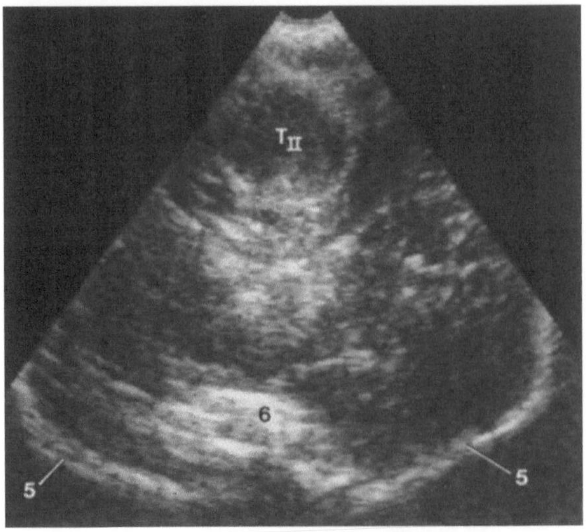

Fig. 143. Coronal US. DRF 100, GPS probe, 5 MHz

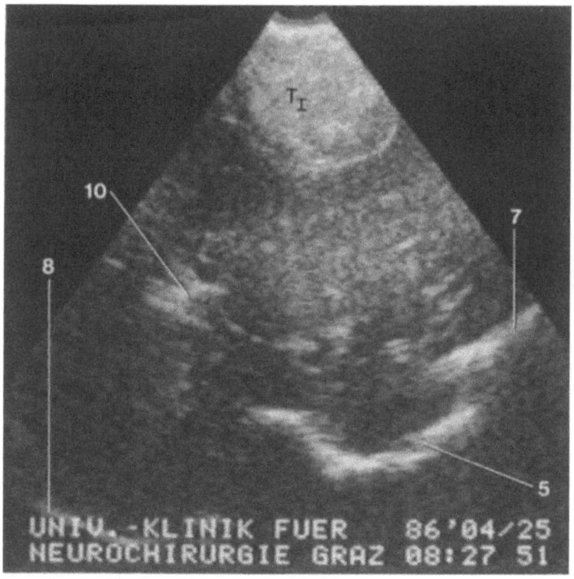

Fig. 144. Sagittal US. DRF 100, GPS probe, 5 MHz

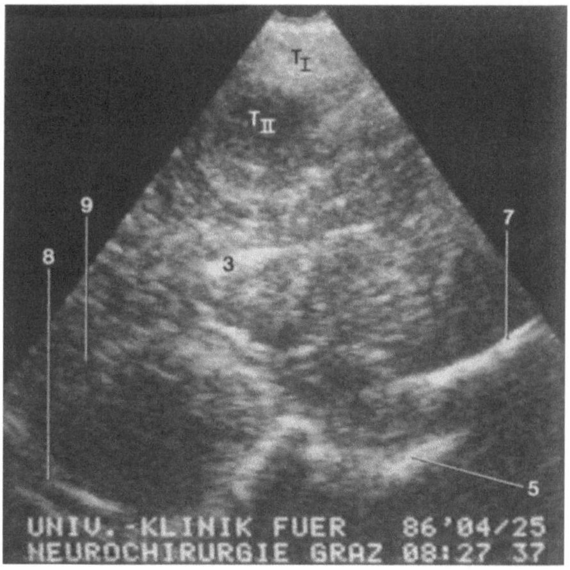

Fig. 145. Sagittal US. DRF 100, GPS probe, 5 MHz

1 Falx
2 Lateral ventricle
3 Choroid plexus
4 Corpus callosum
5 Floor of middle cranial fossa
6 Sella and clivus
7 Floor of anterior cranial fossa
8 Occipital bone
9 Tentorium
10 Trigonal choroid plexus
T_I, T_{II} Two compartments of tumor (see text)

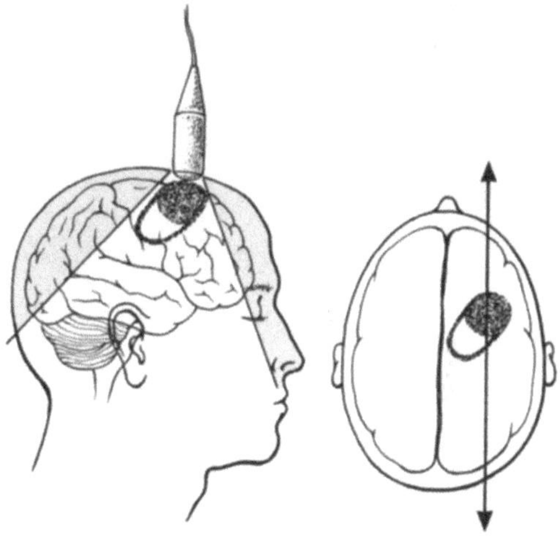

Sector planes for Figs. 144, 145

CASE 24 (Figs. 146, 147)

Frontal *meningioma* in a 62-year-old woman operated upon via bifrontal craniotomy.

The tumor is well delineated and very markedly hyperechoic, although its interior is somewhat variable in echo intensity, agreeing with some differences of density on CT.

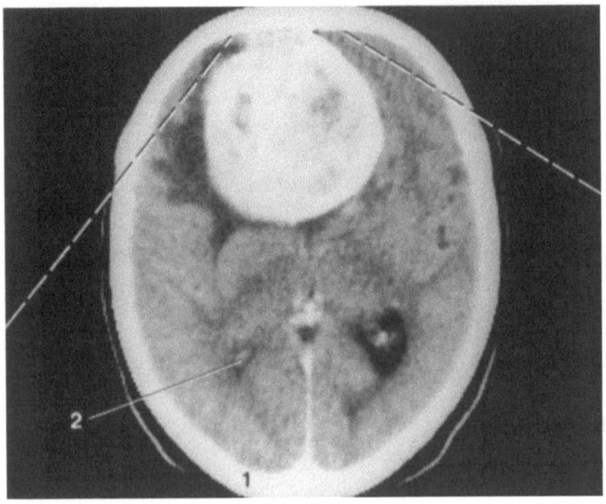

Fig. 146. Horizontal CT

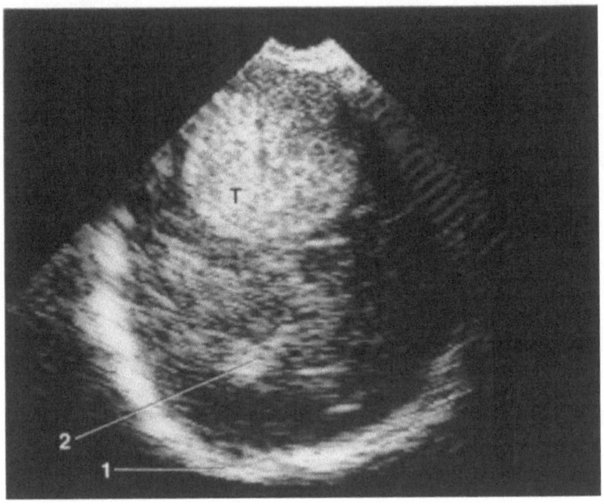

Fig. 147. Horizontal US. NS, 5 MHz

1 Occipital bone
2 Choroid plexus
T Tumor

CASE 25 (Figs. 148–153)

Olfactory groove meningioma in a 53-year-old woman operated upon via bifrontal craniotomy.

On all US sections, the tumor is markedly hyperechoic, homogeneous and well delineated from its surroundings; however, the slit-like CSF space around the tumor surface, as seen on MRI, does not appear clearly on US. Edema around the tumor does not become readily apparent.

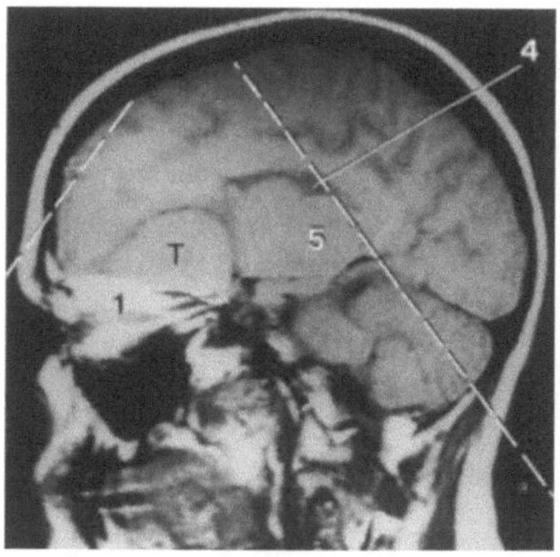

Fig. 148. Sagittal MRI

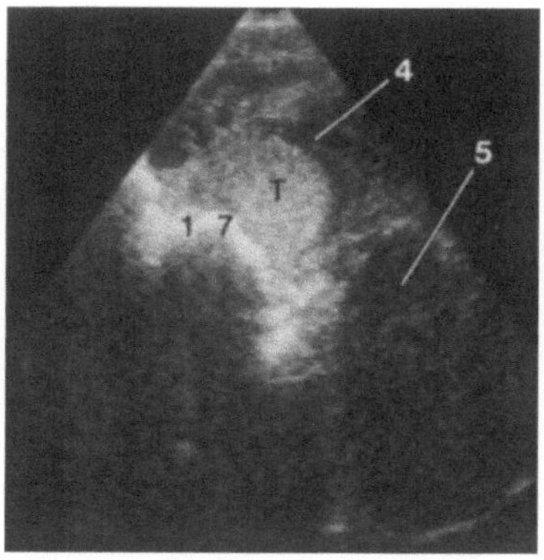

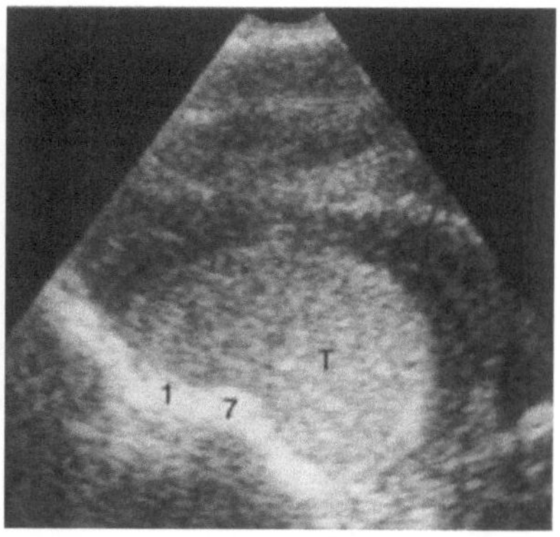

Figs. 149, 150. Sagittal US. DRF 100, GPS probe, 5 MHz

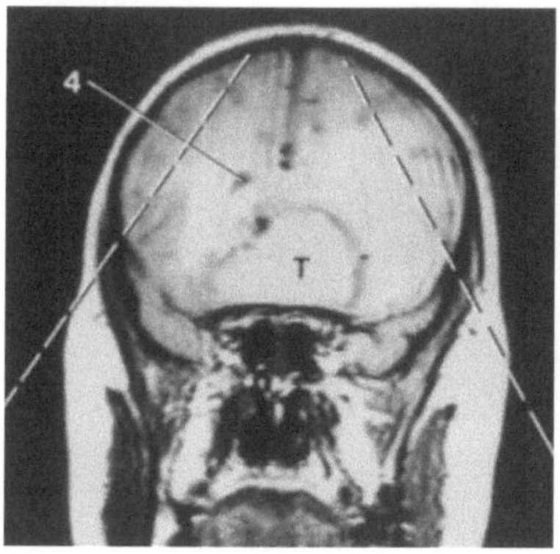

Fig. 151. Coronal MRI

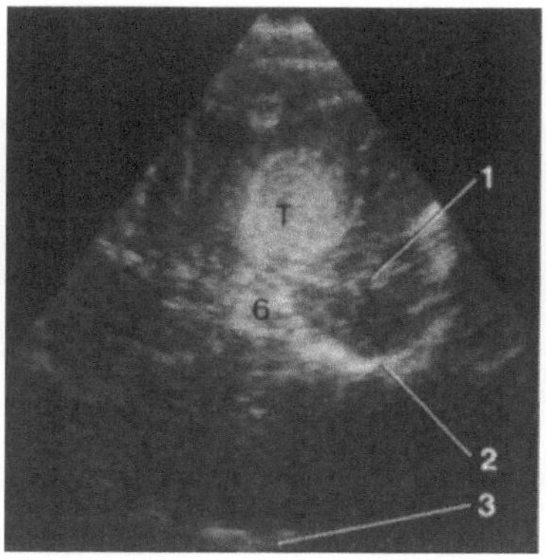

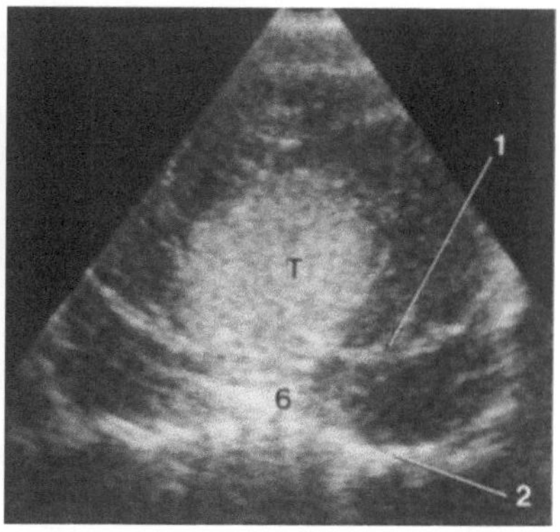

Figs. 152, 153. Diagonal coronal US. DRF 100, GPS probe, 5 MHz

1 Anterior cranial fossa (bony floor) and sphenoid wing
2 Middle cranial fossa (bony floor)
3 Posterior cranial fossa (occipital bone)
4 Lateral ventricle
5 Thalamus
6 Sella turcica
7 Foot of meningioma
T Tumor

CASE 26 (Figs. 154–157)

Medial sphenoid wing meningioma in a 60-year-old woman operated upon via right frontotemporal craniotomy.

The tumor is as hyperdense on contrast-enhanced CT as it is hyperechoic on US, and well demarcated.

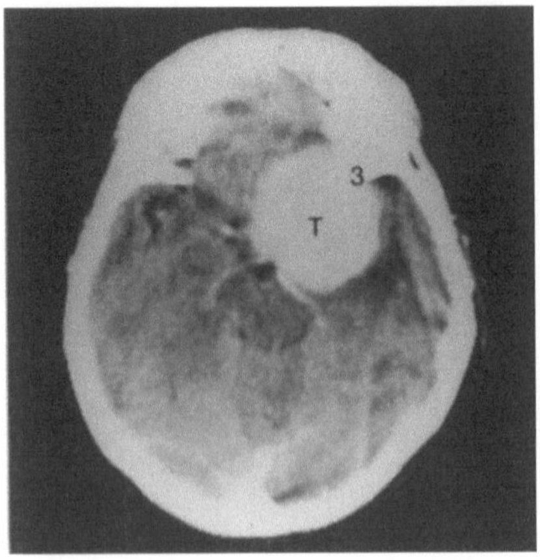

Fig. 154. Horizontal CT

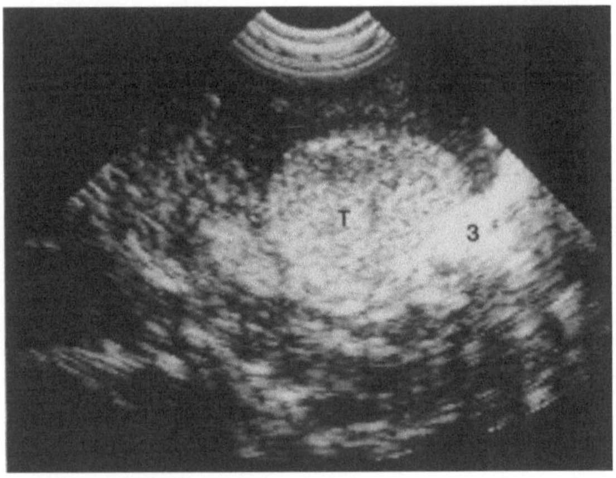

Fig. 155. Diagonal US. NS, 5 MHz

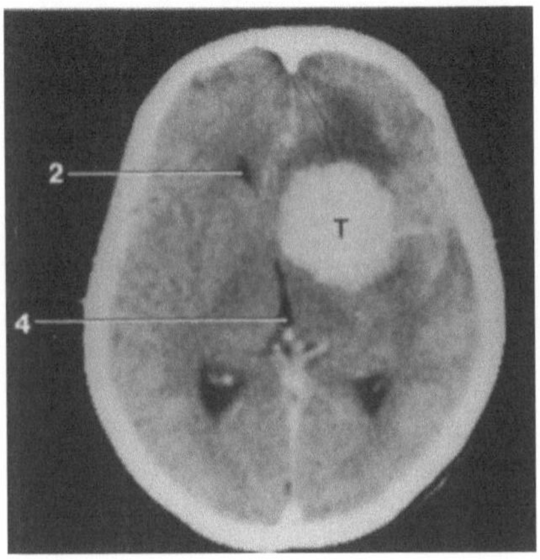

Fig. 156. Horizontal CT

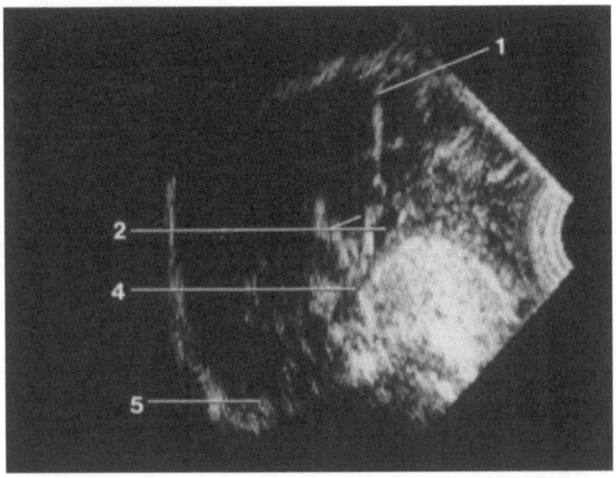

Fig. 157. Coronal US. NS, 5 MHz (see schema)

1 Falx
2 Lateral ventricle
3 Sphenoid wing
4 Third ventricle
5 Contralateral temporal fossa
T Tumor

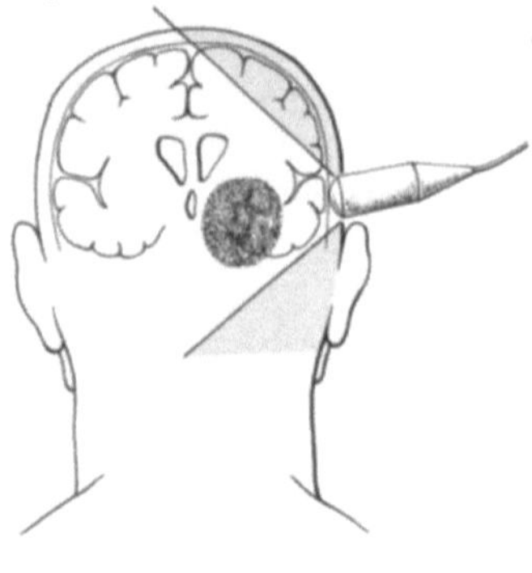

CASE 27 (Figs. 158, 159)

Lateral sphenoid wing meningioma in a 62-year-old man operated upon via right frontotemporal craniotomy.

The tumor, markedly contrast enhanced and well demarcated on CT, is surrounded by extensive edema causing massive midline shift. On US, the meningioma is isoechoic but rather inhomogeneous with a hyperechoic, well-demarcated border. The surrounding edema, hypodense on CT, is rather markedly hypoechoic.

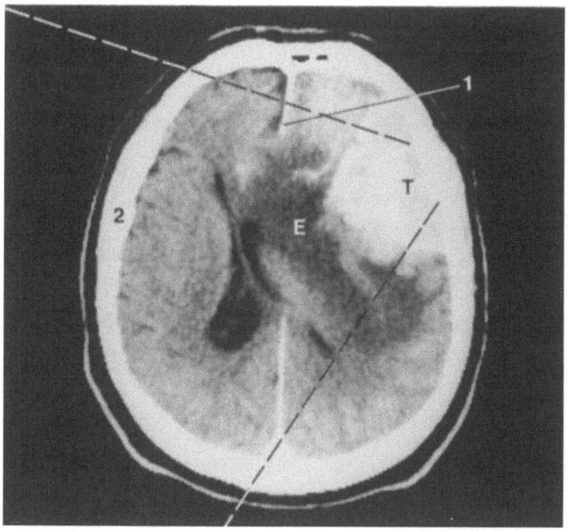

Fig. 158. Horizontal CT

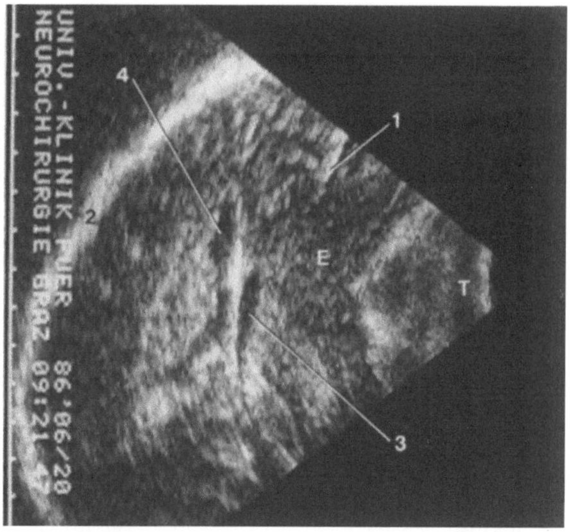

Fig. 159. Horizontal US. DRF 100, GPS probe, 5 MHz

1 Falx
2 Left parietal bone
3 Right lateral ventricle
4 Left lateral ventricle
E Edema
T Tumor

CASE 28 (Figs. 160–163)

Pyramidal (Meckel's cavity) meningioma in a 62-year-old man operated upon via right temporal craniotomy.

The horizontal US image shows the purely supratentorially located, well-demarcated tumor as a hyperechoic lesion with an even more hyperechoic border (the hypoechoic zone toward the probe is an artifact). In this case (Fig. 161), the posterior cranial fossa is also very clearly shown, with the cerebellar lobuli, pons and fourth ventricle.

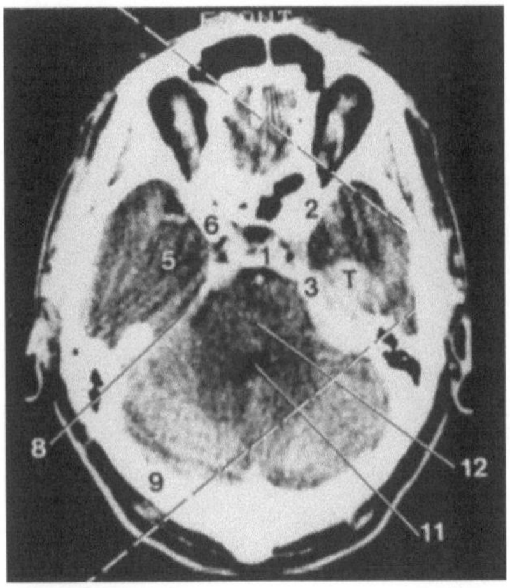

Fig. 160. Horizontal CT

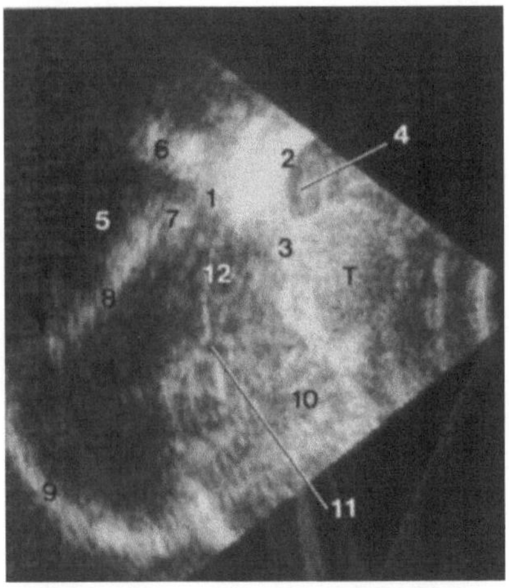

Fig. 161. Horizontal US. DRF 100, GPS probe, 5 MHz

1 Sella turcica
2 Right sphenoid wing
3 Right pyramid
4 Uncus, right temporal lobe
5 Left temporal fossa
6 Left sphenoid wing
7 Left pyramid
8 Left tentorium
9 Left occipital bone
10 Right cerebellar hemisphere
11 Fourth ventricle
12 Pons
13 Lateral ventricle
14 Third ventricle
15 Interpeduncular cistern
E Edema
T Tumor

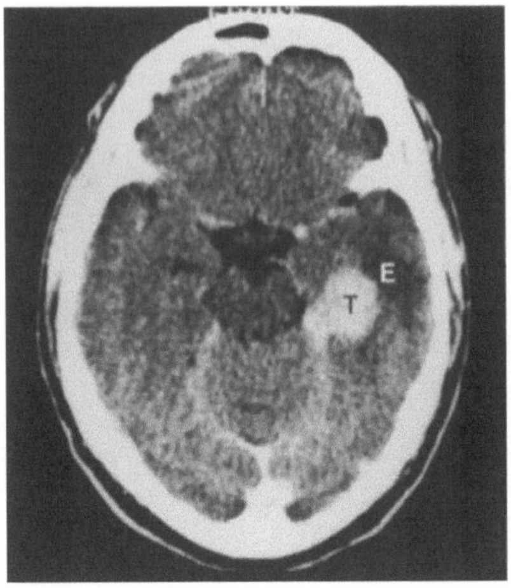

Fig. 162. Horizontal CT

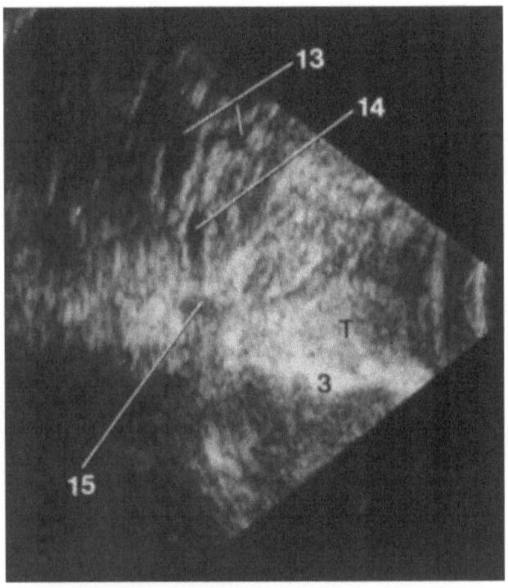

Fig. 163. Coronal US. DRF 100, GPS probe, 5 MHz (see schema)

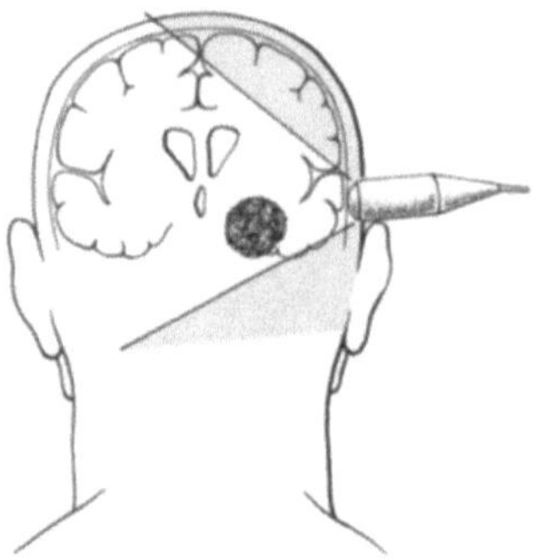

CASE 29 (Figs. 164–167)

Meningioma of Meckel's cavity and cavernous sinus in a 57-year-old woman with diplopia due to abducens nerve palsy.

This tumor was extirpated via a right temporal craniotomy. The tumor, hyperdense on CT, displays high signal intensity on MRI (Fig. 166) and on US (Figs. 165, 167), is clearly demarcated from its surroundings and compresses the right pontomesenphalic region.

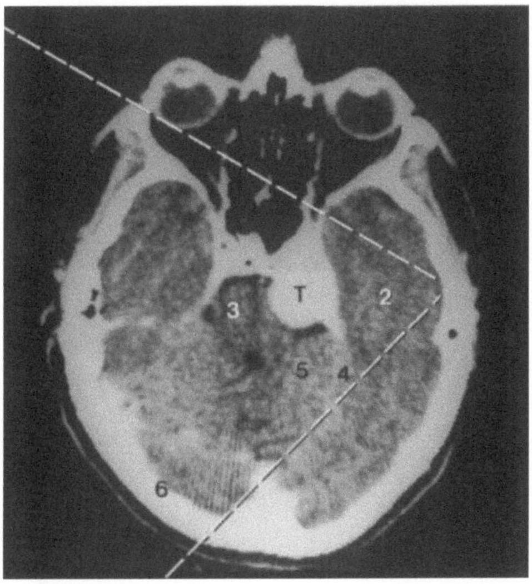

Fig. 164. Horizontal CT

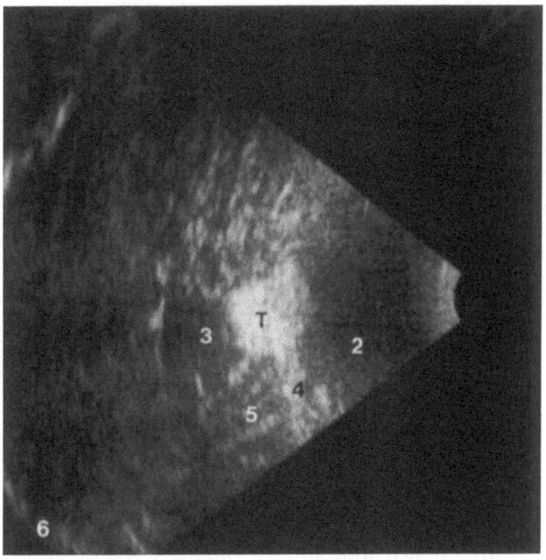

Fig. 165. Horizontal US. DRF 100, GPS probe, 5 MHz

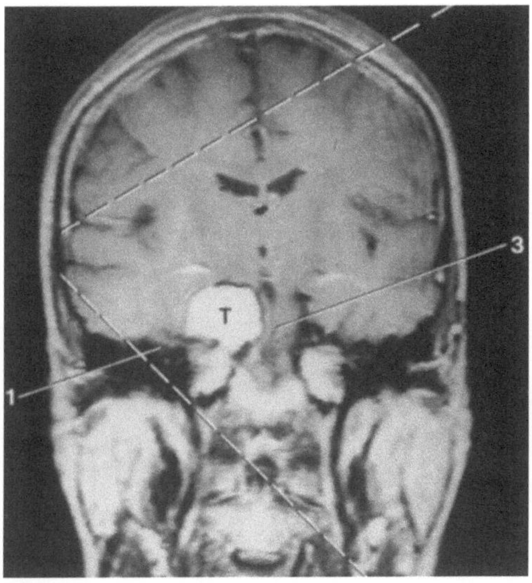

Fig. 166. Coronal MRI

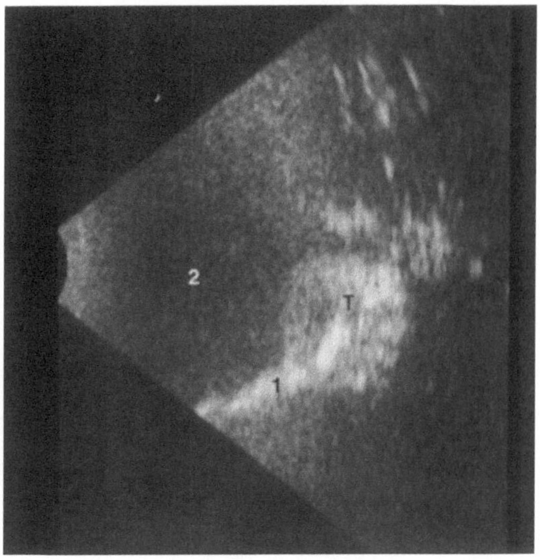

Fig. 167. Coronal US. DRF 100, GPS probe, 5 MHz

1 Surface of pyramid
2 Middle fossa
3 Compressed brainstem
4 Tentorium
5 Cerebellum
6 Contralateral occipital bone
T Tumor

CASE 30 (Figs.168–171)

Meningioma of the left cavernous sinus in a 46-year-old woman operated upon via left pterional approach.

The tumor is hyperechoic and well demarcated from its surroundings. However, US does not fully reproduce the situation as found during operation: the tumor had grown through the inner dural sheet into the middle cranial fossa, there forming a thin meningioma en plaque.

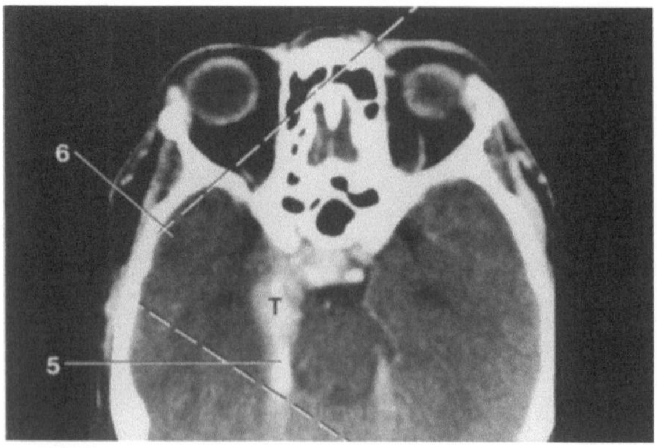

Fig. 168. Horizontal CT

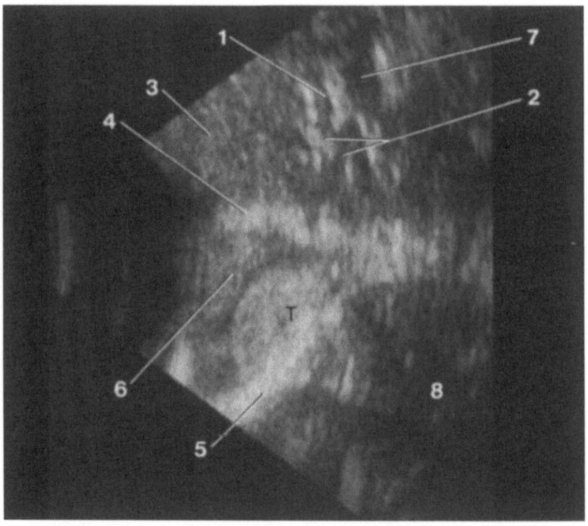

Fig. 169. Horizontal US. DRF 100, GPS probe, 5 MHz

1 Left frontal horn
2 Left foramen of Monro and third ventricle
3 Operculum frontale
4 Sphenoid wing
5 Tentorial edge
6 Inferior temporal gyrus
7 Right frontal horn
8 Posterior cranial fossa
T Tumor

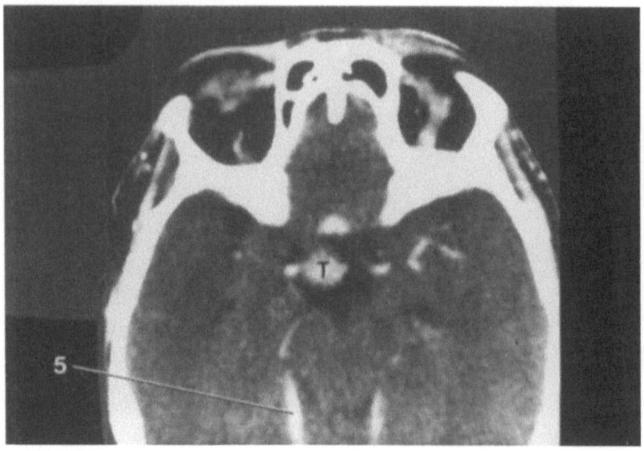

Fig. 170. Horizontal CT

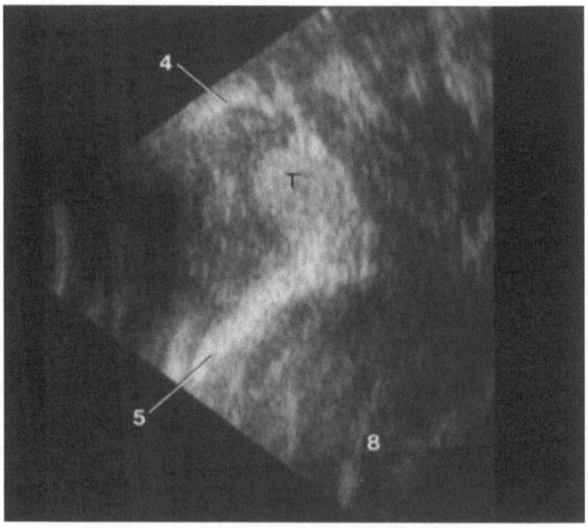

Fig. 171. Horizontal US. DRF 100, GPS probe, 5 MHz

CASE 31 (Figs. 172, 173)

Tentorial meningioma in a 51-year-old woman operated upon via infratentorial and supratentorial occipital craniotomy.

The well-demarcated hyperechoic tumor is seen to fenestrate the tentorium and grow into both directions. It can also be noted that the 3.5-MHz probe ist not adequate to demonstrate anatomical details of the posterior cranial fossa.

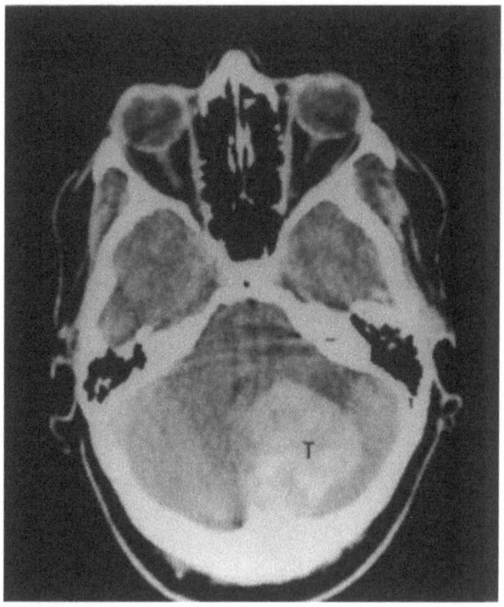

Fig. 172. Horizontal CT

1 Tentorium
2 Cuneus
3 Clivus
4 Parietal bone
T Tumor
T_I Infratentorial part of tumor
T_S Supratentorial part of tumor

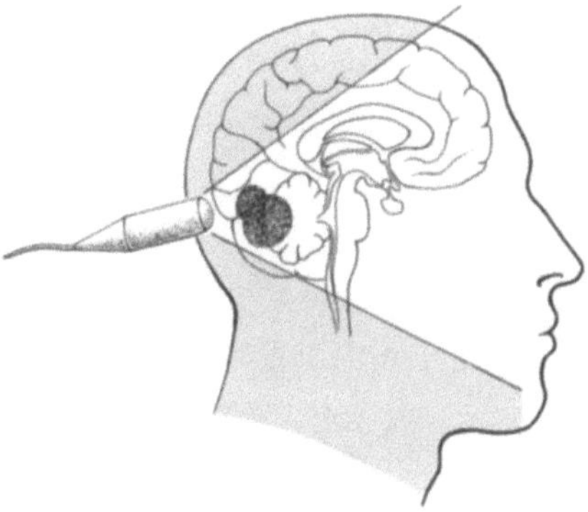

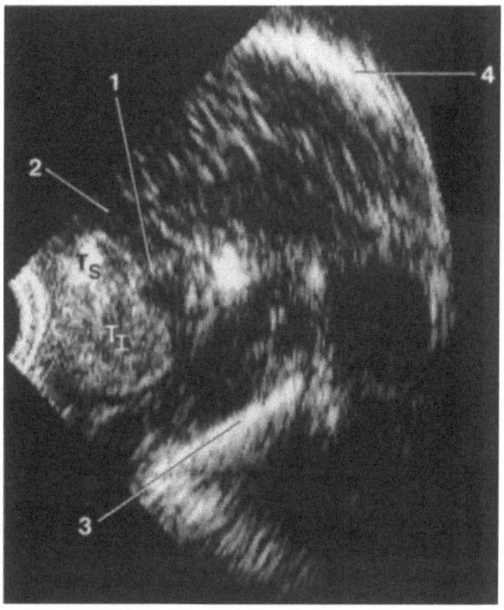

Fig. 173. Sagittal US. NS, 3.5 MHz

CASE 32 (Figs. 174–180)

Tentorial meningioma located in the pineal region in a 62-year-old woman operated upon via left occipital supratentorial craniotomy.

The tumor is only slightly hyperechoic, with a capsule that displays higher signal intensity than the interior.

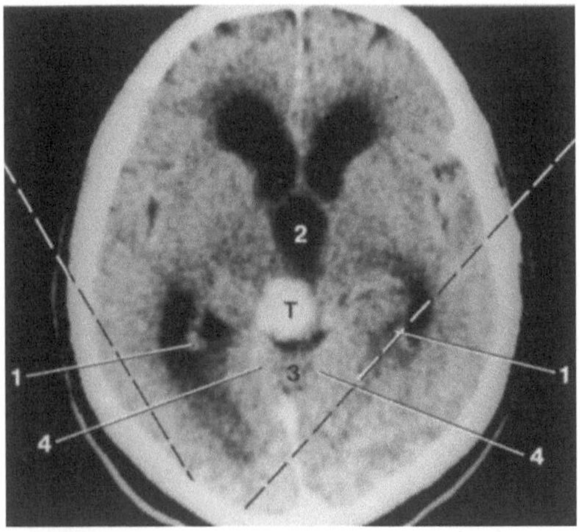

Fig. 174. Horizontal CT

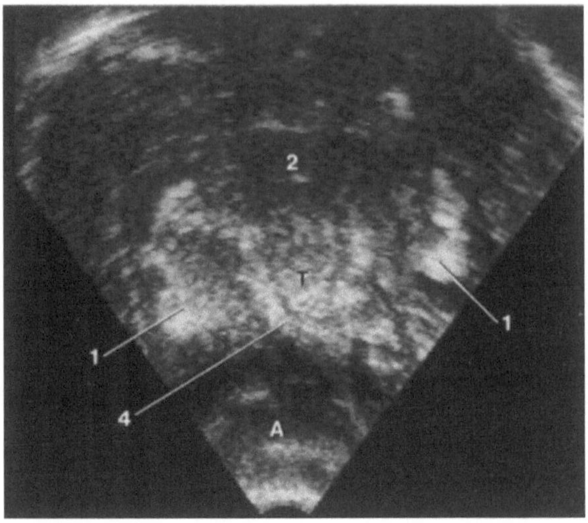

Fig. 175. Horizontal US. DRF 100, GPS probe, 5 MHz

1 Choroid plexus in temporal/trigonal ventricle
2 Third ventricle
3 Upper vermis
4 Tentorial notch
5 Tentorium
6 Crura cerebri
7 Dorsum sellae
8 Interpeduncular cistern
9 Cerebellum
10 Fourth ventricle
11 Occipital bone
12 Petrous bone
14 Clivus
A Hypoechoic artifact
T Tumor

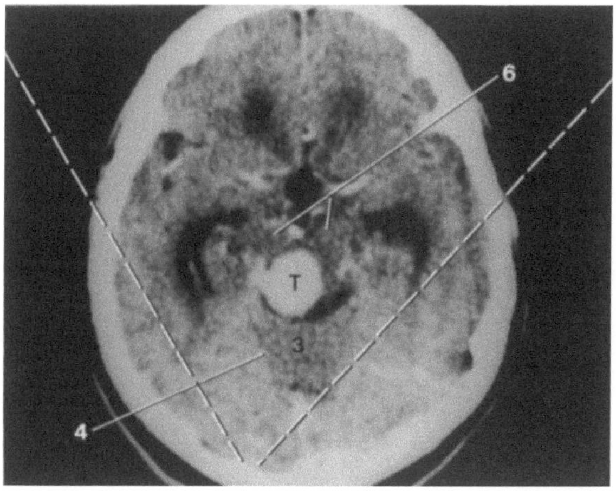

Fig. 176. Horizontal CT

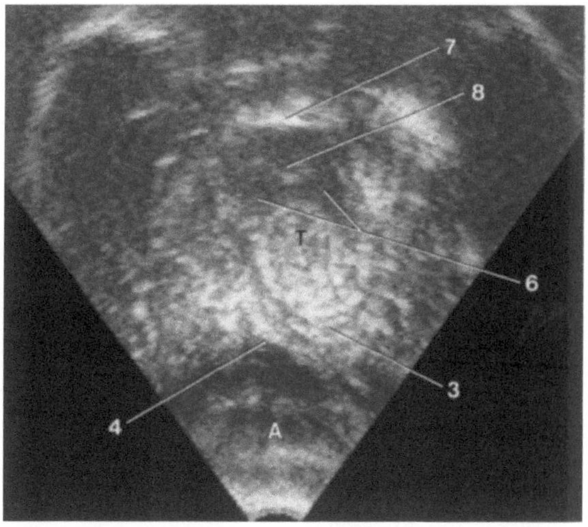

Fig. 177. Horizontal US. DRF 100, GPS probe, 5 MHz

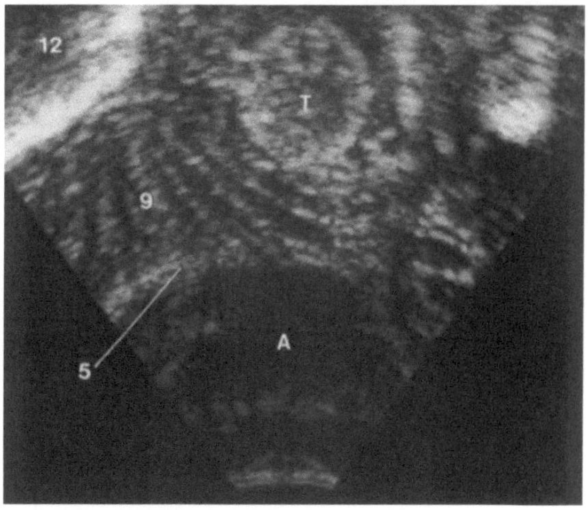

Fig. 178. Horizontal US. DRF 100, GPS probe, 5 MHz

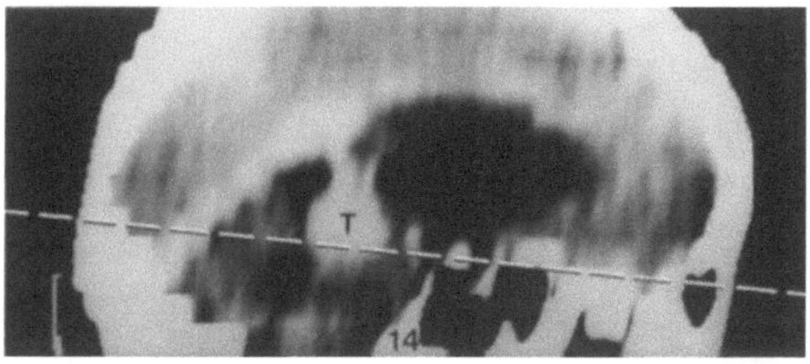

Fig. 179. Sagittal CT. Stippled line = sector plane for Fig. 178

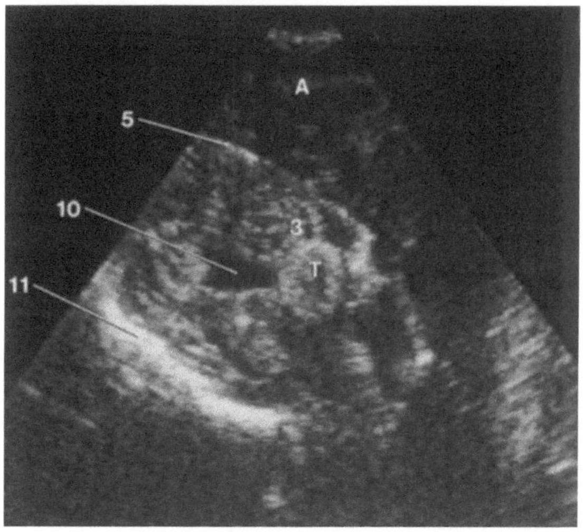

Fig. 180. Midsagittal US. DRF 100, GPS probe, 5 MHz ▷

CASE 33 (Figs. 181, 182)

Tentorial meningioma in a 62-year-old woman operated upon via occipital craniotomy.

Well demarcated hyperechoic tumor on US.

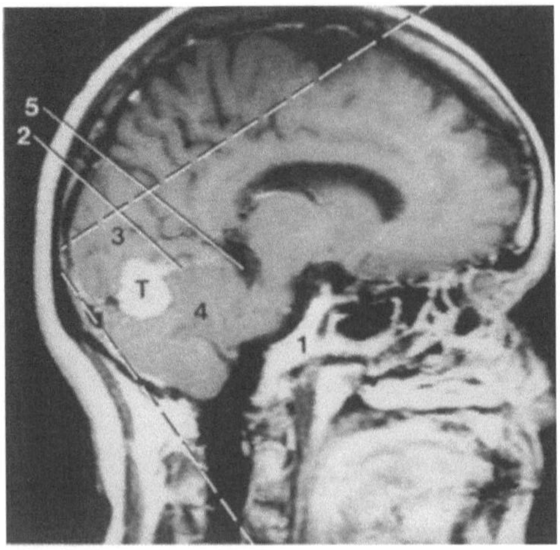

Fig. 181. Sagittal MRI

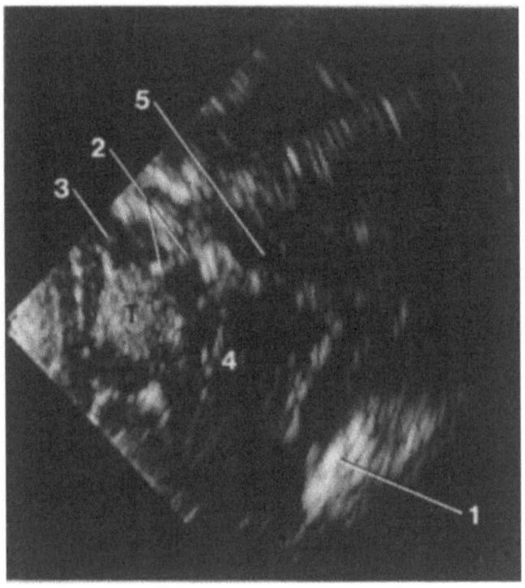

Fig. 182. Sagittal US. SSA 100A, 5 MHz

1 Clivus
2 Tentorium
3 Cuneus
4 Cerebellum
5 Quadrigeminal cistern
T Tumor

Metastases

Cerebral metastases, although of various origins, are rather homogeneously hyperechoic as far as their solid tissue compartments are concerned. Cystic compartments show up very clearly, perhaps even more so than on CT if their content is hypodense with the latter method. Very protein rich fluid mixed with cellular detritus, which gives an isodense appearance on CT, is rather hyperechoic on US, so that the contents of a cyst can be imaged as a mixture of hypoechoic and hyperechoic compartments. Necrotic areas do not always appear as clearly on US as they do on CT. Therefore, a metastasis with unequivocal central necrosis may well appear on US as a homogeneously hyperechoic mass.

Edema around metastases, as around gliomas, is seen on US as a slightly hyperechoic area. On CT, as is well known, edema commonly appears hypodense.

It is important to select the most appropriate US frequency for each investigation (this topic will be discussed in greater detail in the chapter on the practical application of US): when looking for a circumscribed deep-seated metastasis, a 5-MHz probe will be required, because with a 10-MHz probe the lesion may well not be seen. By contrast, a small tumor located in the immediate subcortical region may well be detected with the aid of a 10-MHz probe but missed with a 5-MHz probe. Technical advances will make the selection of a particular frequency less important, but the operating neurosurgeon should nevertheless be aware of the situation.

CASE 34 (Figs. 183-191)

Cystic metastasis from a pulmonary carcinoma in a 76-year-old man operated upon via left frontal craniotomy.

Contrast-enhanced CT shows a markedly hyperdense solid tumor (Fig. 188), and a large hypodense cyst with hyperdense capsule (Fig. 183). US yields a similar picture, i.e., a hyperechoic solid tumor and a cyst with clearly hypoechoic content. The solid hyperechoic tumor is homogeneous throughout; 10-MHz images give very detailed information about the inner surface, toward the cyst, showing caverns and trabeculae (Figs. 190, 191).

The edema originates mostly from the posterior circumference of the cyst capsule and extends into the parietal region on CT (Figs. 183, 188). Exactly the same distribution of edema can be recognized on US; there, however, edema is hyperechoic and thereby blurs the border between the capsule of the cyst and the surroundings (Figs. 184, 189).

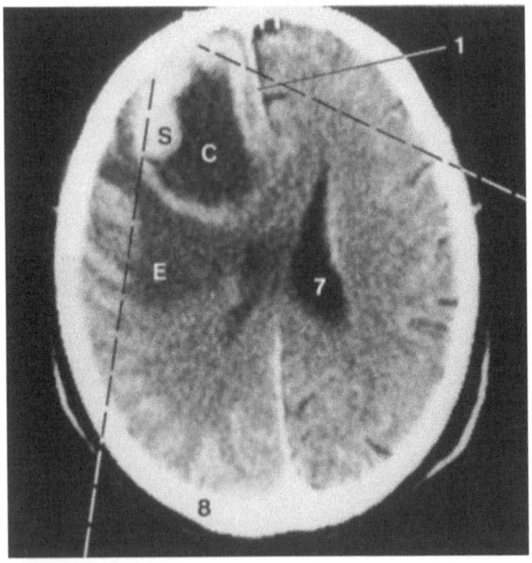

Fig. 183. Horizontal CT

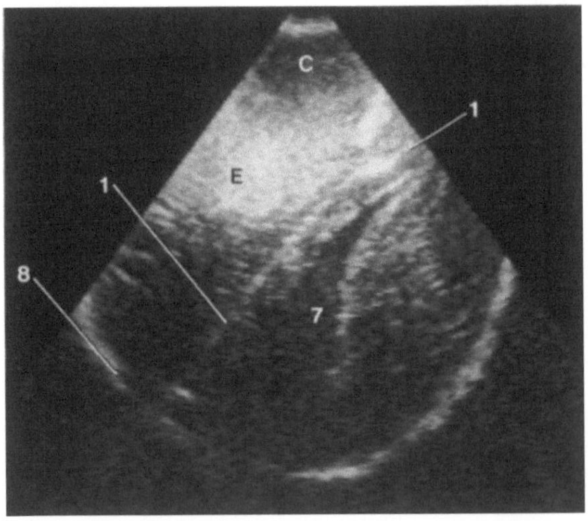

Fig. 184. Horizontal US. DRF 100, GPS probe, 5 MHz

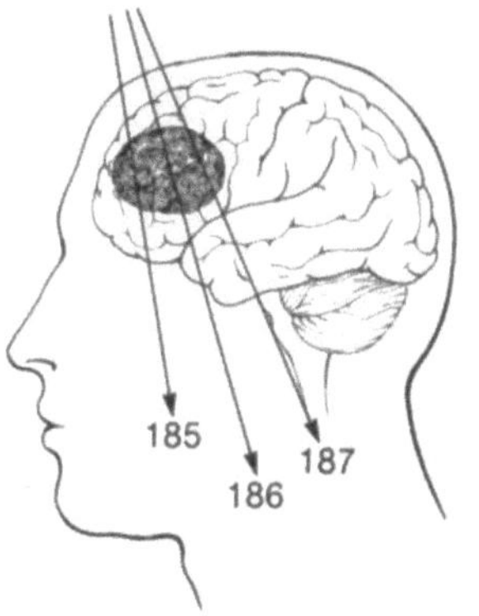

1 Falx
2 Frontal base of skull
3 Sphenoid wing
4 Sella turcica
5 Temporal fossa
6 Contralateral temporal bone
7 Right lateral ventricle
8 Occipital bone
E Edema
C Cystic part of tumor
S Solid part of tumor

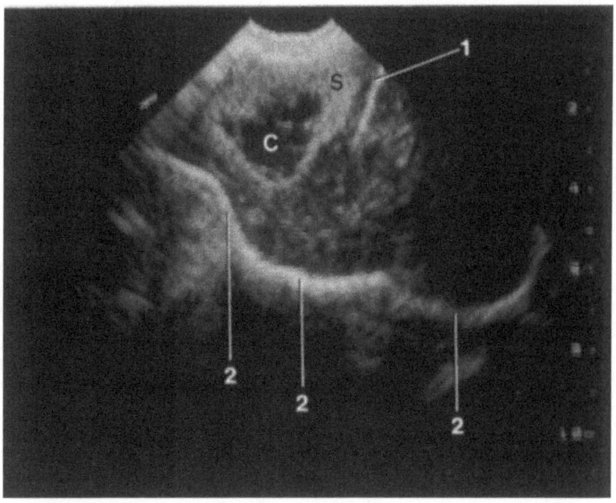

Fig. 185. Coronal US. UM 8, annular array probe, 5 MHz

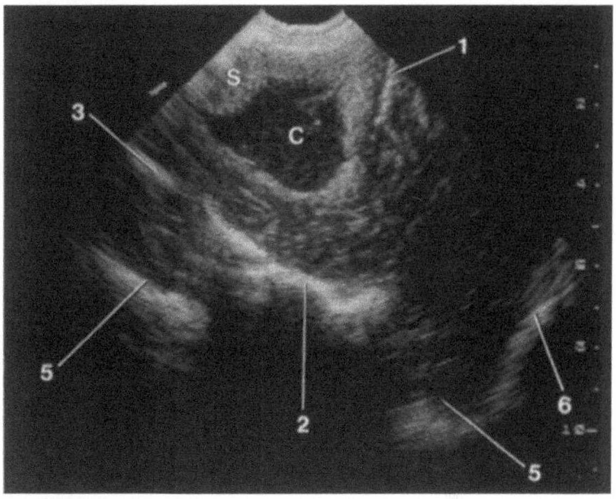

Fig. 186. Coronal US. UM 8, annular array probe, 5 MHz

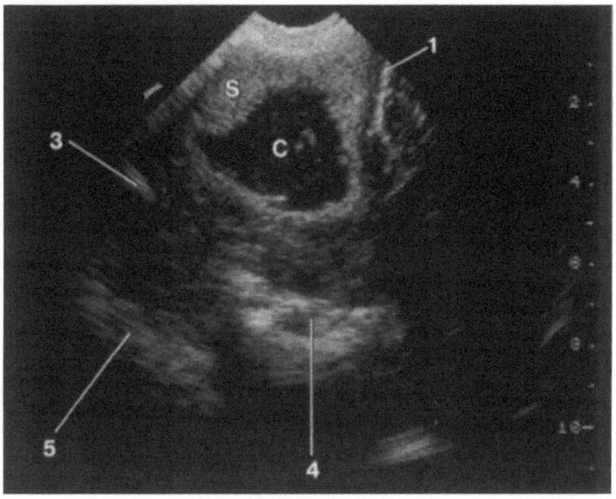

Fig. 187. Coronal US. UM 8, annular array probe, 5 MHz

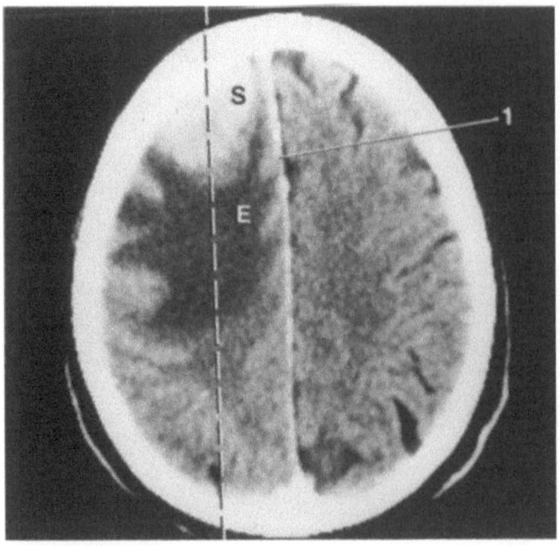

Fig. 188. Horizontal CT. Stippled line = sector plane for Figs. 189–191

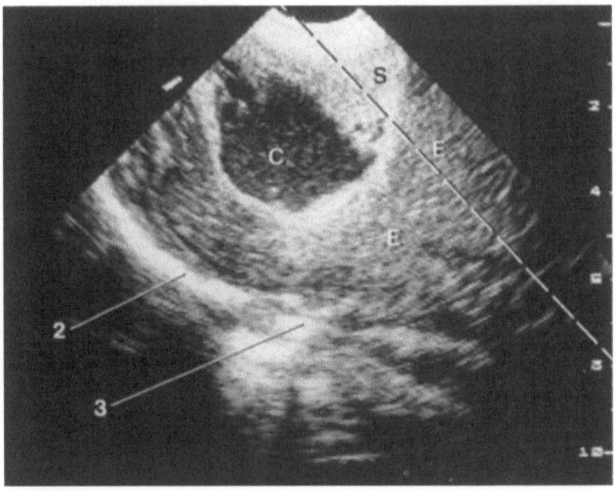

Fig. 189. Sagittal US. UM 8, annular array probe, 5 MHz (see schema). Stippled line = CT-plane

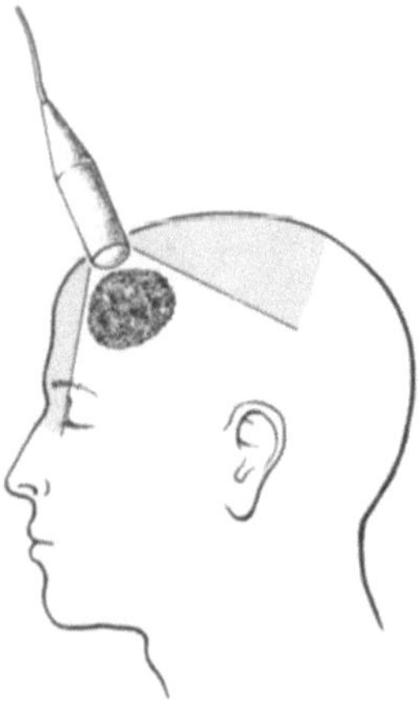

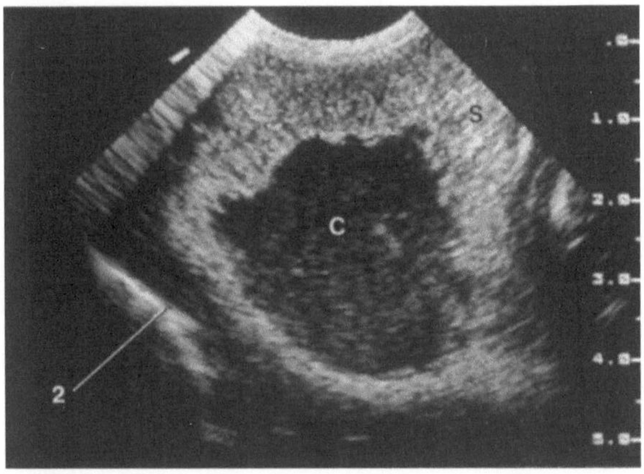

Fig. 190. Sagittal US. UM 8, annular array probe, 10 MHz (see schema)

1 Falx
2 Frontal base of skull
3 Sphenoid wing
E Edema
C Cystic part of tumor
S Solid part of tumor

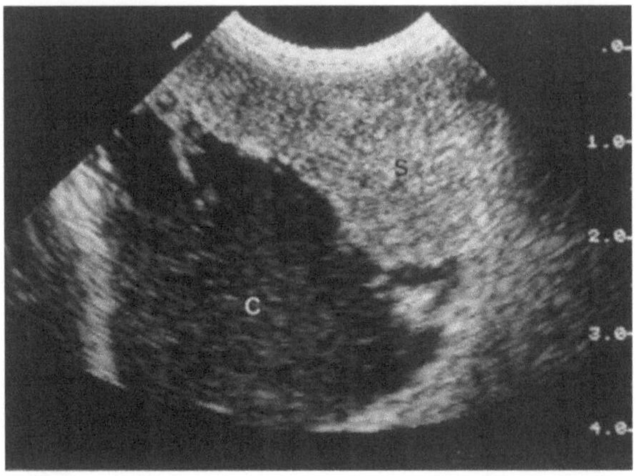

Fig. 191. Sagittal US. UM 8, annular array probe, 10 MHz (see schema)

CASE 35 (Figs. 192, 193)

Metastasis of unknown origin in a 60-year-old woman operated upon via left temporoparietal craniotomy.

The tumor is homogeneously hyperechoic and well demarcated. The surrounding edema, hypodense on CT, is slightly hyperechoic on US.

1 Falx
E Edema
T Tumor

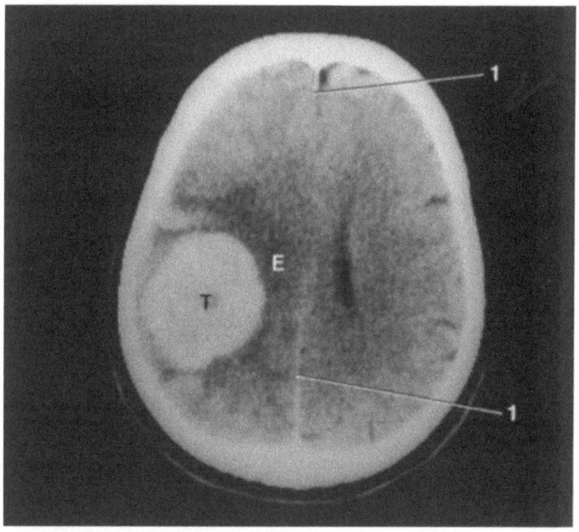

Fig. 192. Horizontal CT

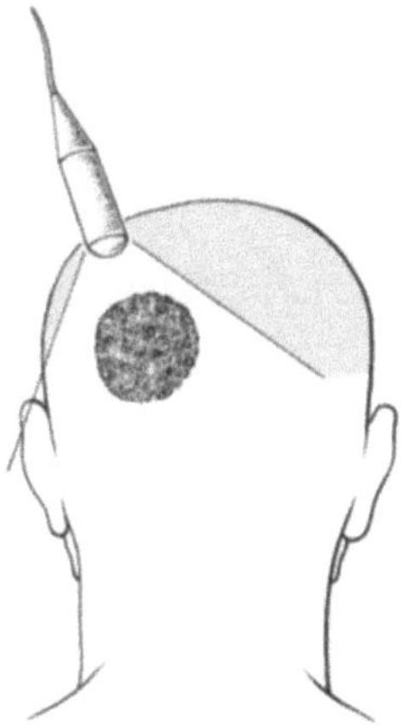

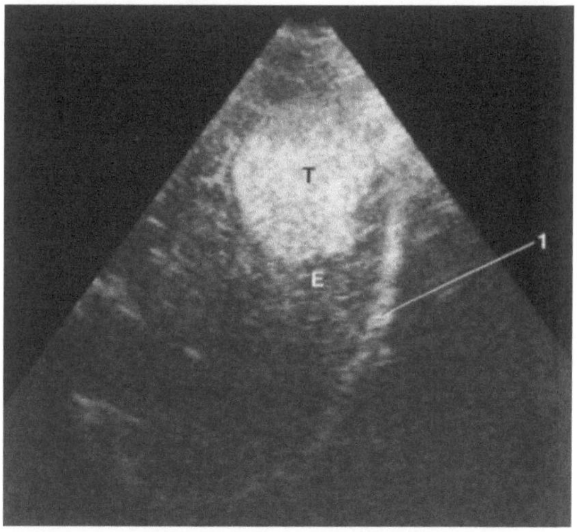

Fig. 193. Coronal US. DRF 100, GPS probe, 5 MHz

CASE 36 (Figs. 194–198)

Cystic metastasis from osteosarcoma in a 24-year-old man.

US-guided drainage of the cyst was done as a first operative step. The compartmentalized nature of the cyst is recognized both on preoperative CT (Fig. 194) and US (Figs. 195, 196). However, the hypodense compartment is isoechoic on US, the isodense part is markedly hyperechoic. Both imaging procedures show the level between the two compartments. The patient was in a supine position during CT, while the head was turned 45° to the right during operation (Fig. 195 corresponds to preoperative CT, Fig. 196 shows a coronal US view from left temporal). The thin capsule is hyperechoic. On control US toward the end of the operation (Fig. 198, coronal view corresponding to Fig. 196), the massive midline shift seen before drainage is now reduced, as shown particularly clearly by the left frontal horn. The cyst is markedly smaller, and its remaining content is homogeneously hyperechoic due to some blood staining of the fluid. The lateral ventricles are wider than in Fig. 196.

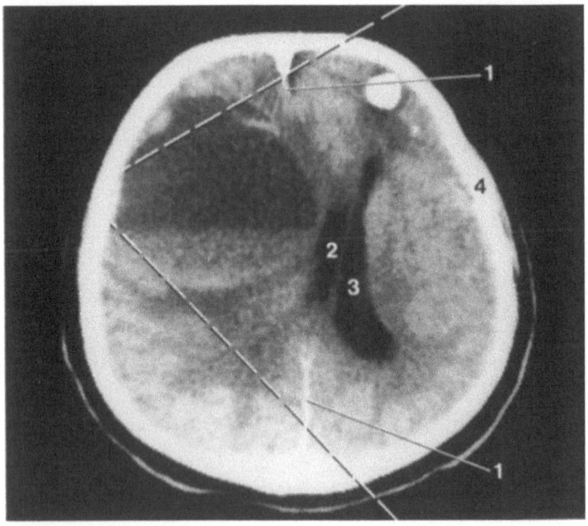

Fig. 194. Preoperative horizontal CT

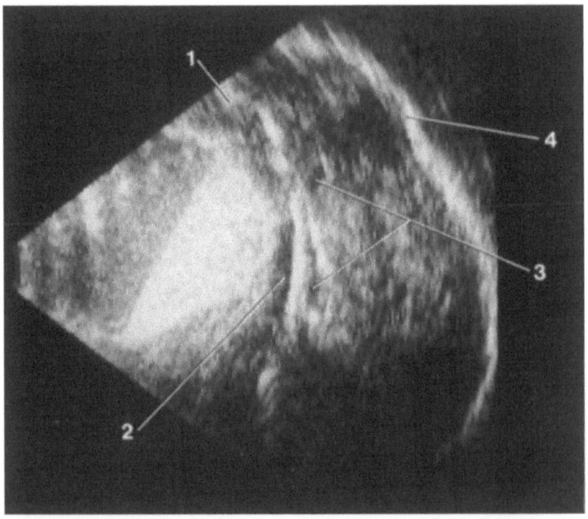

Fig. 195. Horizontal US. DRF 100, GPS probe, 5 MHz

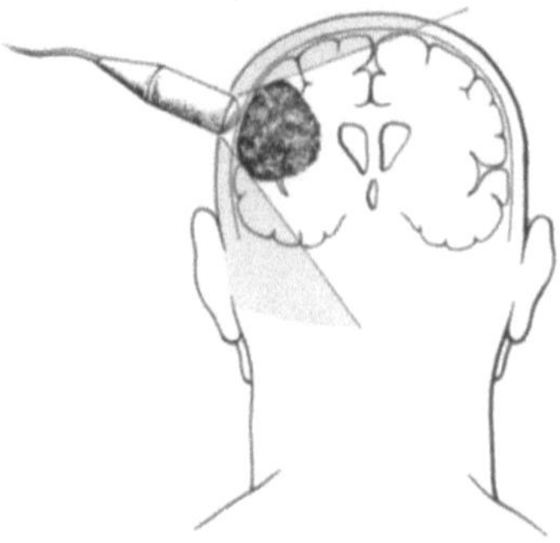

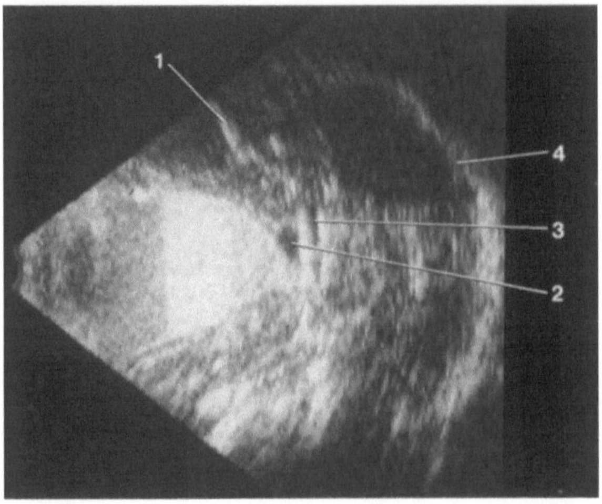

Fig. 196. Coronal US. DRF 100, GPS probe, 5 MHz (see schema)

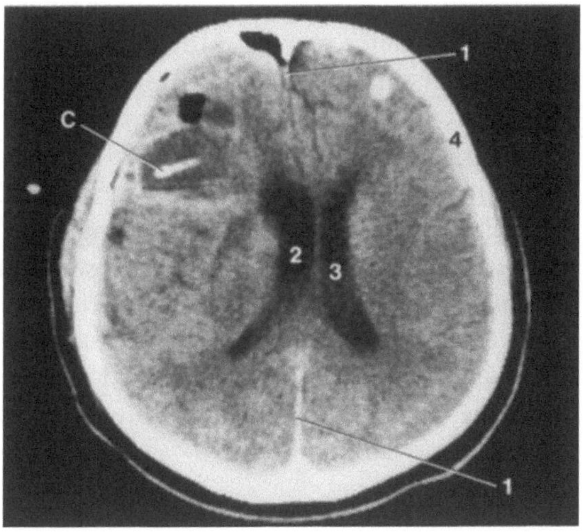

Fig. 197. Postoperative horizontal CT

1 Falx
2 Left lateral ventricle
3 Right lateral ventricle
4 Right frontotemporal bone
C Catheter in tumor cavity

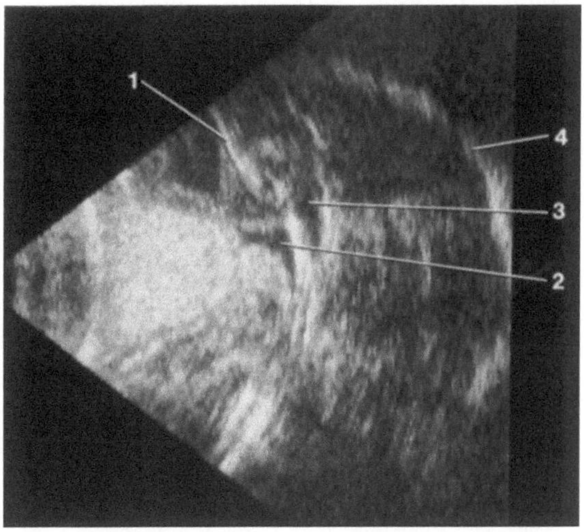

Fig. 198. Coronal US near end of operation. DRF 100, GPS probe, 5 MHz

CASE 37 (Figs. 199-205)

Metastasis from pulmonary carcinoma in a 65-year-old man operated upon via right parietal craniotomy.

The globular tumor is slightly hyperechoic in its interior and has a markedly hyperechoic capsule. The extensive collateral edema, seen as a big hypodense area on CT, is shown on US as a slightly hyperechoic area which makes the white matter appear brighter in the right hemisphere than on the left side (Fig. 200) and depresses the ipsilateral pars centralis (Fig. 202). Due to the hyperechoicity of the surrounding edema, the border of the tumor is blurred (Figs. 202-205). Circumscribed tumors such as this in the depth of the white matter may be difficult to find with a very small surgical exposure (instead of a larger exposure involving considerable tissue destruction). Fig. 205 shows the use of US guidance in this situation: the surgeon introduces a Cushing needle or similar toward the tumor with one hand, and with the other hand checks the track of the needle with the US probe until it is seen to move the tumor. The surgeon can now, in the knowledge of the exact position of the tumor, select the smallest possible transcortical exposure for its removal.

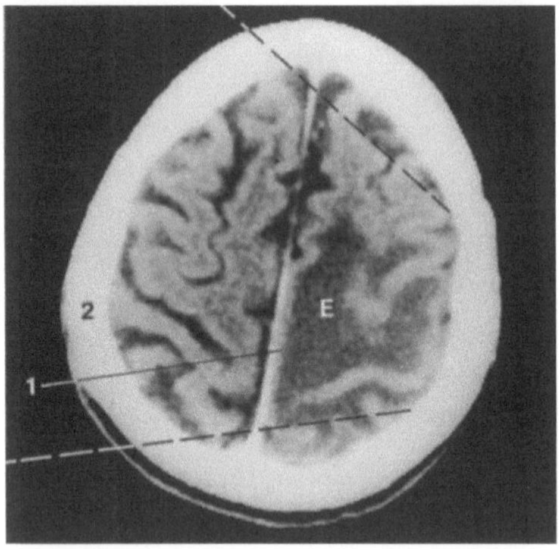

Fig. 199. Horizontal CT (see schema)

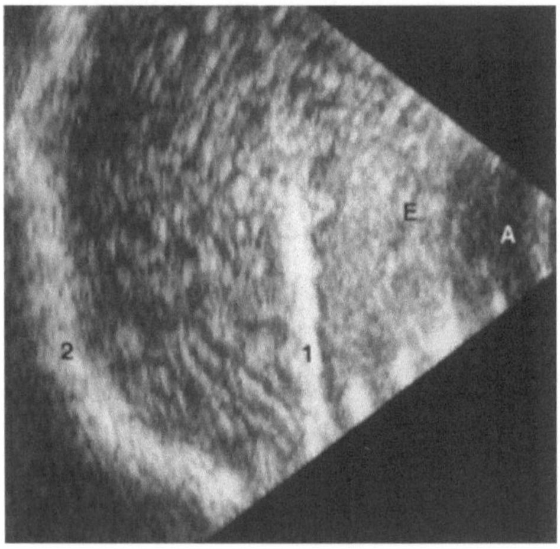

Fig. 200. Horizontal US. DRF 100, GPS probe, 5 MHz (see schema)

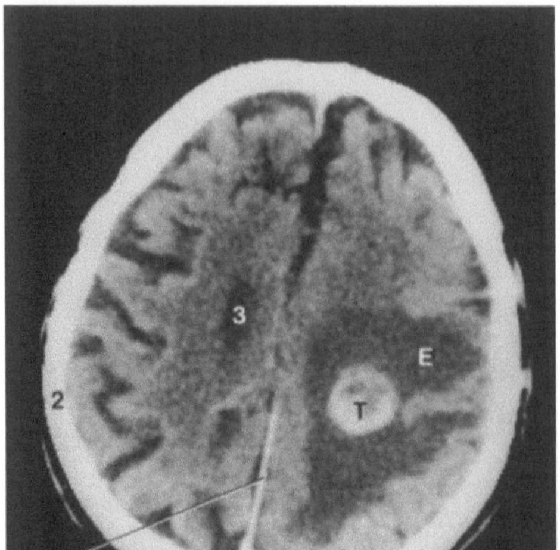

Fig. 201. Horizontal CT (see schema)

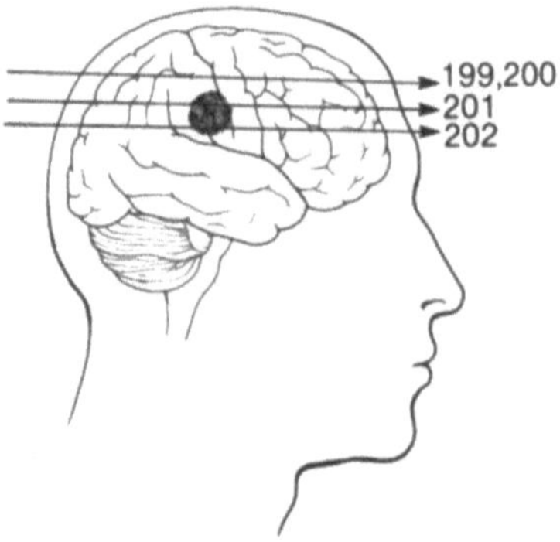

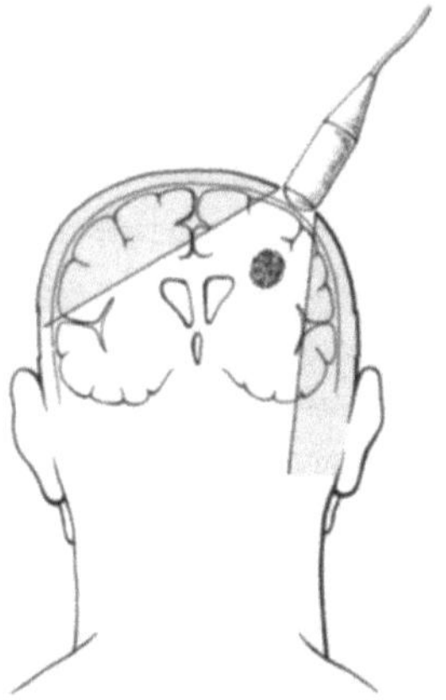

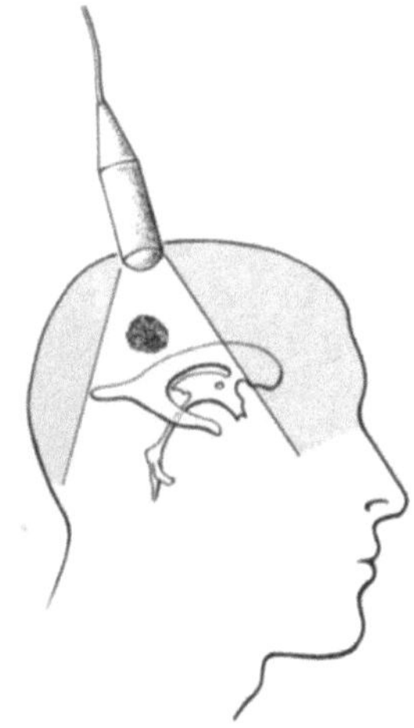

1 Falx
2 Left parietal bone
3 Left lateral ventricle
4 Compressed right lateral ventricle
5 Choroid plexus
A Artifact
E Edema
N Cushing needle
T Tumor

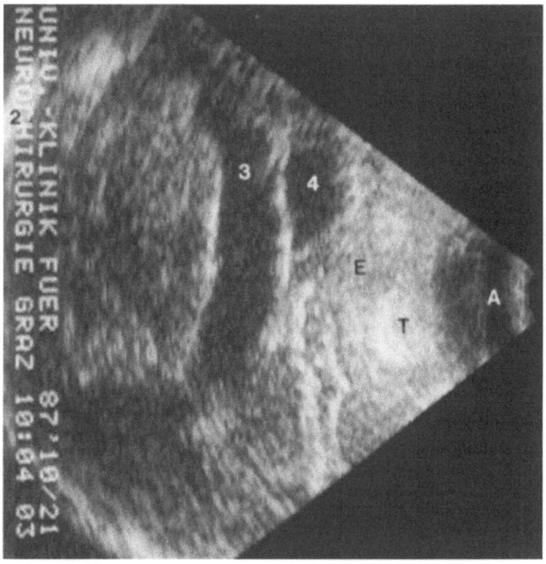

Fig. 202. Horizontal US. DRF 100, GPS probe, 5 MHz (see schema, p. 72)

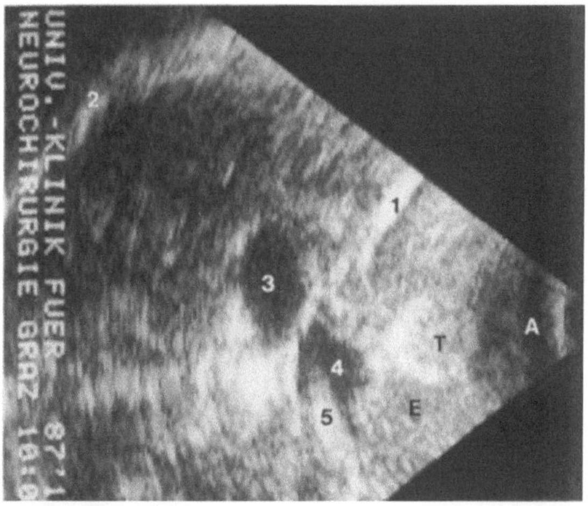

Fig. 203. Coronal US. DRF 100, GPS probe, 5 MHz (see schema)

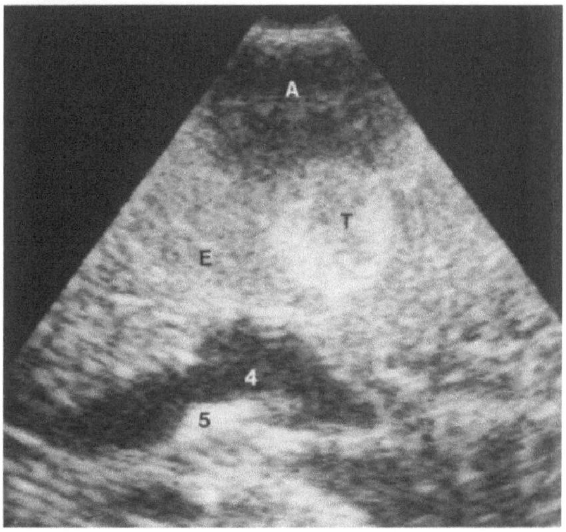

Fig. 204. Sagittal US. DRF 100, GPS probe, 5 MHz (see schema)

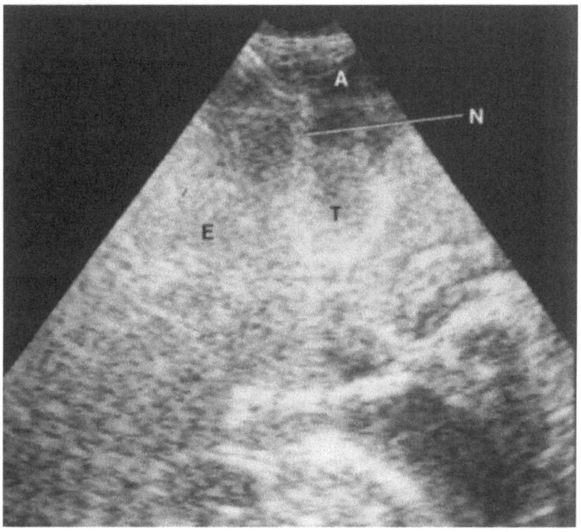

Fig. 205. Diagonal US. DRF 100, GPS probe, 5 MHz

CASE 38 (Figs. 206–209)

Metastasis from malignant melanoma in a 59-year-old man operated upon via right temporal craniotomy.

Contrast-enhanced CT shows a partly hyperdense, partly isodense or hypodense lesion surrounded by massive edema. On US the tumor is hyperechoic with an isoechoic border. The collateral edema is hyperechoic [see especially the coronal US image in Fig. 209, where the hyperechoic zone of edema corresponds to the hypodense area of edema on the horizontal CT section taken above the tumor (Fig. 208)].

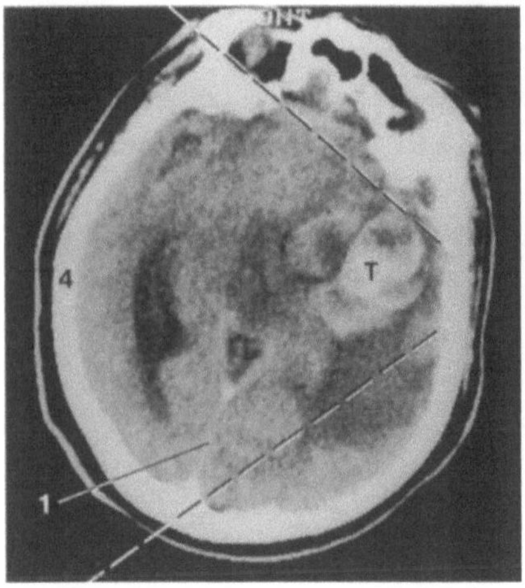

Fig. 206. Horizontal CT

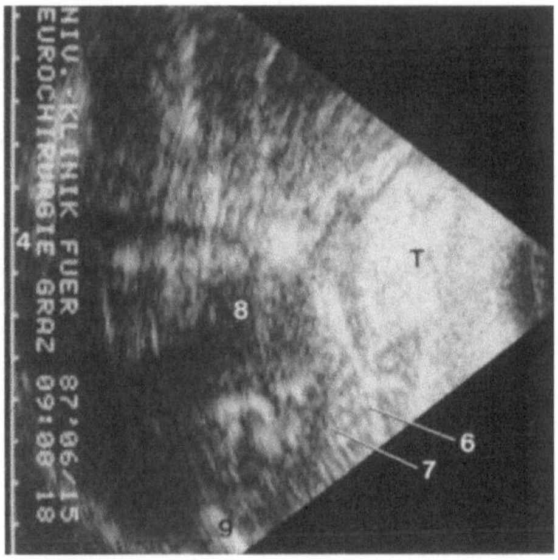

Fig. 207. Horizontal US. DRF 100, GPS probe, 5 MHz

1 Falx
2 Lateral ventricle
4 Left parietal bone
6 Tentorium
7 Cerebellum
8 Pontomesencephalic region
9 Internal occipital crest
E Edema
T Tumor

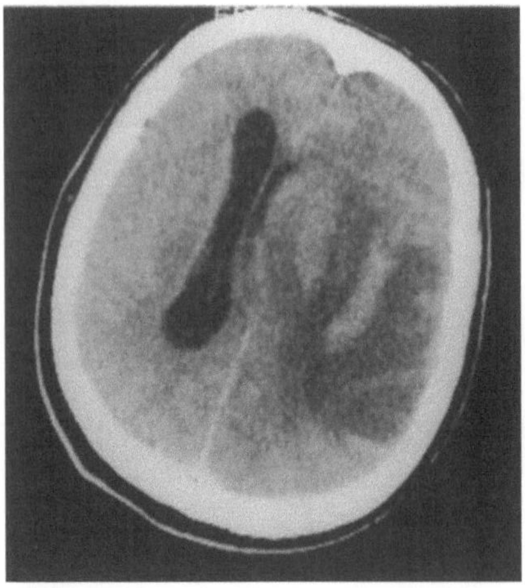

Fig. 208. Horizontal CT

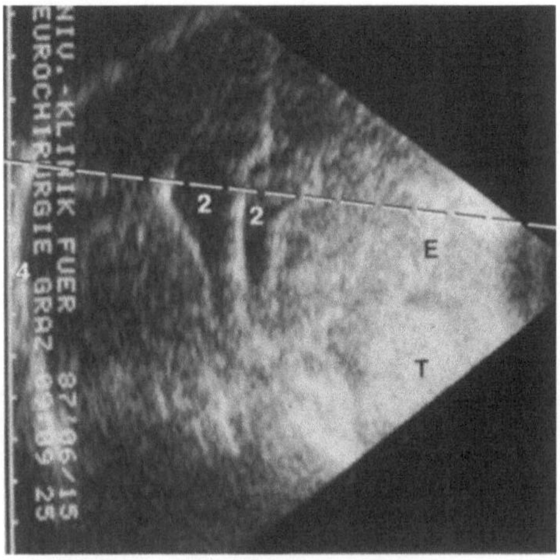

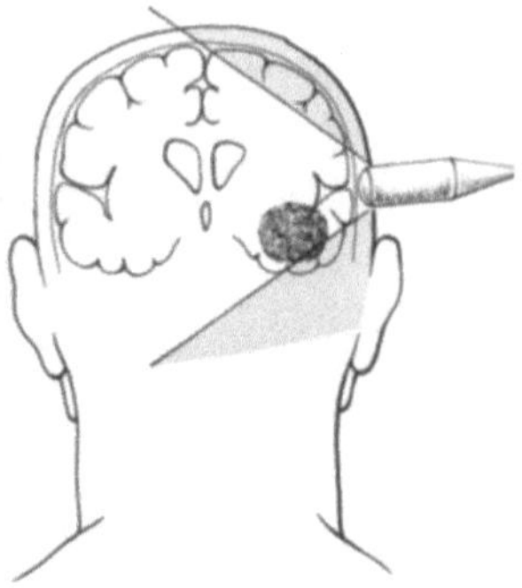

Fig. 209. Slightly diagonal coronal US. DRF 100, GPS probe, 5 MHz (see schema). Stippled line = CT-plane for Fig. 208

CASE 39 (Figs. 210-215)

Occipito-central *metastasis from hypernephroma* in a 51-year-old man operated upon via left occipital craniotomy.

The tumor is hyperechoic on US with several areas of hypoechoicity due to necrosis (also visible on CT as hypodense center). The part of the tumor within the trigonum of the left lateral ventricle is in close contact with the choroid plexus (Figs. 211, 215). The surrounding brain edema, hypodense on CT, displays slightly higher echoicity than normal white matter.

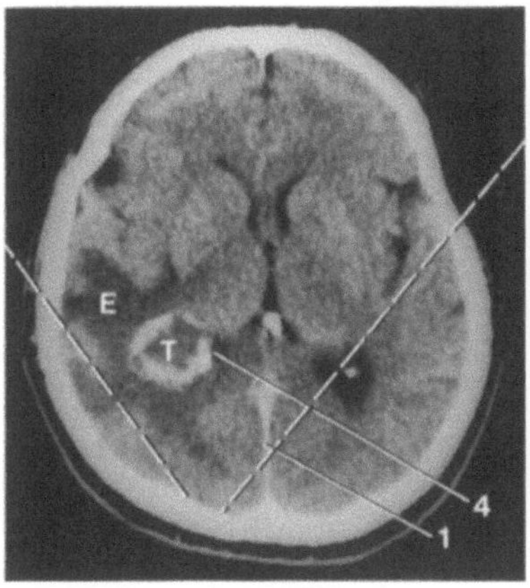

Fig. 210. Horizontal CT

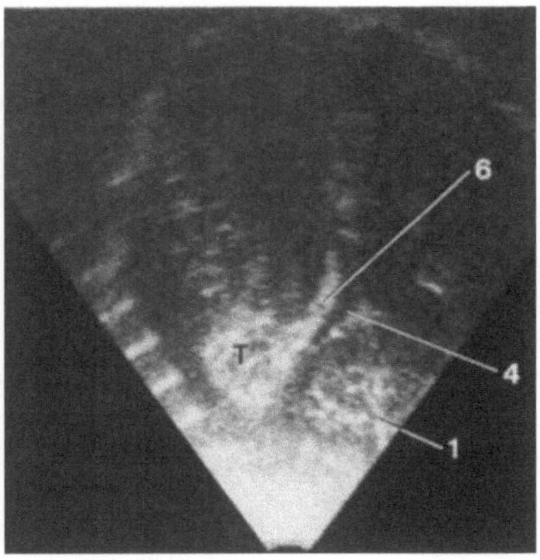

Fig. 211. Horizontal US. DRF 100, GPS probe, 5 MHz

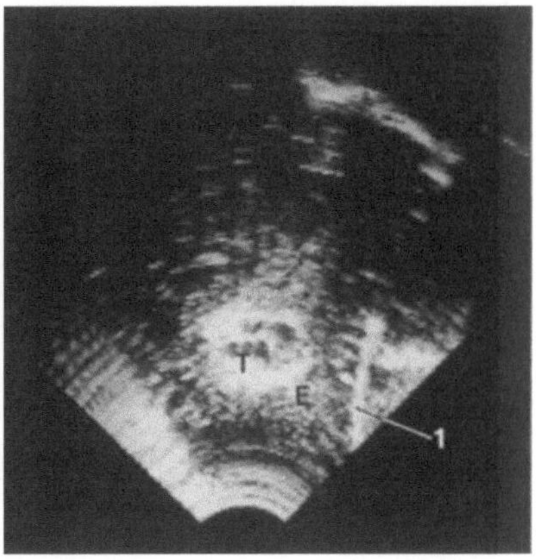

Fig. 212. Horizontal US. NS, 5 MHz

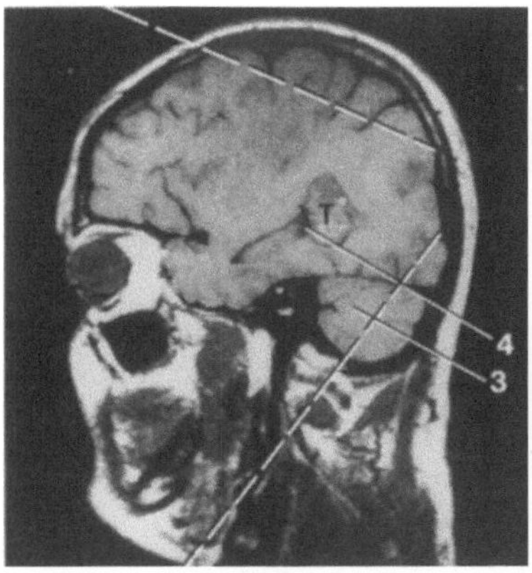

Fig. 213. Sagittal MRI

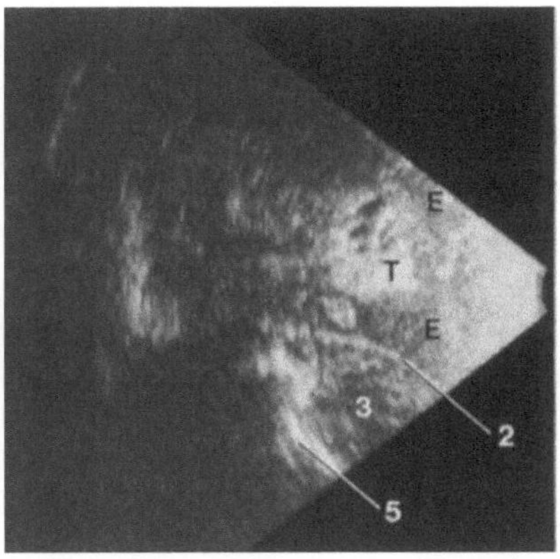

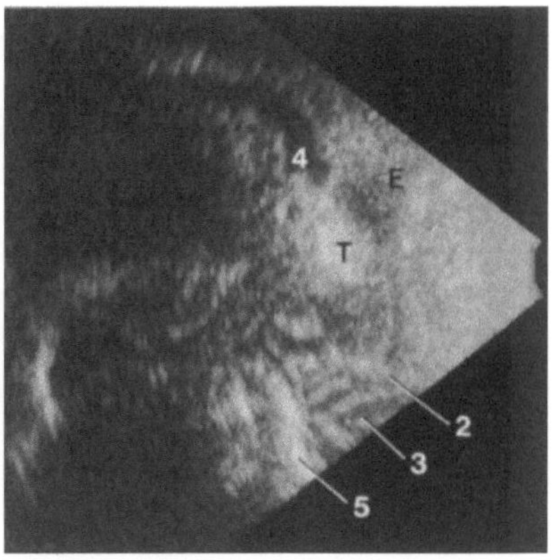

Figs. 214, 215. Sagittal US. DRF 100, GPS probe, 5 MHz

1 Falx
2 Tentorium
3 Cerebellum
4 Left trigonum
5 Base of skull
6 Choroid plexus
E Edema
T Tumor

CASE 40 (Figs. 216-222)

Deep-seated *metastasis from bronchial carcinoma* in a 64-year-old man operated upon via left occipital craniotomy.

On US the tumor is homogeneously hyperechoic, and the central necrosis, hypodense on CT (Fig. 216), is not visible. As is apparent from a series of horizontal sections (Figs. 219-222), the lower circumference of the tumor is tightly adherent to the choroid plexus in the trigonum (Figs. 221-222) and the tumor grows from there above the roof of the ventricle into the occipital white matter (Figs. 219-220). The perifocal edema, hypodense on CT as usual, is slightly hyperechoic on US (Figs. 219-221). The sagittal US sections (Figs. 217-218) give satisfactory anatomical orientation in the posterior fossa.

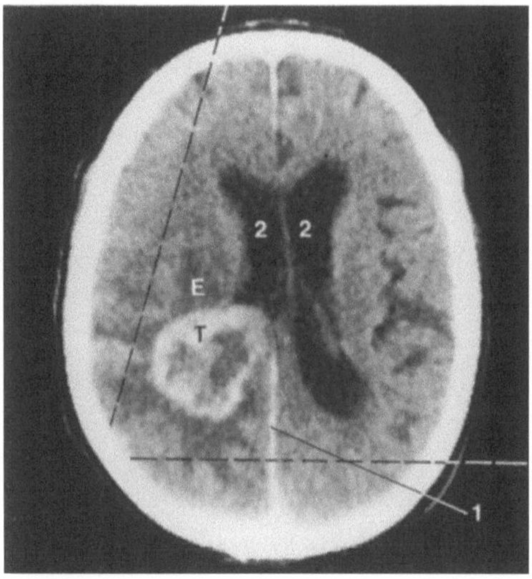

Fig. 216. Horizontal CT. Stippled line = sector plane for Fig. 220

1 Falx
2 Lateral ventricles
3 Choroid plexus
4 Third ventricle
5 Right occipital horn
6 Left occipital horn
7 Tentorium
8 Fourth ventricle
9 Cerebellar hemisphere
10 Clivus
11 Pons
12 Quadrigeminal plate
13 Occipital bone
14 Cisterna magna
15 Vermis
16 Quadrigeminal cistern
17 Thalamus
18 Frontal bone
19 Sphenoid bone
20 Parietooccipital fissure
A Hypoechoic artifact
E Edema
T Tumor

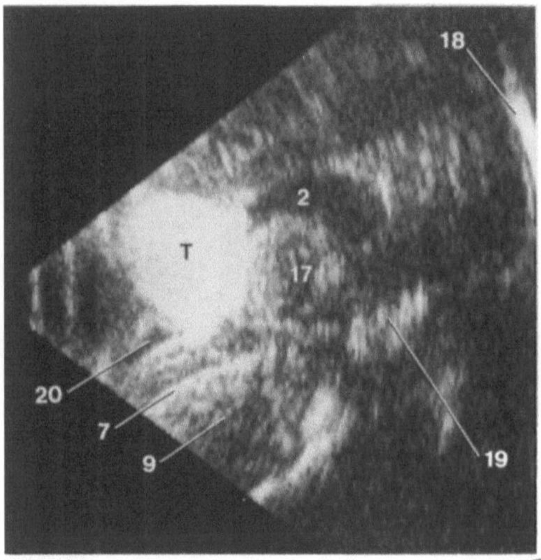

Fig. 217. Sagittal US. DRF 100, GPS probe, 5 MHz

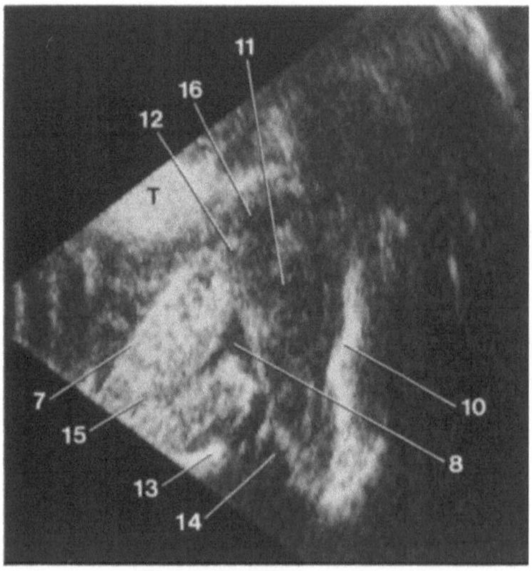

Fig. 218. Sagittal US. DRF 100, GPS probe, 5 MHz

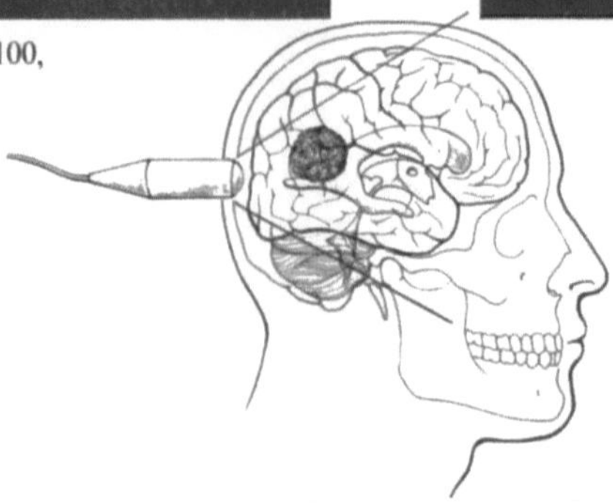

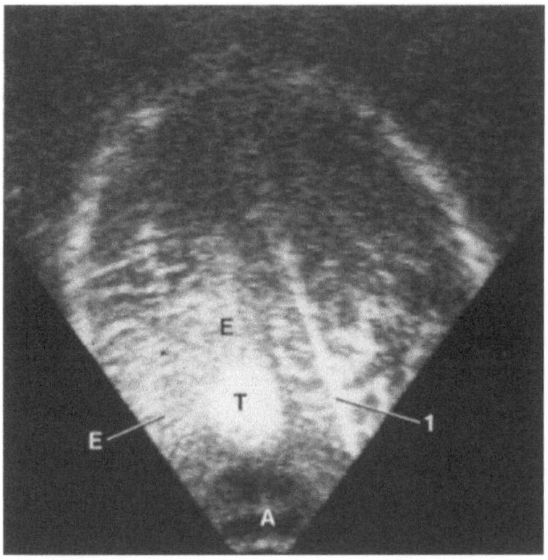

Fig. 219. Horizontal US. DRF 100, GPS probe, 5 MHz

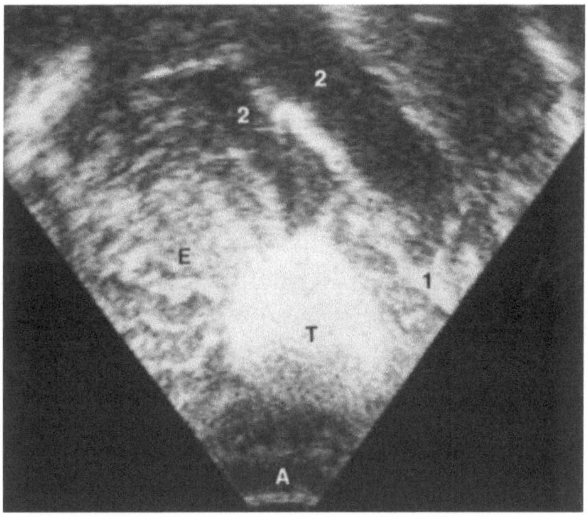

Fig. 220. Horizontal US. DRF 100, GPS probe, 5 MHz

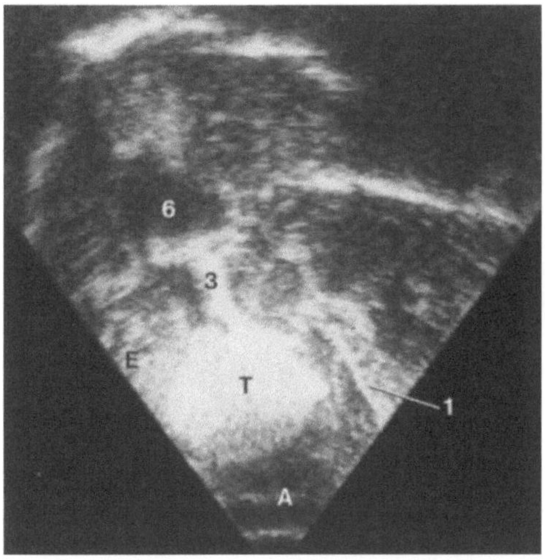

Fig. 221. Horizontal US. DRF 100, GPS probe, 5 MHz

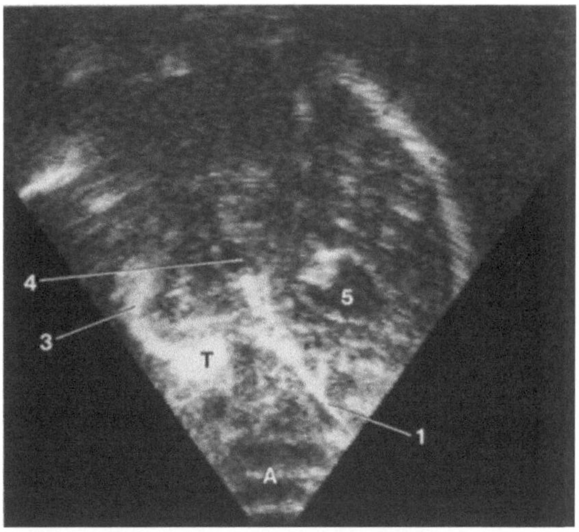

Fig. 222. Horizontal US. DRF 100, GPS probe, 5 MHz

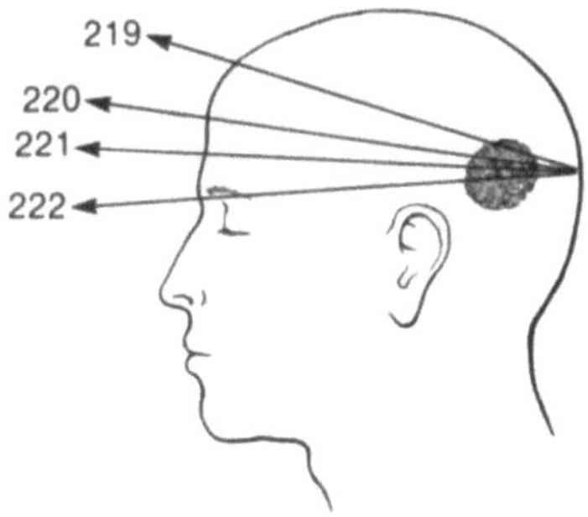

Ventricular Tumors

Tumors in, or bulging into, the ventricular system do not differ from tumors elsewhere in the brain as far as their pathomorphological appearance is concerned. Their intraventricular border is obviously very well delineated against the anechoic CSF. The interior of craniopharyngioma cysts is mostly isoechoic, surrounded by a markedly hyperechoic capsule; the same is true for colloid cysts. Calcified areas in solid craniopharyngiomas are very hyperechoic and throw a shadow. The case of medulloblastoma described in this section displayed a homogeneous, markedly hyperechoic appearance on US. Intraventricular tissue of pituitary adenomas also appeared homogeneous and slightly hyperechoic. A cavernous hemangioma extending intraventricularly appeared as a large hypoechoic cyst with a slightly hyperechoic capsule.

CASE 41 (Figs. 223, 224)

Cystic craniopharyngioma of the third ventricle in a 38-year-old woman operated upon by endoscopy via a right frontal burrhole.

The interior of the cyst is isoechoic, the capsule is hyperechoic. Most markedly hyperechoic on this coronal US section is the bottom of the cyst, probably indicating a small solid part with calcification.

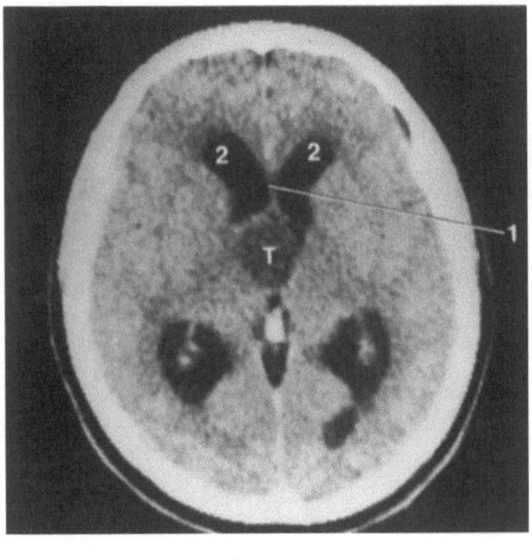

Fig. 223. Horizontal CT

1 Septum pellucidum
2 Lateral ventricle
3 Temporal lobe
T Tumor

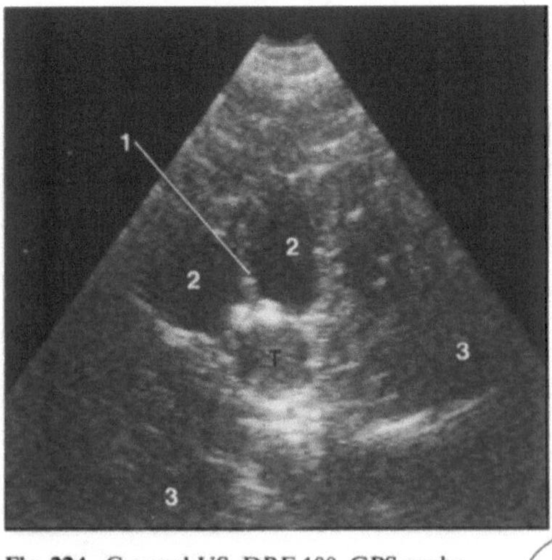

Fig. 224. Coronal US. DRF 100, GPS probe, 5 MHz (see schema)

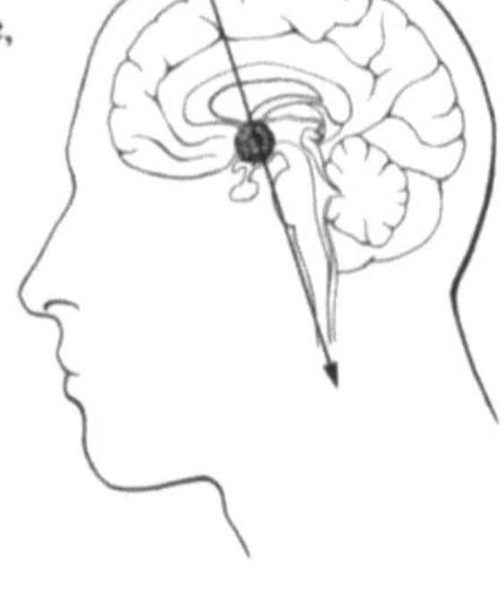

CASE 42 (Figs. 225–229)

Metastasis of a medulloblastoma in a 34-year-old woman operated upon by endoscopy via a right frontal burrhole.

The US sections show a hyperechoic, well-demarcated tumor attached to the septum pellucidum and the right head of the caudate nucleus.

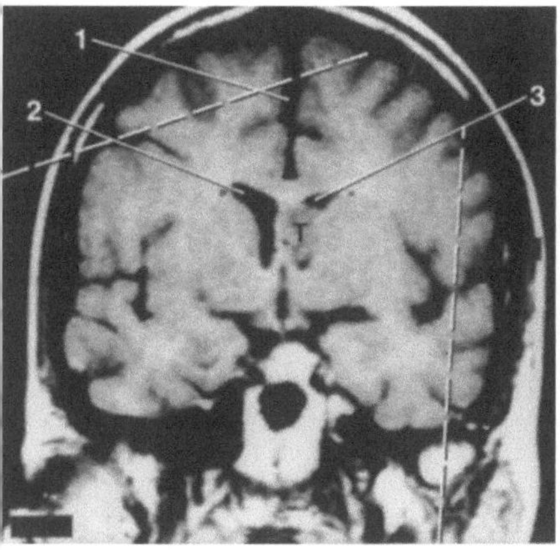

Fig. 225. Coronal MRI

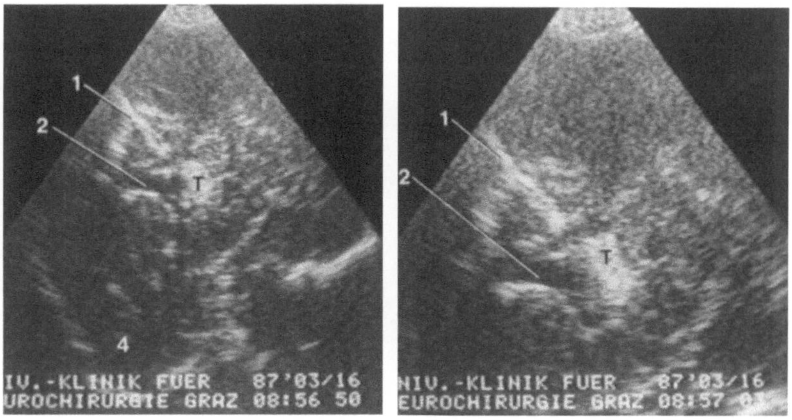

Figs. 226, 227. Coronal US. DRF 100, GPS probe, 5 MHz

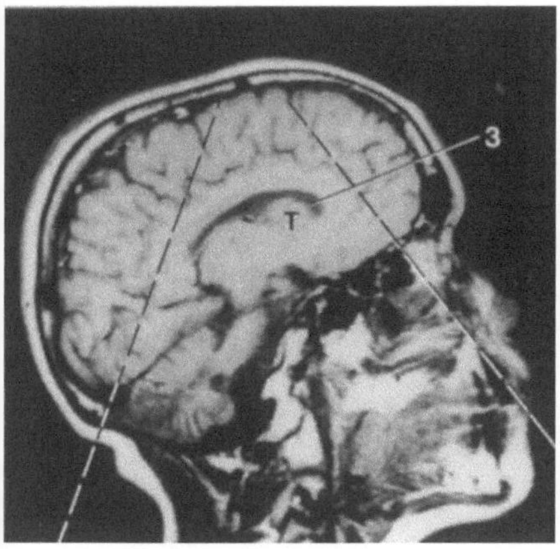

Fig. 228. Sagittal MRI

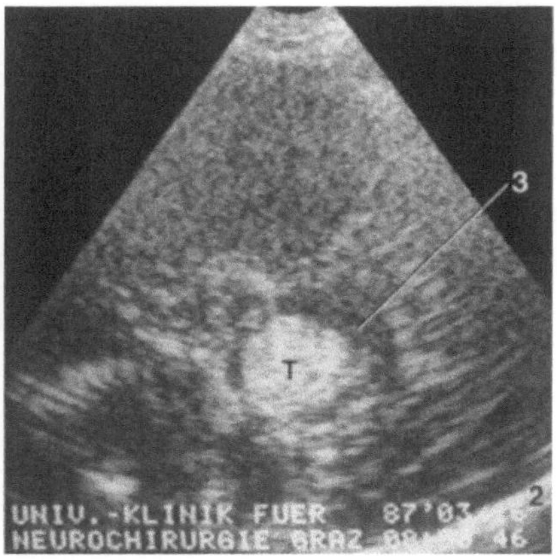

Fig. 229. Sagittal US. DRF 100, GPS probe, 5 MHz

1 Interhemispheric space
2 Lateral ventricle
3 Frontal horn of right lateral ventricle
4 Temporal lobe
T Tumor

CASE 43 (Figs. 230–234)

Astrocytoma grade 2 involving the septum pellucidum and the fornices reaching deep into the third ventricle, the anterior part of which is entirely occupied by tumor.

The coronal US sections taken through a right frontal burrhole for endoscopic biopsy and resection provide a precise anatomical picture of the frontal horns, the septum pellucidum with a cavum vergae and the columnae fornicis, which are invaded by the tumor. The tumor is homogeneously hyperechoic and rather ill defined in the depth of the third ventricle.

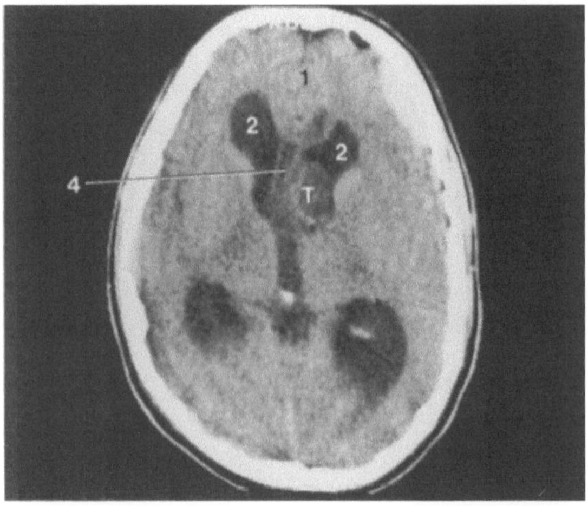

Fig. 230. Horizontal CT

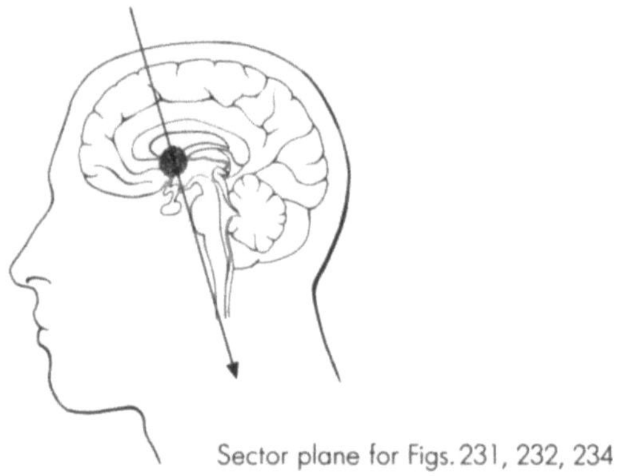

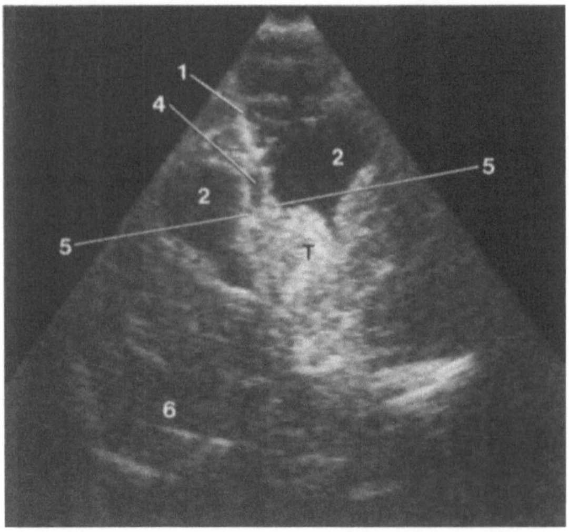

Fig. 231. Coronal US. DRF 100, GPS probe, 5 MHz

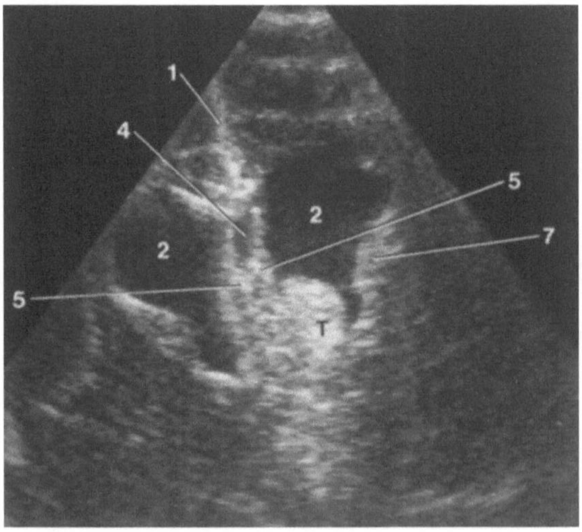

Fig. 232. Coronal US. DRF 100, GPS probe, 5 MHz

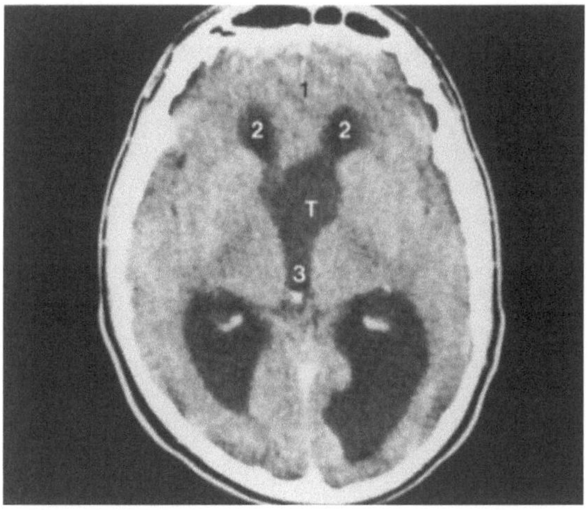

Fig. 233. Horizontal CT

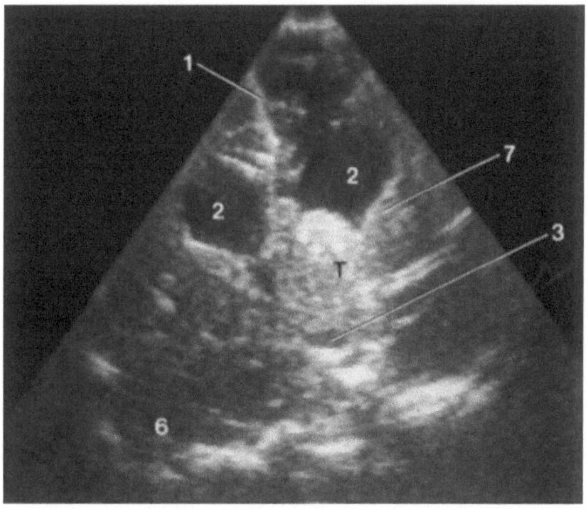

Fig. 234. Coronal US. DRF 100, GPS probe, 5 MHz

1 Interhemispheric space
2 Lateral ventricle
3 Third ventricle
4 Cavum vergae
5 Columnae fornicis
6 Left temporal fossa
7 Caudate nucleus
T Tumor

CASE 44 (Figs. 235, 236)

Ependymoma in the right lateral ventricle extending into the third ventricle in a 35-year-old man operated upon via a right frontal craniotomy.

The partly calcified lesion is well delineated on US, distinctly hyperechoic but rather inhomogeneous.

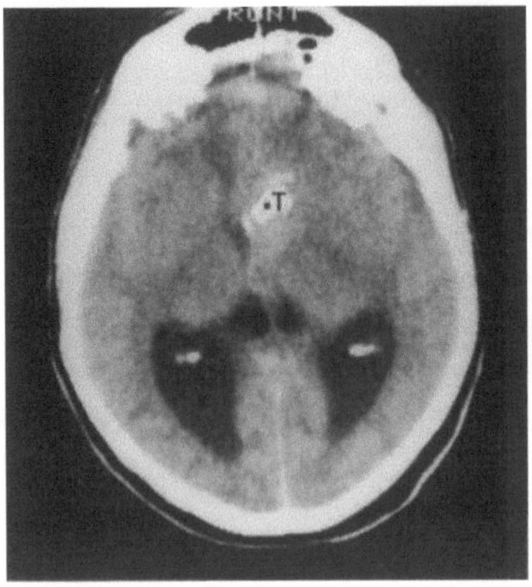

Fig. 235. Horizontal CT

1 Frontal falx
2 Left lateral ventricle
3 Choroid plexus
T Tumor

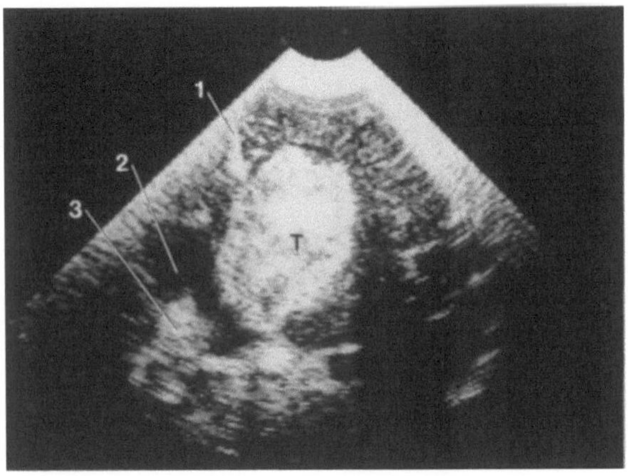

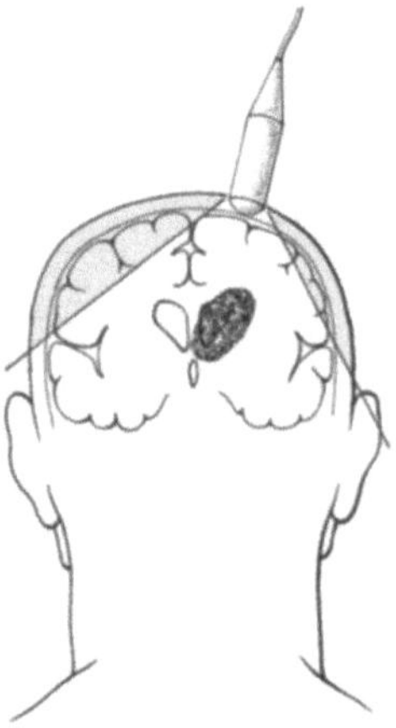

Fig. 236. Coronal US. NS, 5 MHz (see schema)

Posterior Fossa Lesions

The US appearance of tumors, cysts and hematomas of the posterior fossa is the same as those of the supratentorial space. The posterior fossa lesions are treated together in this section for two practical reasons: one is that neurosurgeons are accustomed to see infratentorial lesions as a separate entity due to the different surgical approaches, the other is the different pattern of landmarks for orientation on US (see p. 20).

Besides neurinoma and meningioma, some examples of hemangioblastoma with its isoechoic or hypoechoic cysts and the markedly hyperechoic vascular nodus are shown, as well as a solid hemangioblastoma.

CASE 45 (Figs. 237, 238)

Partly cystic, partly solid acoustic neurinoma in a 52-year-old woman operated upon via a suboccipital approach.

The area of lower density within the solid part on CT is not apparent on US. The whole solid tumor displays higher echo intensity than the cerebellar tissue, although the interior is rather inhomogeneous. The cystic part is clearly hypoechoic. The internal acoustic meatus can be well appreciated.

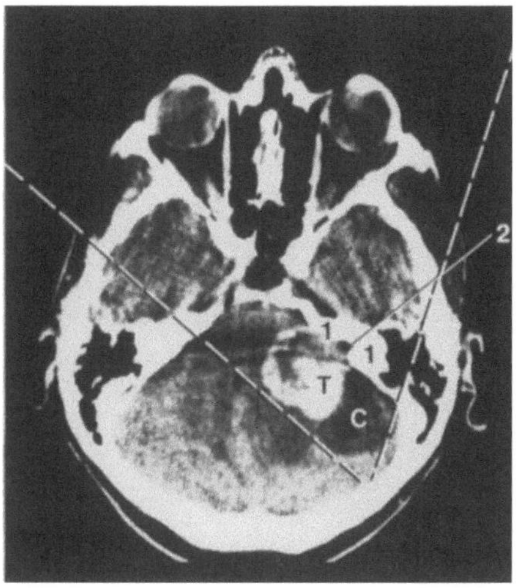

Fig. 237. Horizontal CT

1 Petrous bone
2 Internal acoustic meatus
C Cyst
T Solid tumor

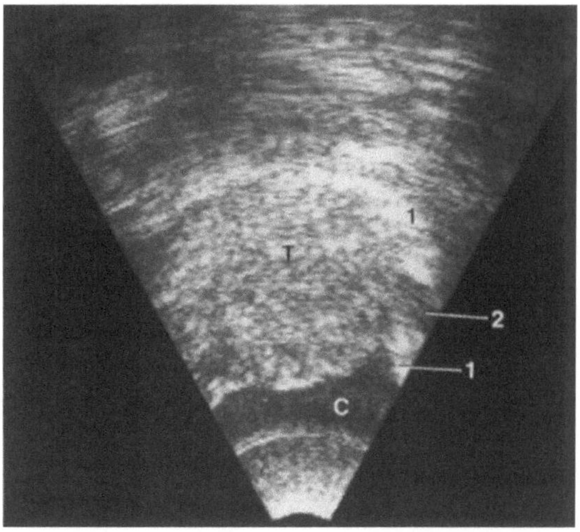

Fig. 238. Horizontal US. DRF 100, IOP probe, 5 MHz

CASE 46 (Figs. 239–243)

Small *acoustic neurinoma* in a 50-year-old man operated upon via a right lateral suboccipital approach.

On US, the globular tumor has a markedly hyperechoic capsule and an interior whose signal intensity is lower, only slightly above that of the surrounding cerebellar tissue.

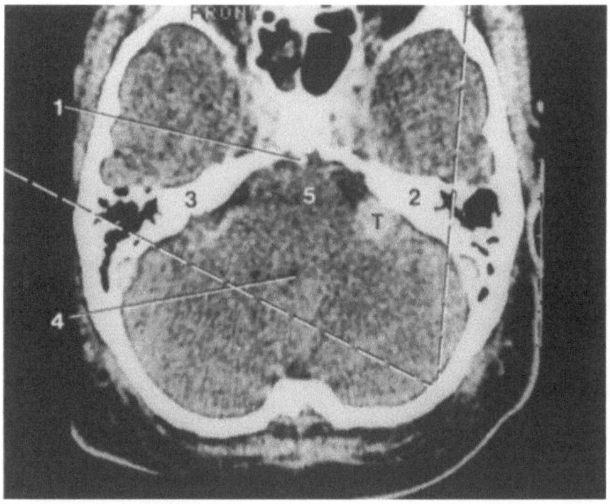

Fig. 239. Horizontal CT

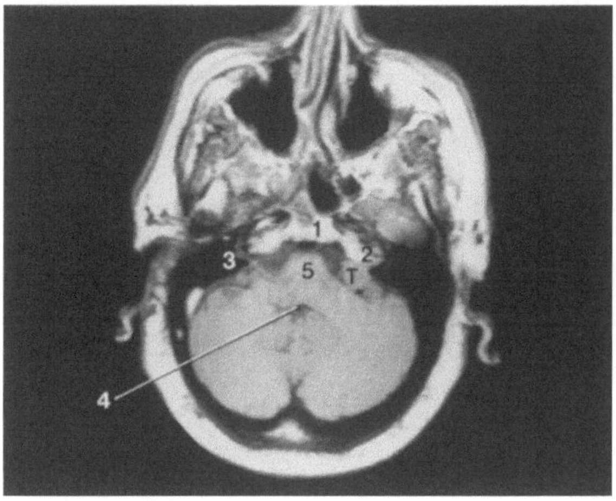

Fig. 240. Horizontal MRI

1 Clivus
2 Right petrous bone
3 Left petrous bone
4 Fourth ventricle
5 Pons
7 Internal acoustic meatus
T Tumor

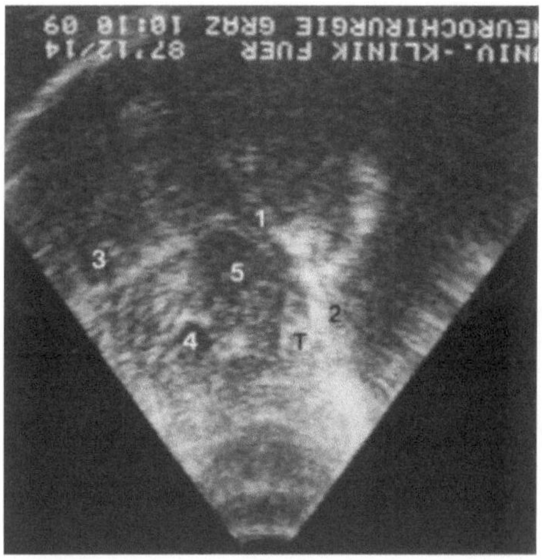

Fig. 241. Horizontal US. DRF 100, GPS probe, 5 MHz

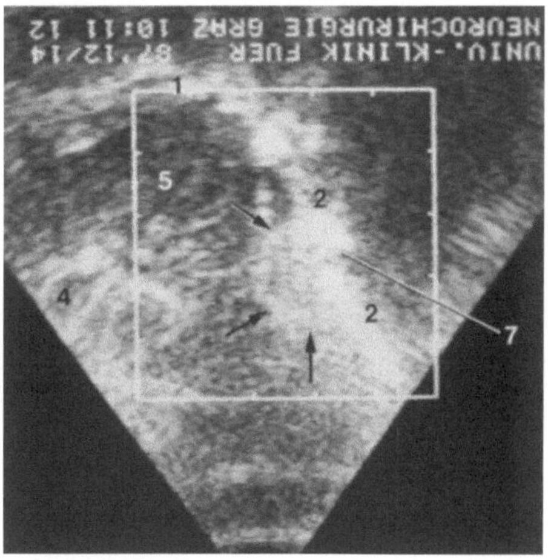

Fig. 242. Horizontal US. DRF 100, GPS probe, 5 MHz

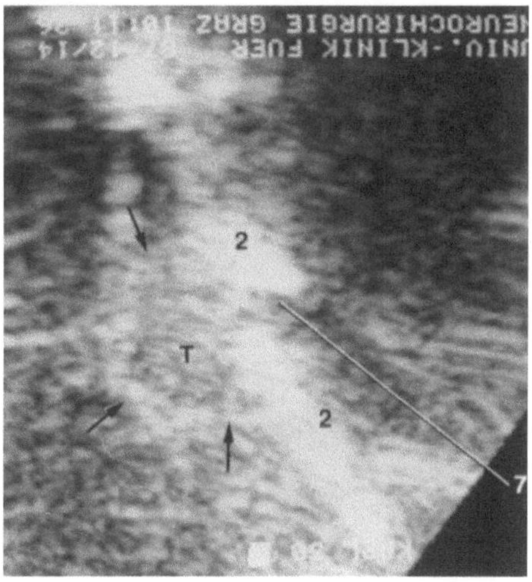

Fig. 243. Horizontal US. DRF 100, GPS probe, 5 MHz

CASE 47 (Figs. 244–247)

Cerebellopontine angle meningioma in a 58-year-old woman operated upon via a right suboccipital approach.

The hyperechoic tumor is rather homogeneous in its interior and well demarcated from the surroundings. The sagittal image shows the upward-displaced tentorium and the enlargement of the lateral ventricle due to the displacement and compression of the fourth ventricle.

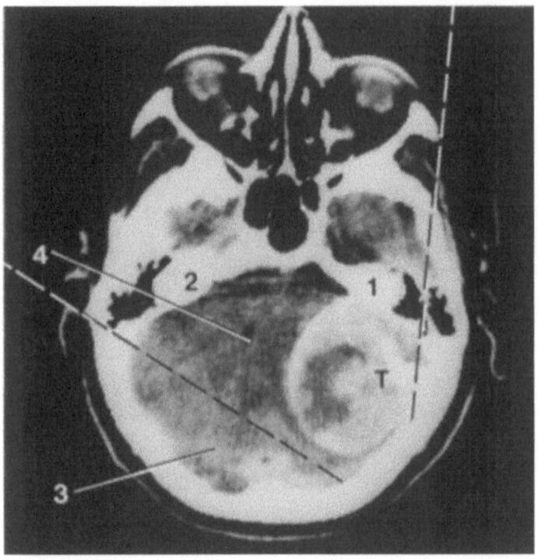

Fig. 244. Horizontal CT

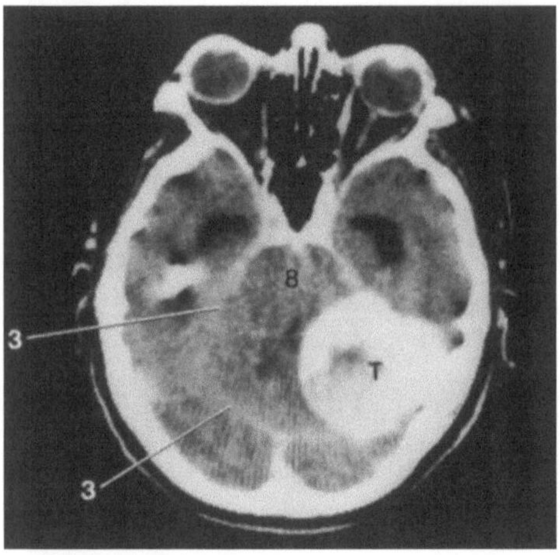

Fig. 245. Horizontal CT

1 Right petrous bone
2 Left petrous bone
3 Tentorium
4 Fourth ventricle
5 Clivus
6 Lateral ventricle
7 Choroid plexus
8 Pons
T Tumor

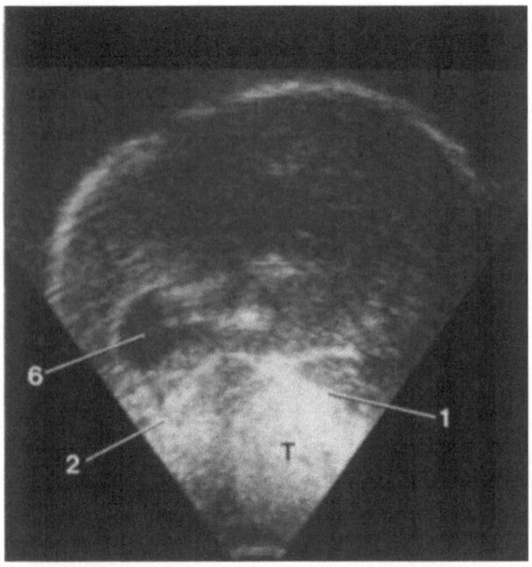

Fig. 246. Diagonal horizontal US. DRF 100, GPS probe, 5 MHz (see schema)

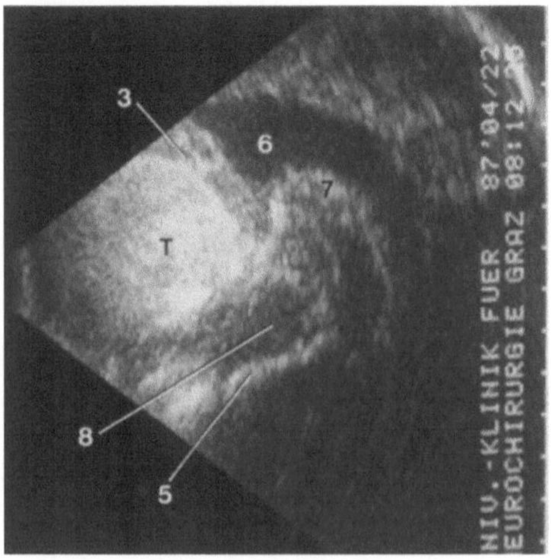

Fig. 247. Sagittal US. DRF 100, GPS probe, 5 MHz (see schema)

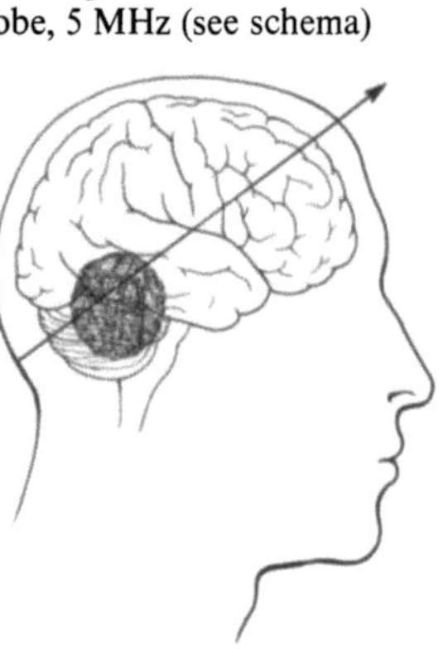

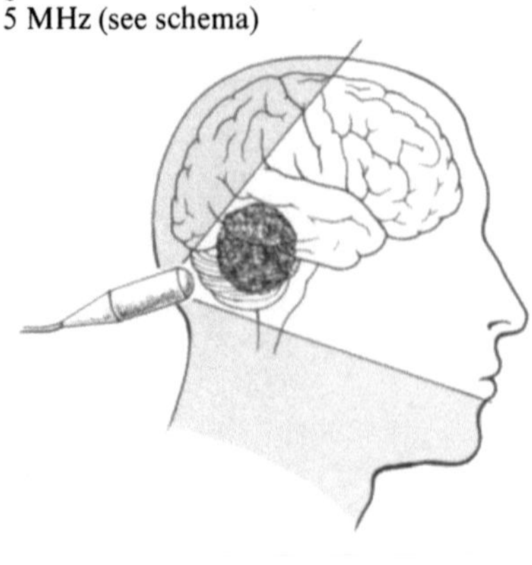

CASE 48 (Figs. 248-251)

Hemangioblastoma (Hippel-Lindau tumor) in a 49-year-old man operated upon via suboccipital craniotomy.

The interior of the cyst is rather isoechoic compared with the tissue of the pons, whereas it is markedly hypodense on CT and displays low signal intensity on MRI. The vascular nodus, hyperdense on CT, is hyperechoic.

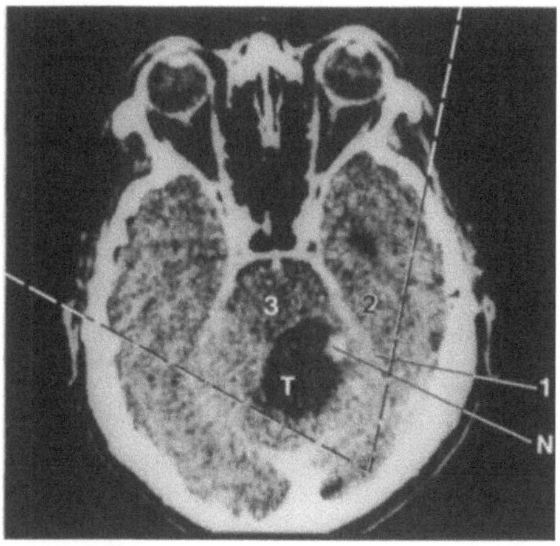

Fig. 248. Horizontal CT

1 Tentorium
2 Temporal lobe
3 Pons
N Vascular nodus
T Tumor

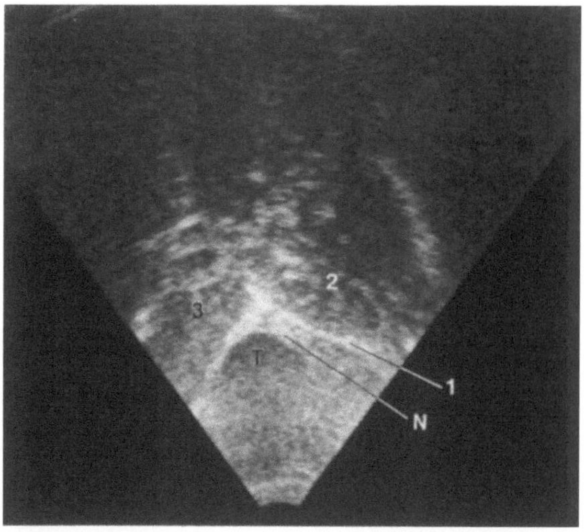

Fig. 249. Horizontal US. DRF 100, GPS probe, 5 MHz

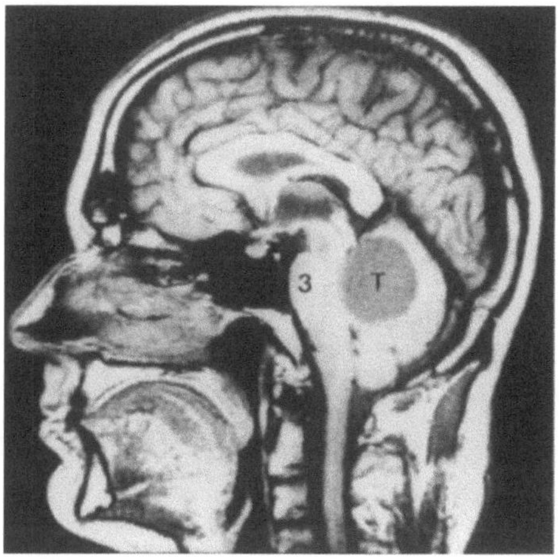

Fig. 250. Sagittal MRI

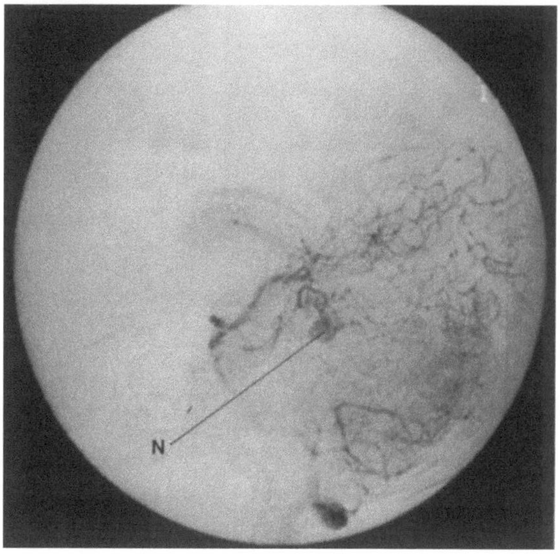

Fig. 251. Lateral vertebral angiogram

CASE 49 (Figs. 252-256)

Hemangioblastoma (Hippel-Lindau tumor) in a 49-year-old woman operated upon via suboccipital craniotomy.

On CT, the hypodense cyst has a slightly hyperdense and rather thick capsule on the left side. On US, mainly the anterior part of the cyst is markedly hypoechoic; the thick capsule is slightly hyperechoic and not very well delineated. By slanting the US plane upward from the horizontal, the enlarged lateral ventricles can be demonstrated.

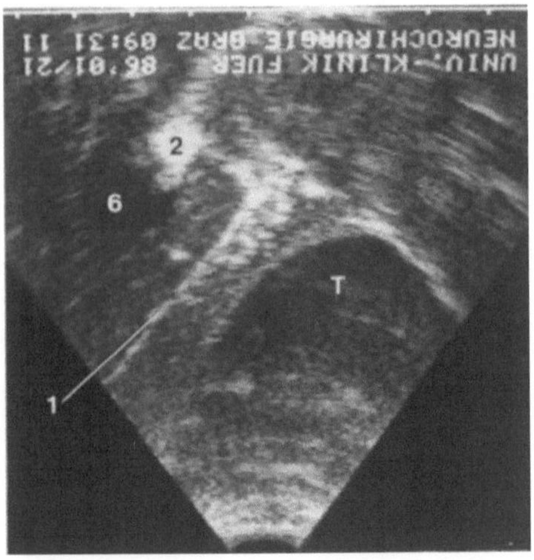

Fig. 254. Diagonal US. DRF 100, GPS probe, 5 MHz

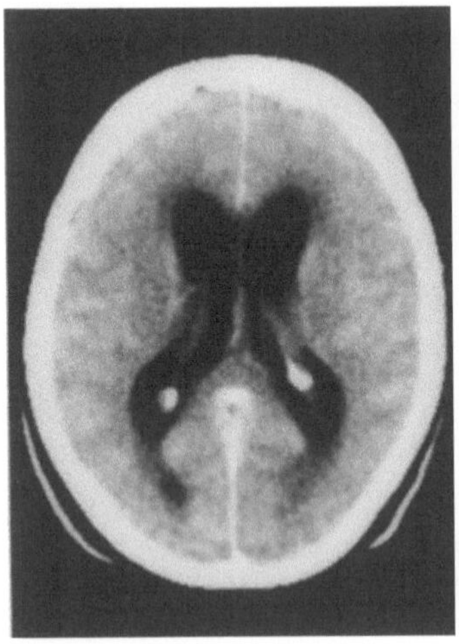

Fig. 252. Horizontal CT

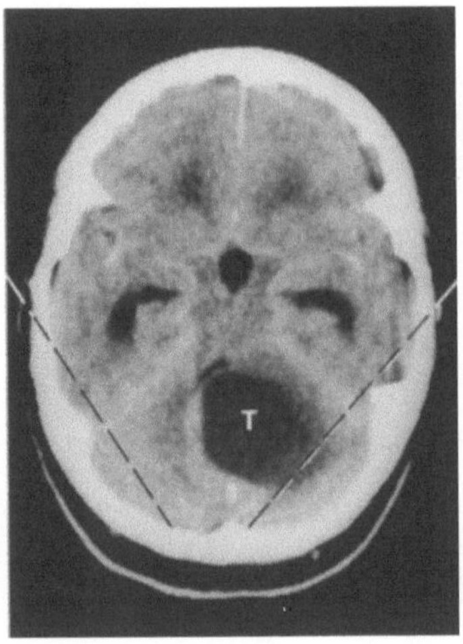

Fig. 253. Horizontal CT

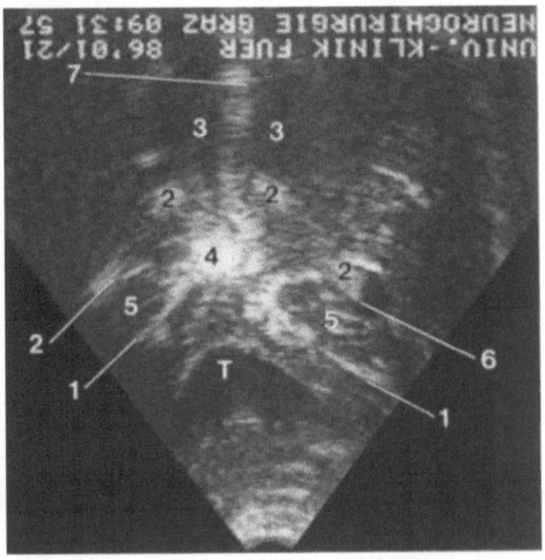

Fig. 255. Diagonal US. DRF 100, GPS probe, 5 MHz

1 Tentorium
2 Choroid plexus
3 Lateral ventricle
4 Pineal body
5 Temporal lobe
6 Temporal horn
7 Septum pellucidum
8 Upper vermis
9 Splenium of corpus callosum
T Tumor

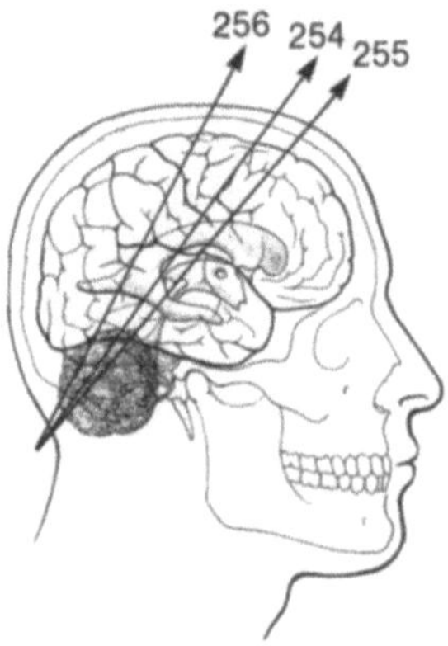

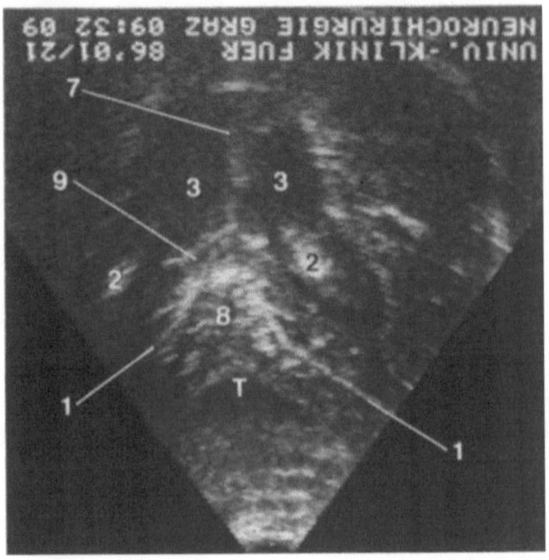

Fig. 256. Diagonal US. DRF 100, GPS probe, 5 MHz

CASE 50 (Figs. 257-261)

Cerebellar *hemangioblastoma* in a 52-year-old man operated upon via suboccipital craniotomy.

The lesion is markedly hyperdense on contrast-enhanced CT with several small hypodense areas; the collateral edema is hypodense. On T2-weighted MRI, the area of edema is even larger than on CT. US shows a slightly hyperechoic tumor with a clearly hyperechoic, rather well demarcated capsule; the edema is also hyperechoic, like the interior of the tumor.

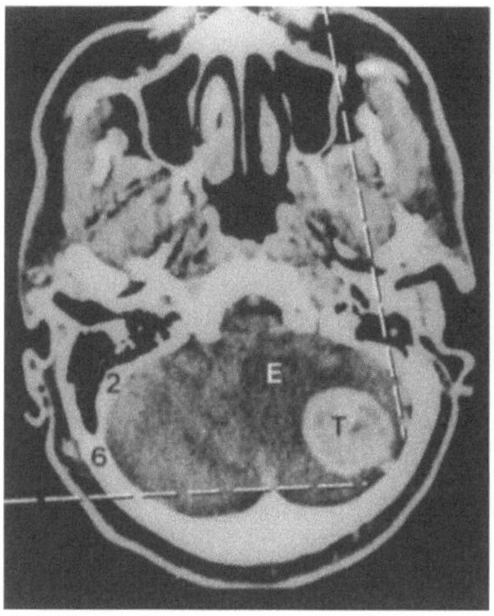

Fig. 257. Horizontal CT

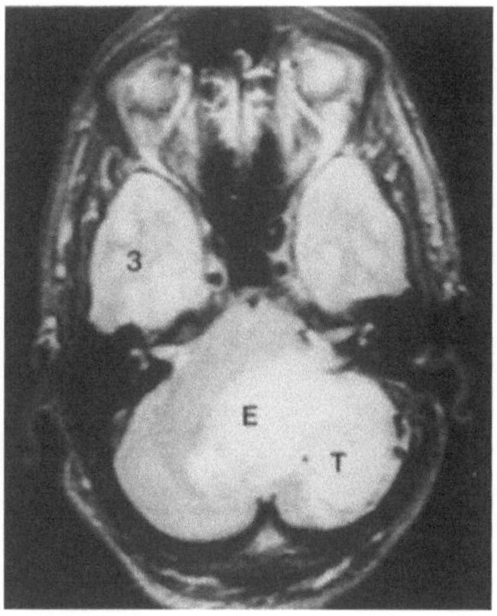

Fig. 258. Horizontal MRI

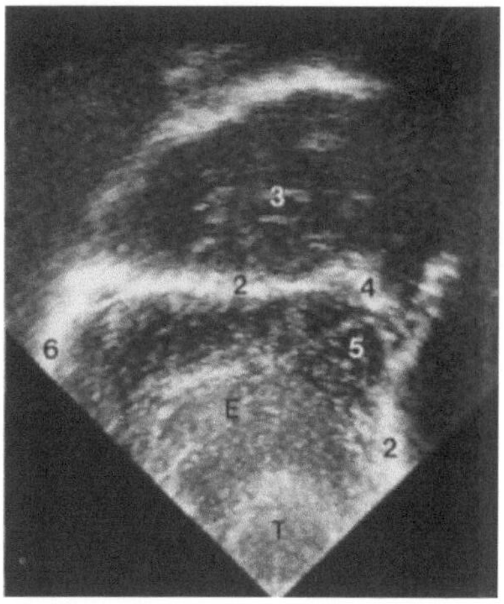

Fig. 259. Horizontal US. SSA 100A, 5 MHz

1 Tentorium
2 Petrosal edge
3 Temporal lobe
4 Clivus
5 Pons
6 Lateral occipital bone
7 Choroid plexus
8 Temporal horn of lateral ventricle
E Edema
T Tumor

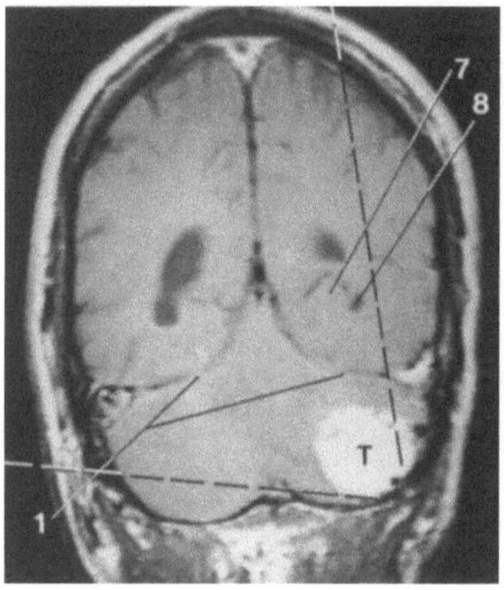

Fig. 260. Coronal MRI

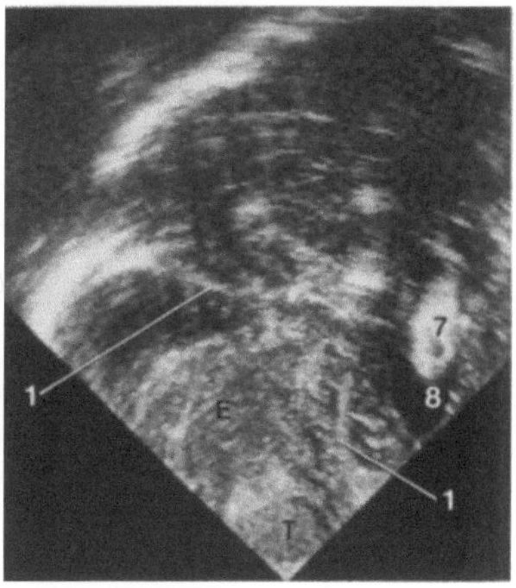

Fig. 261. Diagonal coronal US. SSA 100A, 5 MHz

CASE 51 (Figs. 262-265)

Chronic subdural hematoma over the left cerebellar hemisphere in a 13-year old girl operated upon via a leftsided burrhole.

The interior is hypoechoic like CSF. The dura and the cerebellar lobuli can be very clearly recognized.

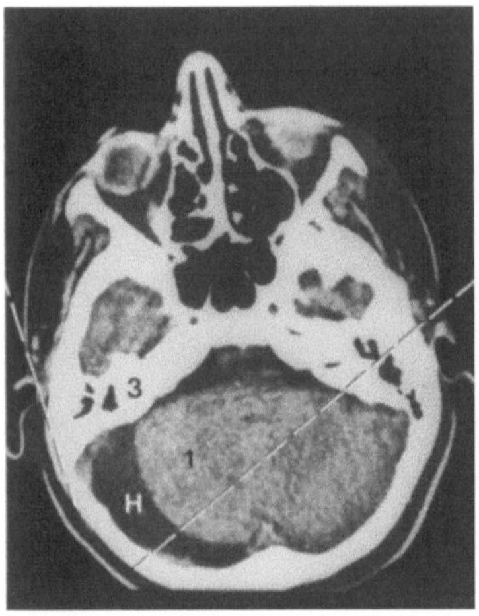

Fig. 262. Horizontal CT

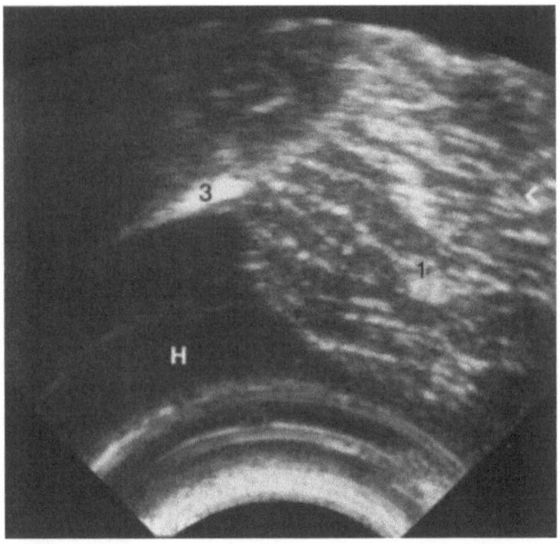

Fig. 263. Horizontal US. SPA 1000, GPWA probe, 5 MHz

1 Cerebellar hemisphere
2 Dura
3 Petrous bone
H Chronic subdural hematoma

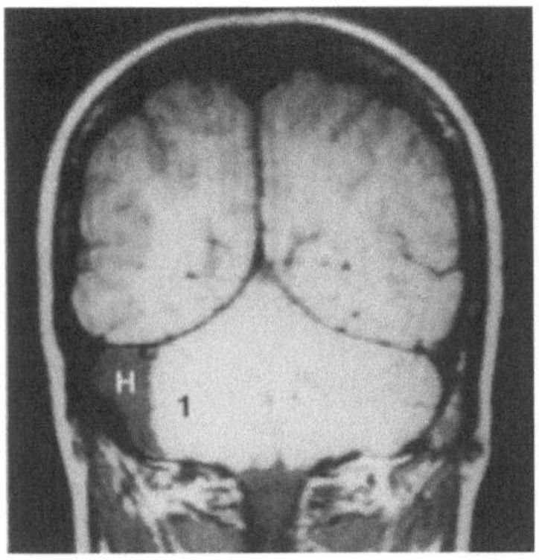

Fig. 264. Coronal MRI

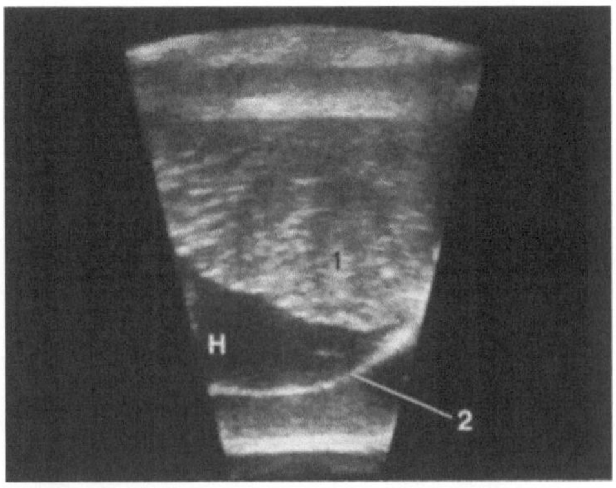

Fig. 265. Horizontal US. SPA 1000, NF probe, 10 MHz

CASE 52 (Figs. 266, 267)

Cerebellar hematoma which has ruptured into the fourth ventricle.

US-guided endoscopic evacuation was performed through a left occipital burrhole. On US, the hematoma appears as a markedly hyperechoic mass.

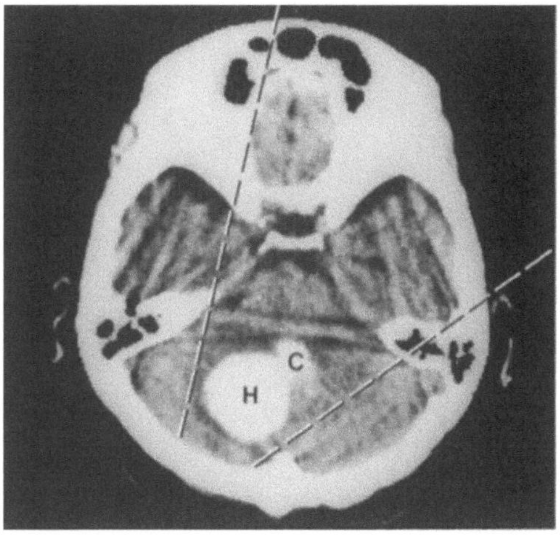

Fig. 266. Horizontal CT

C Clot in fourth ventricle
H Hematoma

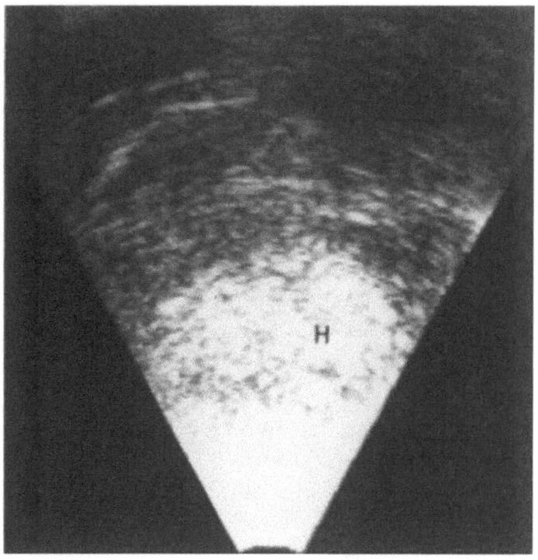

Fig. 267. Horizontal US. DRF 100, IOP probe, 5 MHz

Other Tumors

Described below are one example each of

periarteritis nodosa,
cavernous hemangioma of the orbit,
suprasellar dysgerminoma and
arachnoid cyst

CASE 53 (Figs. 268-270)

Periarteritis nodosa in a 64-year-old woman operated upon via left frontal craniotomy.

The markedly hyperdense tumor on contrast-enhanced CT is clearly hypoechoic on US with an isoechoic to slightly hyperechoic capsule. The surrounding edema is also very slightly hyperechoic.

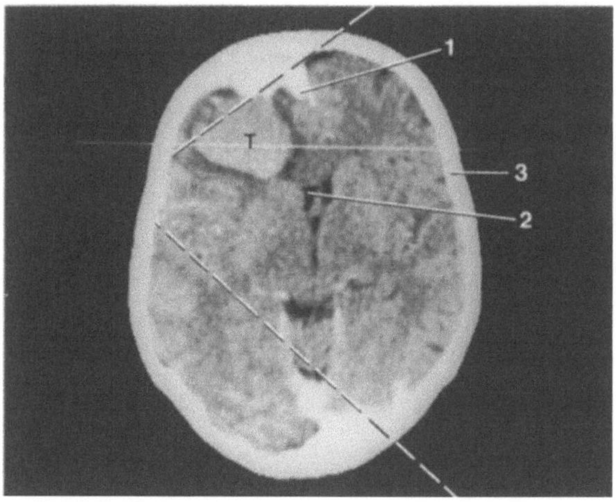

Fig. 268. Horizontal CT

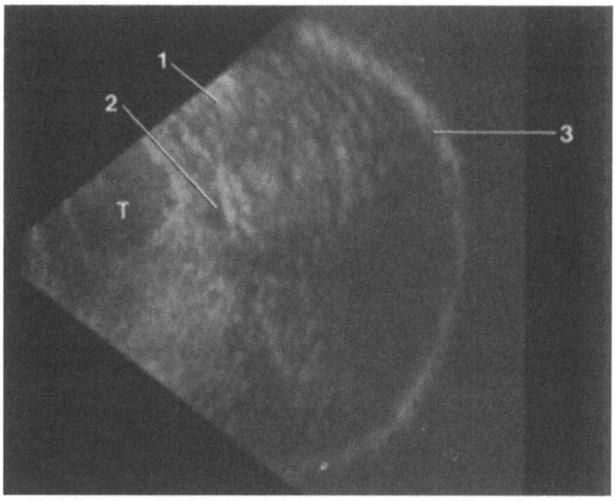

Fig. 269. Horizontal US. DRF 100, GPS probe, 5 MHz

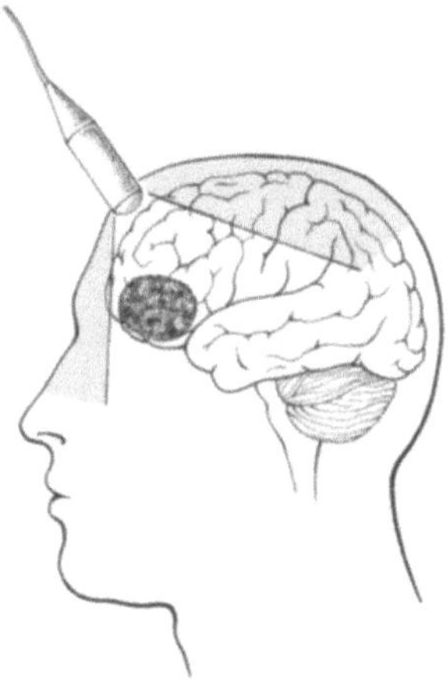

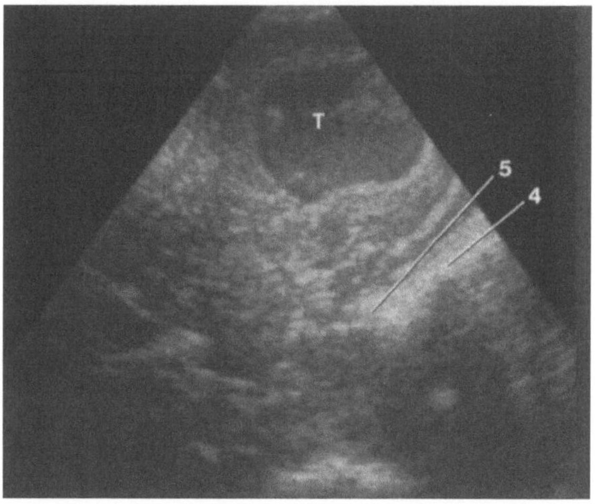

1 Falx
2 Displaced left frontal horn
3 Right temporal bone
4 Frontal base of skull
5 Sphenoid wing
T Tumor

Fig. 270. Sagittal US. DRF 100, GPS probe, 5 MHz (see schema)

CASE 54 (Figs. 271–273)

Cavernous hemangioma of the right orbit in a 58-year-old man operated upon via a right subfrontal extradural approach.

The tumor is homogeneously hyperechoic in its upper half and has a capsule with even higher echoicity. In the lower half, cavities with a lower echo intensity can be seen.

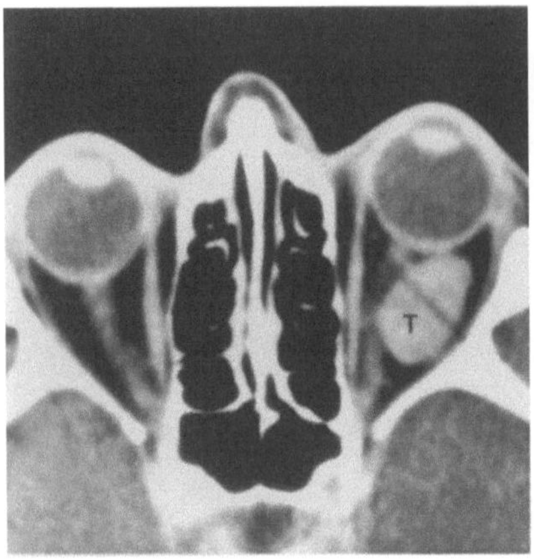

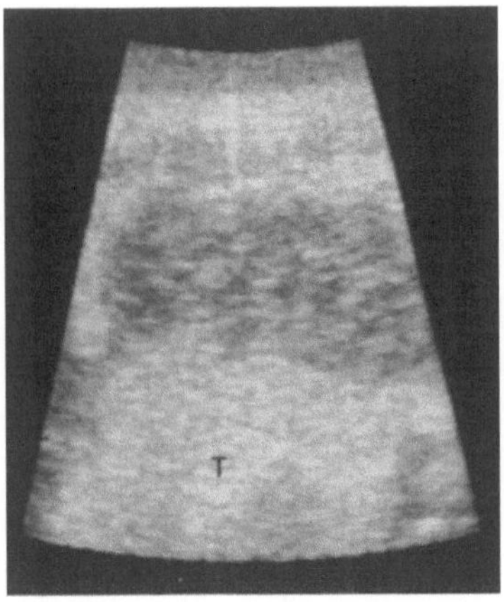

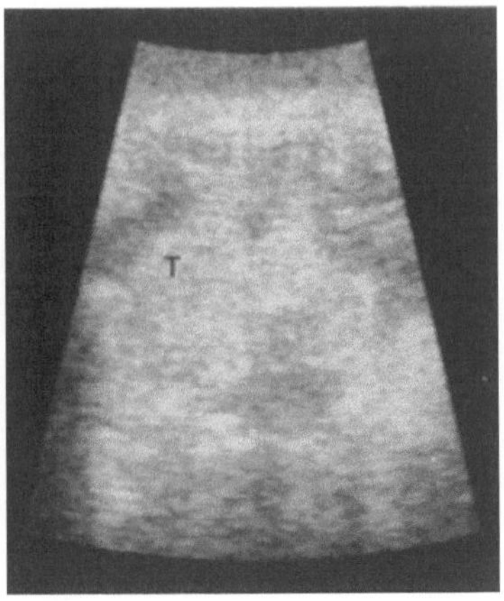

Fig. 271. Horizontal CT

Figs. 272, 273. Slightly diagonal sagittal US of the orbit, parallel to the course of the optic nerve. DRF 100, NF probe, 10 MHz

T Tumor

CASE 55 (Figs. 274, 275)

Suprasellar *dysgerminoma* in a 15-year-old boy operated upon via a pterional approach.

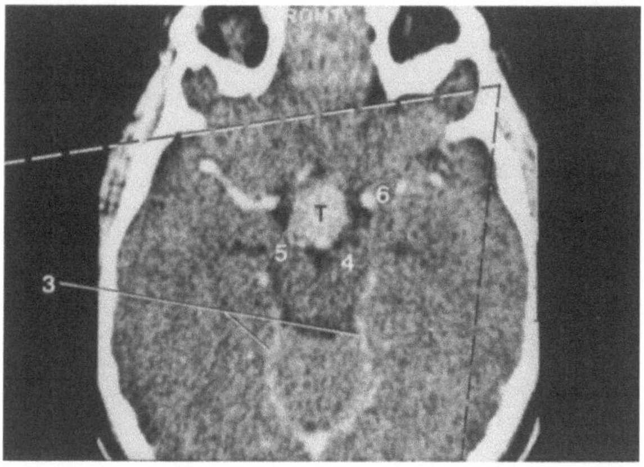

Fig. 274. Horizontal CT

1 Cerebellum
2 Occipital bone
3 Tentorium
4 Right crus cerebri
5 Left crus cerebri
6 Right sylvian fissure
7 Right uncus
T Tumor

The US image shows a homogeneously hyperechoic tumor completely occupying the interpeduncular cistern and attached to the right uncus.

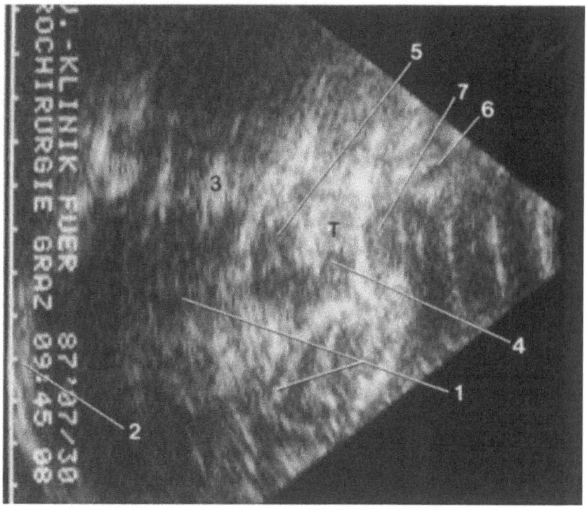

Fig. 275. Horizontal US. DRF 100, GPS probe, 5 MHz

CASE 56 (Figs. 276, 277)

Left frontal *arachnoid cyst* in a 61-year-old woman operated upon via a frontal burrhole.

On US, the lesion is anechoic like ventricular CSF, although it is less hypodense on CT than the lateral ventricles are.

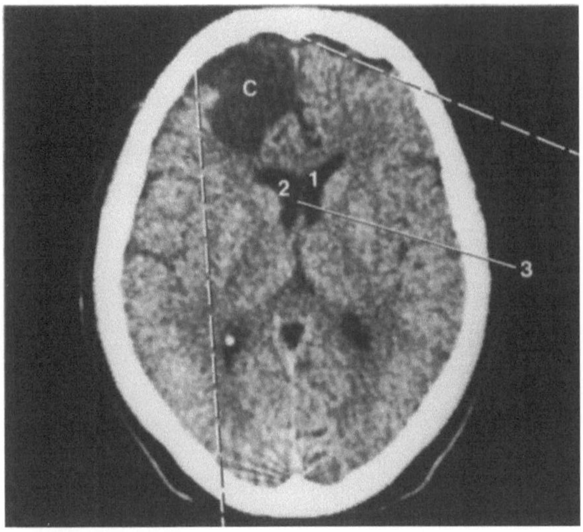

Fig. 276. Horizontal CT

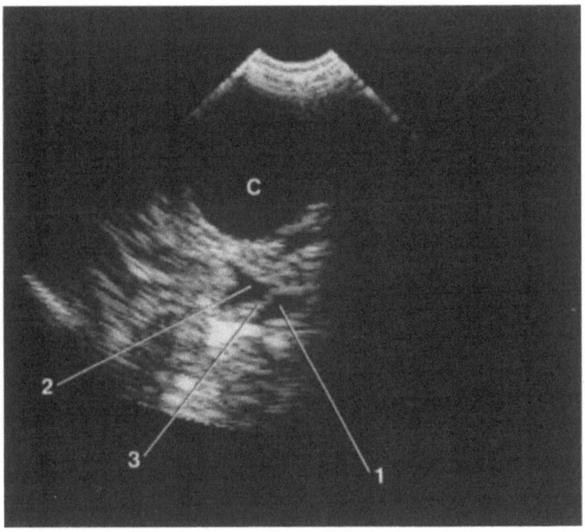

Fig. 277. Diagonal horizontal US. NS, 5 MHz

1 Right frontal horn
2 Left frontal horn
3 Septum pellucidum
C Cyst

Brain Abscesses

The most frequent appearance of a brain abscess on US is that of an isoechoic to slightly hypoechoic lesion surrounded by a strongly hyperechoic capsule and an ill-defined, slightly hyperechoic zone of edema outside of the capsule. Sometimes, the interior contains a markedly hypoechoic ring of fluid content. Clear-cut diagnosis is not, however, possible on the basis of US alone, because a similar pattern may occur with other lesions, especially gliomas with a central necrosis (see case 2).

Further reading: references [16, 17].

CASE 57 (Figs. 278, 279)

Right occipital *brain abscess* in a 79-year-old woman operated upon via a burrhole.

The interior of the abscess is hypoechoic on US and hypodense on CT. The capsule, hyperdense on CT, appears as a rather ill-demarcated hyperechoic structure. The collateral edema is hyperechoic on US, but hypodense on CT.

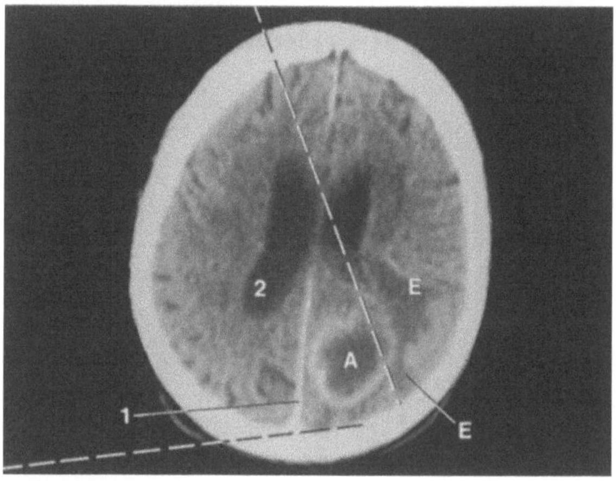

Fig. 278. Horizontal CT

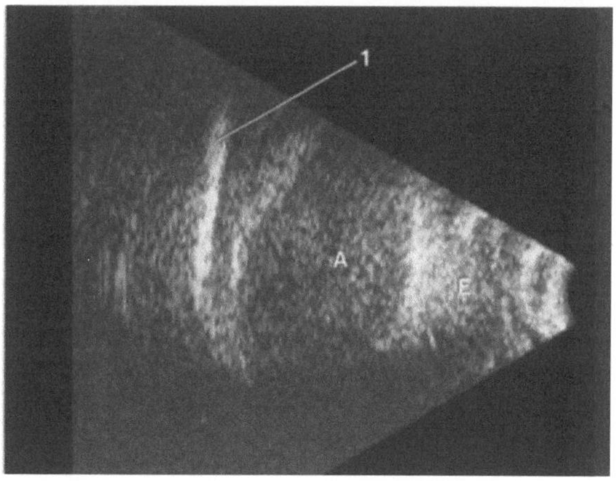

Fig. 279. Horizontal US, DRF 100, GPS probe, 5 MHz

1 Falx
2 Left lateral ventricle
A Abscess cavity
E Collateral edema

CASE 58 (Figs. 280, 281)

Right frontal *brain abscess* in a 47-year-old man operated upon by drainage via a frontal burr-hole.

The distinctly hypoechoic cavity lacks, on US, the well-defined capsule seen on CT. The collateral massive edema is hypodense on CT, but hyperechoic on US.

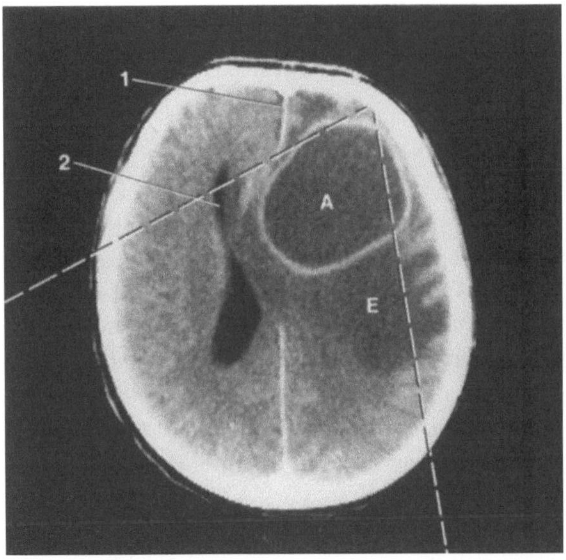

Fig. 280. Horizontal CT

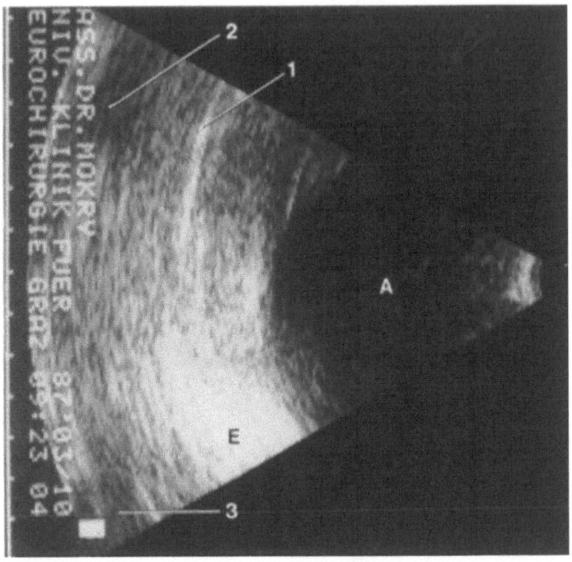

Fig. 281. Horizontal US. DRF 100, IOP probe, 5 MHz

1 Falx
2 Left frontal horn
3 Left trigonum
A Abscess cavity
E Collateral edema

Hydrocephalus

Ultrasound imaging in neurosurgery really began with the diagnosis and follow-up of hydrocephalus and hemorrhage in children through open fontanelles. This procedure, now a matter of clinical routine, was then extended to neurosurgical interventions in hydrocephalic children, where the ventricular catheter was implanted under US control.

Since the normal ventricles have been shown to be important anatomical landmarks for orientation during intracranial US imaging in general, it will already be obvious that US provides an excellent overview of hydrocephalic ventricular systems as well as related porencephalic cysts. Large ventricles will thus always appear as wide dark spaces, their choroid plexus as a very markedly hyperechoic structure. In the case of porencephalic cysts it may be helpful to use US during shunting procedures, because septal structures may be visualized better than by other imaging techniques, allowing the surgeon better to differentiate whether the tip of the shunt catheter is in a lateral ventricle or a porencephalic cyst. The following examples provide a survey of different pathologies encountered in daily routine. Several examples of the practical application of US for shunt implantation under US guidance will be presented in the appropriate section of the next chapter (p. 131).

CASE 59 (Figs. 282-284)

Occlusive supratentorial hydrocephalus in a 16-day-old boy.

A birth trauma had led to hemorrhage in the quadrigeminal cistern (*) and cerebellum (Fig. 282, CT on day 6 after birth). Control CT, 2 weeks after birth, shows that the hemorrhage has been mostly resorbed; however, there is also hydrocephalus due to aqueduct stenosis (Fig. 283). The hematoma in resorption is seen on US (Fig. 284) as a hypoechoic area (*).

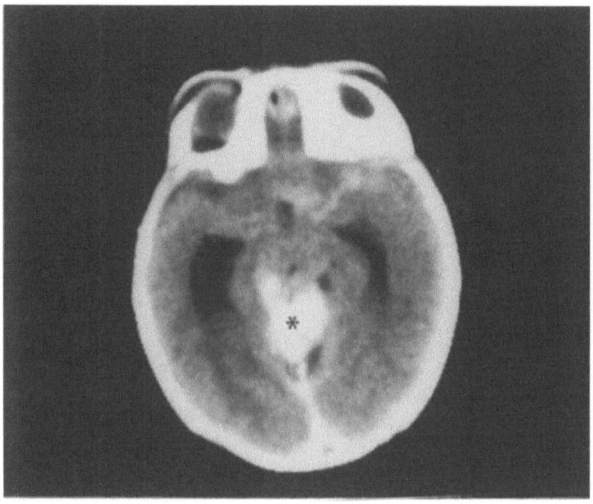

Figs. 282. Horizontal CT

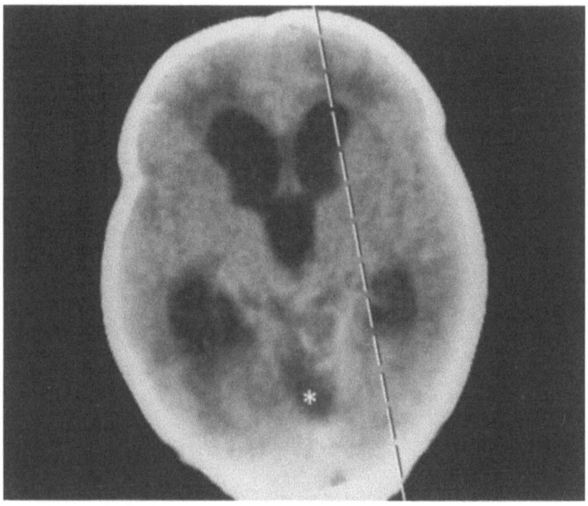

Fig. 283. Horizontal CT. Stippled line = plane for Fig. 284

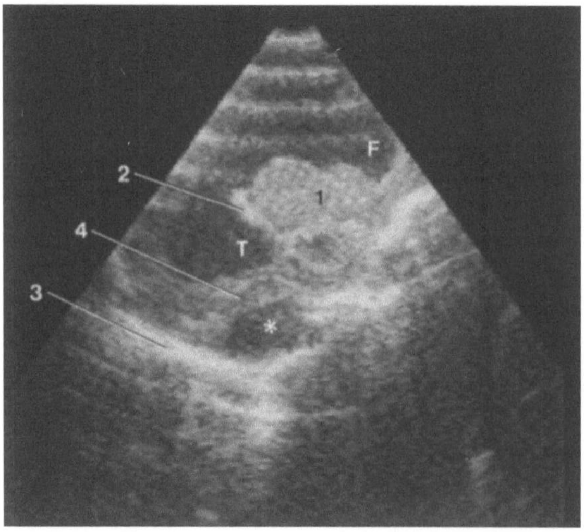

Fig. 284. Sagittal US. DRF 100, GPS probe, 5 MHz

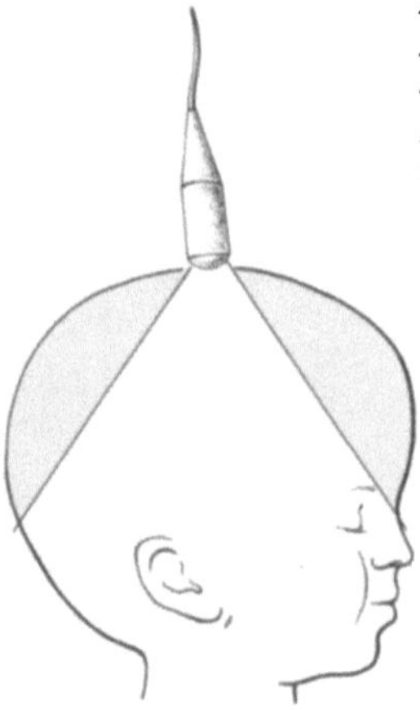

1 Basal ganglia
2 Choroid plexus
3 Occipital bone
4 Area of tentorium
F Frontal horn
T Temporal horn
* Hemorrhage from birth trauma

CASE 60 (Figs. 285, 286)

Hydrocephalus as a consequence of ventricular bleeding grade 3 in a 5-week-old boy following premature birth in the 29th gestational week.

A 10-MHz image taken through the frontal fontanelle shows hydrocephalic enlargement of both frontal horns (Fig. 286). A 5-MHz coronal section through the frontal fontanelle shows irregular hydrocephalic enlargement of ventricles (Fig. 285). The hyperechoic dot in the right pars centralis represents the ventricular catheter.

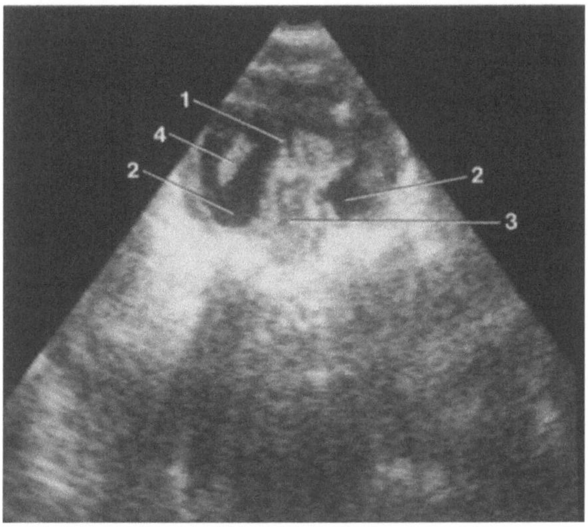

Fig. 285. Coronal US. DRF 100, GPS probe, 5 MHz

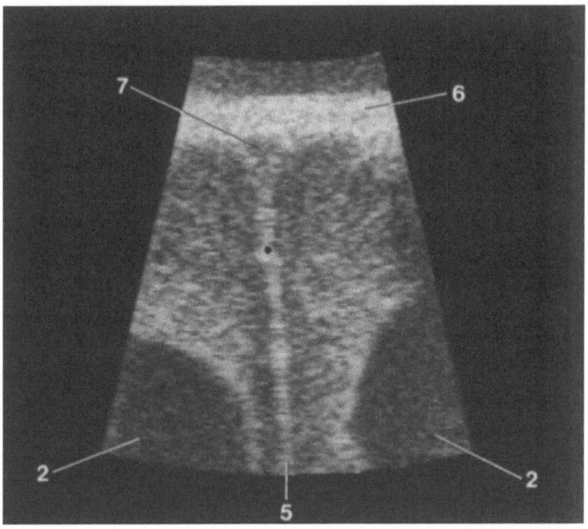

Fig. 286. Coronal US. DRF 100, NF probe, 10 MHz

1 Septum pellucidum
2 Lateral ventricle
3 Brainstem
4 Shunt catheter
5 Falx
6 Parietal dura
7 Superior sagittal sinus

CASE 61 (Figs. 287-289)

Porencephaly and *hydrocephalus* in a 5-day-old boy.

US imaging was performed through the frontal fontanelle. The asymmetry can be appreciated particularly well in Figs. 287 and 288, where the right pars centralis, occipital horn and temporal horn are seen to be markedly wider than the corresponding structures on the left side.

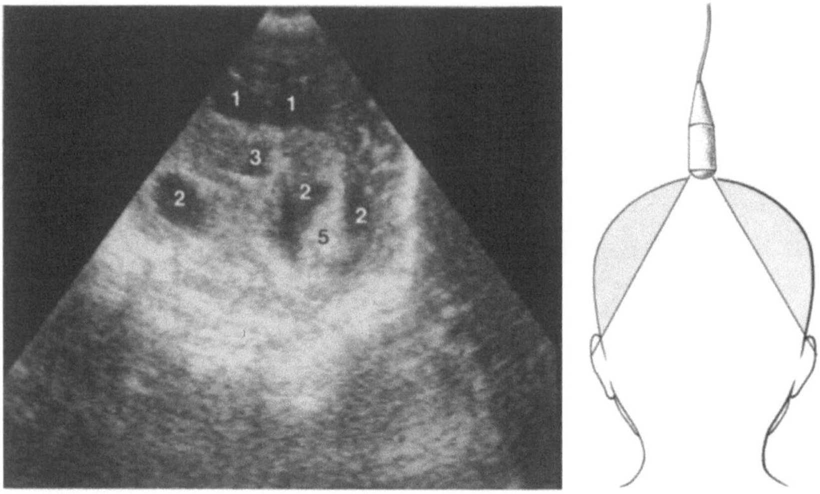

Fig. 287. Coronal US. DRF 100, GPS probe, 5 MHz

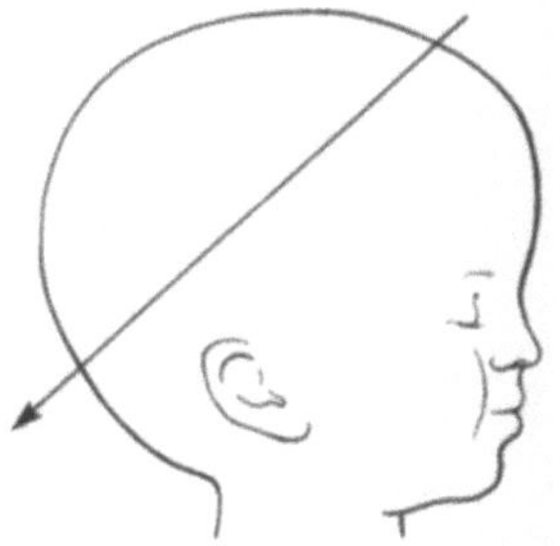

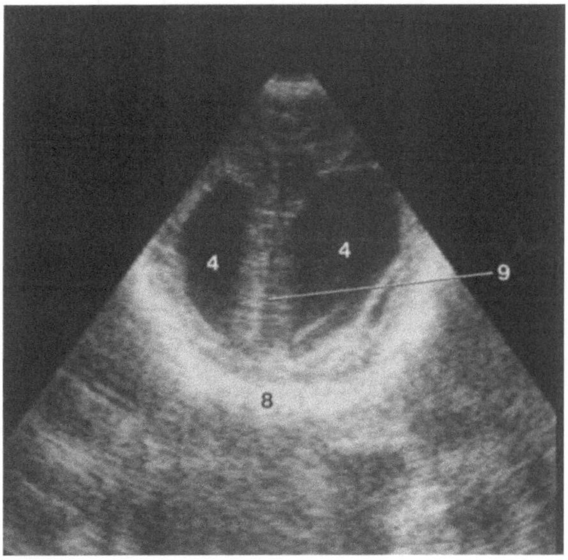

Fig. 288. Diagonal (coronal/horizontal) US. DRF 100, GPS probe, 5 MHz

1 Frontal horn
2 Temporal horn
3 Third ventricle
4 Pars centralis and occipital horn
5 Choroid plexus
6 Thalamus
7 Pars centralis/trigonum of lateral ventricle
8 Occipital bone
9 Interhemispheric space

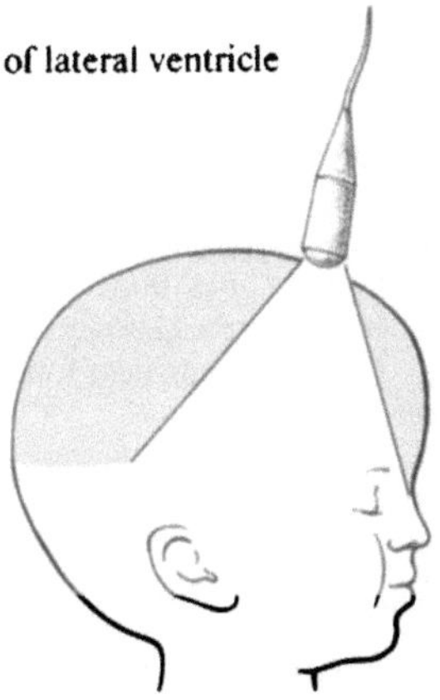

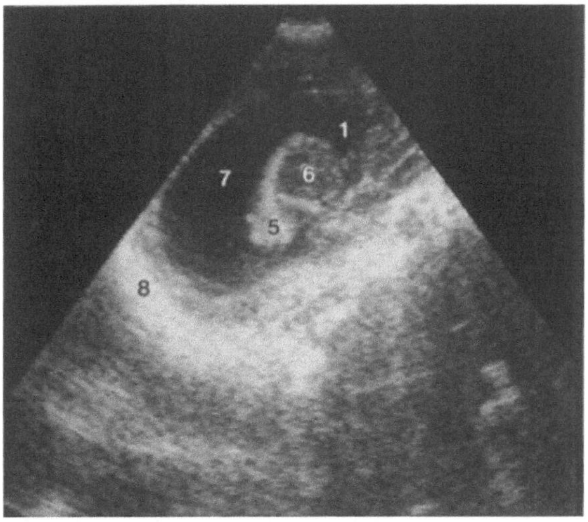

Fig. 289. Parasagittal US. DRF 100, GPS probe, 5 MHz

CASE 62 (Figs. 290-293)

Asymmetrical posthemorrhagic *hydrocephalus* in a baby 3 weeks after premature birth (in the 35th gestational week).

Especially the posterior horn of the left lateral ventricle is significantly enlarged.

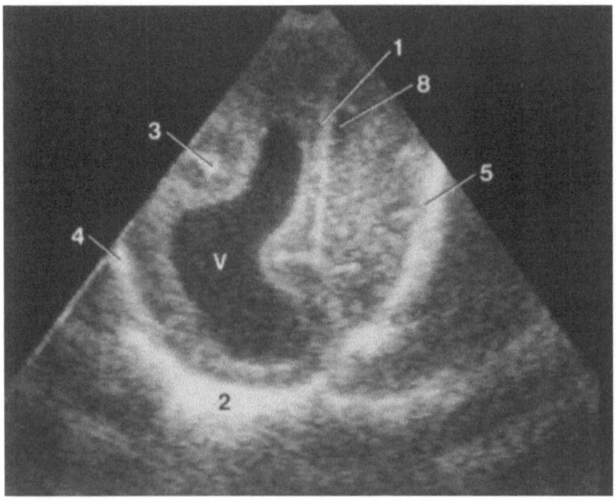

Fig. 290. Slightly diagonal horizontal US through fontanelle. DRF 100, GPS probe, 5 MHz

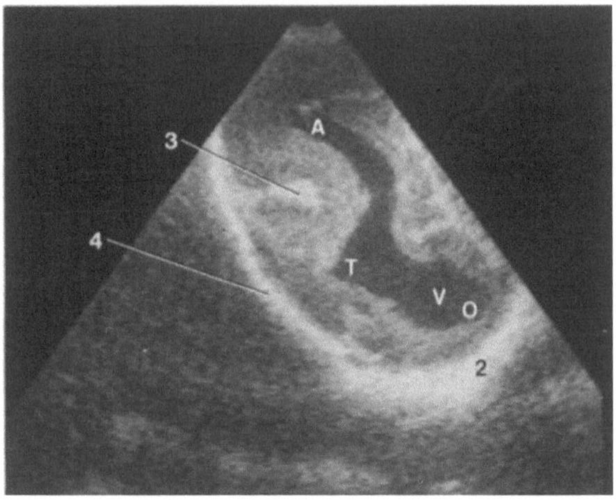

Fig. 291. Slightly diagonal horizontal US. DRF 100, GPS probe, 5 MHz

1 Interhemispheric space
2 Occiput
3 Sylvian fissure
4 Left temporal bone
5 Right temporal bone
6 Occipital bone near foramen magnum
7 Thalamus
8 Right frontal horn
9 Choroid plexus
A Anterior horn
O Occipital horn
T Temporal horn
V Enlarged left lateral ventricle

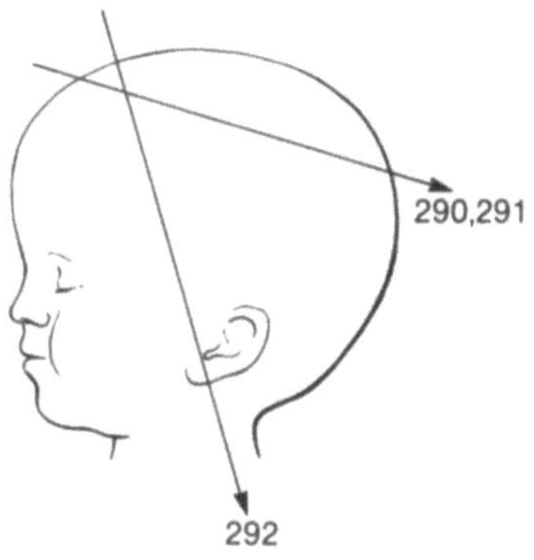

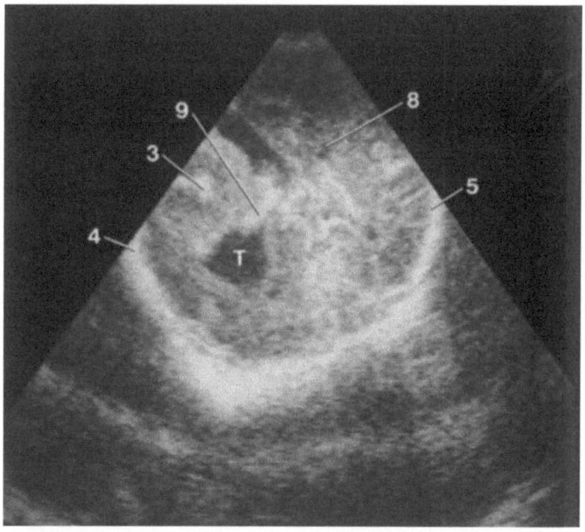

Fig. 292. Diagonal coronal US. DRF 100, GPS probe, 5 MHz

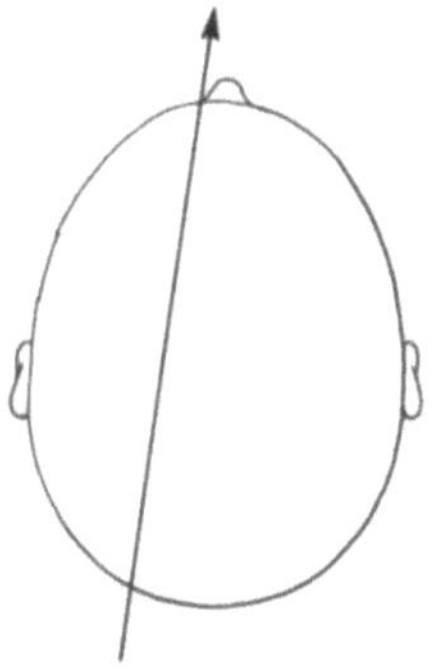

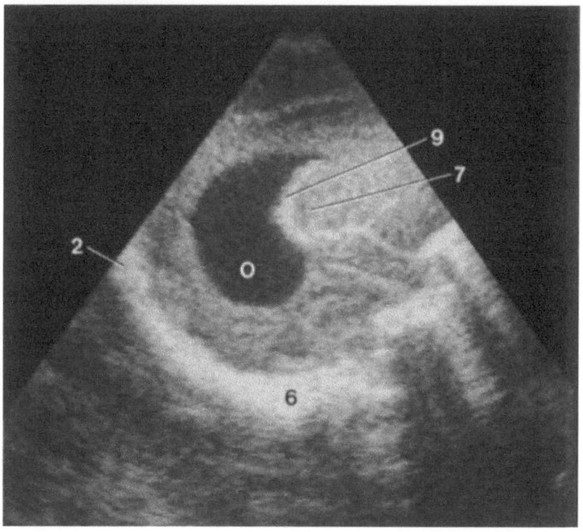

Fig. 293. Parasagittal US. DRF 100, GPS probe, 5 MHz

CASE 63 (Figs. 294, 295)

Occlusive *hydrocephalus* due to aqueduct stenosis caused by a tumor of the pineal region in a 62-year-old woman operated upon via left occipital supratentorial craniotomy.

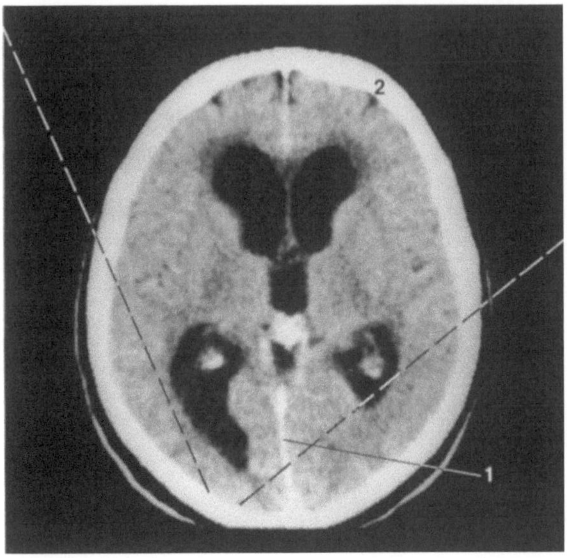

Fig. 294. Horizontal CT

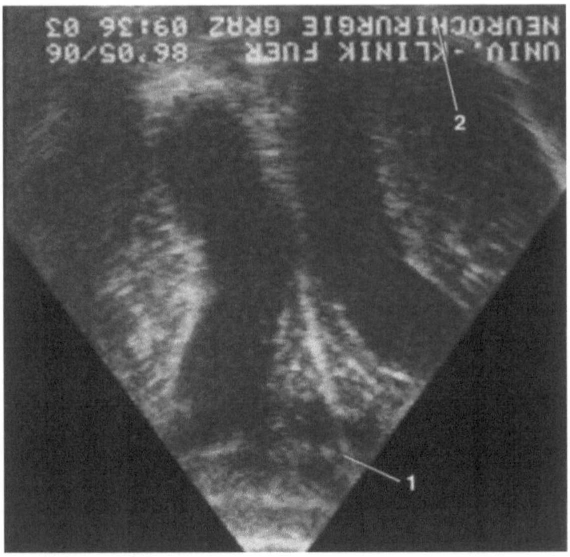

Fig. 295. Horizontal US. DRF 100, GPS probe, 5 MHz

1 Falx
2 Right frontal bone

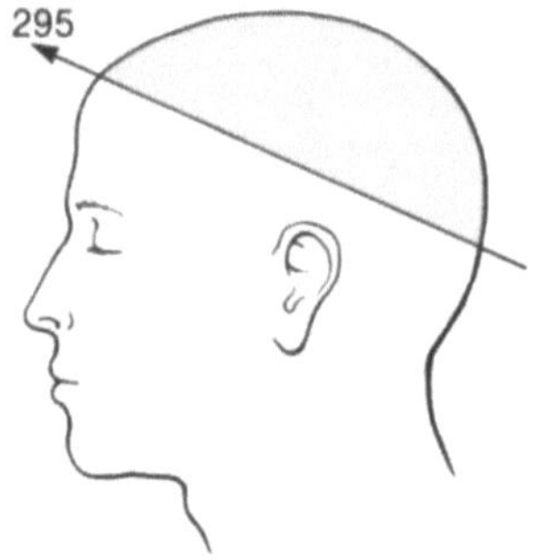

CASE 64 (Figs. 296–298)

Posttraumatic *hydrocephalus* in a young man with left temporal trauma and right temporal contrecoup lesion.

The US imaging was done through a left temporal bone defect after the ventriculoatrial shunt implanted via the left occipital horn had become inoperative: the images show that the ventricular shunt catheter perforates the septum pellucidum and reaches the contralateral ventricle, suggesting occlusion of the catheter at the site of perforation of the septum, where the catheter can be seen thickened by surrounding tissue. Occlusion was verified on revision of the ventricular catheter.

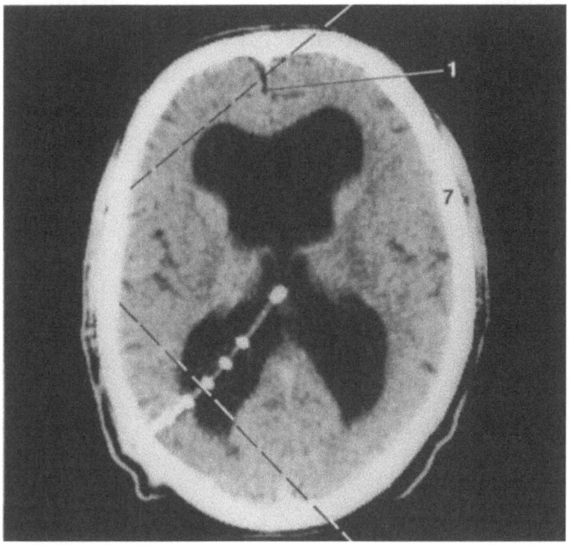

Fig. 296. Horizontal CT

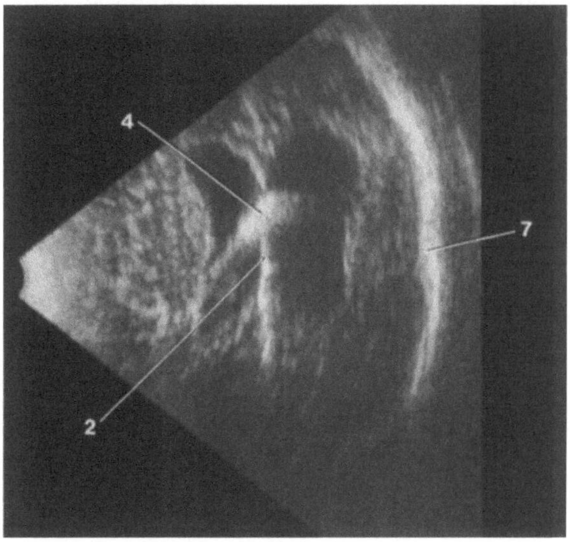

Fig. 297. Horizontal US. DRF 100, GPS probe, 5 MHz

1 Falx
2 Septum pellucidum
3 Third ventricle
4 Shunt catheter perforating septum pellucidum
5 Temporal horn
6 Clivopetrosal area
7 Right temporoparietal **bone**
→ Foramen of Monro

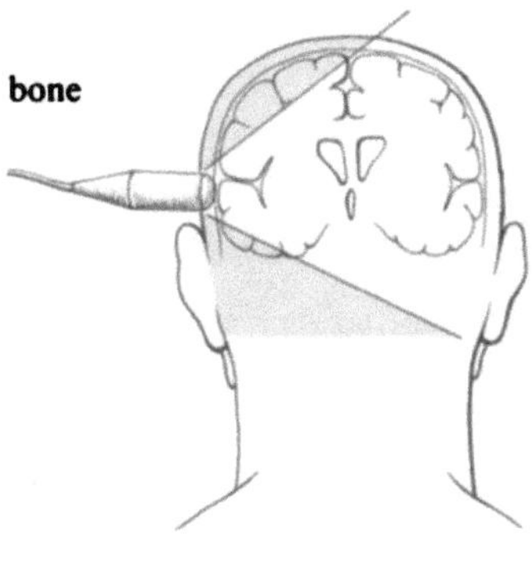

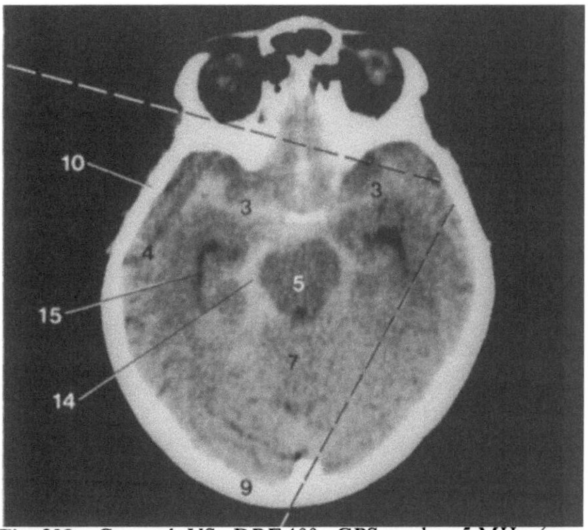

Fig. 298. Coronal US. DRF 100, GPS probe, 5 MHz (see schema)

Subarachnoid Hemorrhage, Aneurysms and Arteriovenous Malformations

Recent hemorrhage into the subarachnoid space can be recognized by hyperechoicity of cisternal CSF spaces, which would normally appear as hypoechoic or anechoic areas like the ventricles.

Aneurysms are not very well visualized on static US images, especially when they are small; on real-time imaging, however, they can be clearly recognized by virtue of the turbulent blood flow within them, although at all times the swirling blood is hypoechoic [30]. The thrombosed component of an aneurysm is mostly hyperechoic; when the interior is isoechoic, then the wall is visualized as a clearly delineated hyperechoic ring. In the following examples, the first aim is to show the landmarks for topographical orientation in the area surrounding blood-filled basal cisterns. In addition, the appearance of hypoechoic perfused vs hyperechoic thrombosed aneurysms will be shown.

Arteriovenous malformations (AVMs) of the brain show two characteristic features on US: the nidus is usually detectable as a hyperechoic or isoechoic mass, and vessels which are large enough can be seen as an irregular mixture of longitudinally or transversally sectioned hypoechoic structures. Small subcortical or deep-seated AVMs are visualized as hyperechoic lesions clearly delineated from the surrounding brain tissue.

CASE 65 (Figs. 299-301)

Subarachnoid hemorrhage from a small basilar artery aneurysm in a 69-year-old woman operated upon 1 day after the bleeding via a right pterional approach.

The lower horizontal US section (Fig. 301) shows the base of the temporal lobes, the posterior fossa (pons and cerebellum) and the gyri recti. The basal cisterns are filled with blood, showing up as hyperechoicity. The higher horizontal US section (Fig. 300) which corresponds to the CT image (Fig. 299), shows the left sylvian fissure, the cisterna ambiens and the frontal interhemispheric space filled with blood, i.e., hyperechoic.

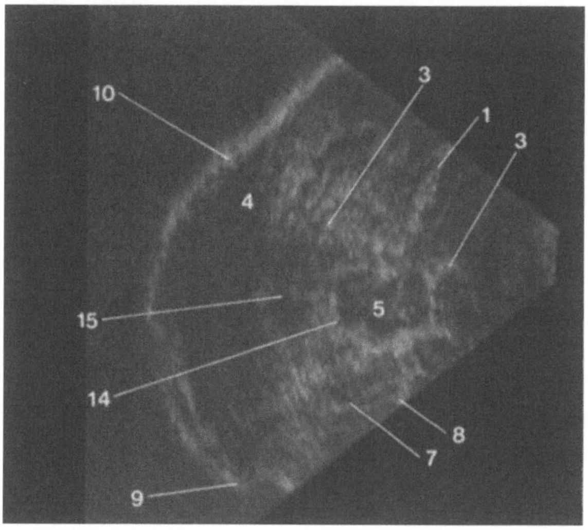

Fig. 299. Horizontal CT

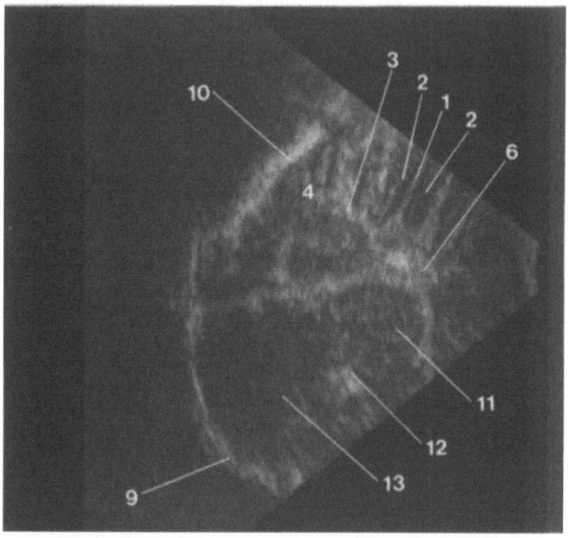

Fig. 300. Horizontal US. DRF 100, GPS probe, 5 MHz

1 Interhemispheric space
2 Gyrus rectus
3 Sylvian fissure
4 Temporal lobe
5 Midbrain
6 Suprasellar and interpeduncular cisterns
7 Vermis
8 Tentorium
9 Occipital bone
10 Left temporal bone
11 Pons
12 Fourth ventricle
13 Cerebellum
14 Cisterna ambiens
15 Temporal horn

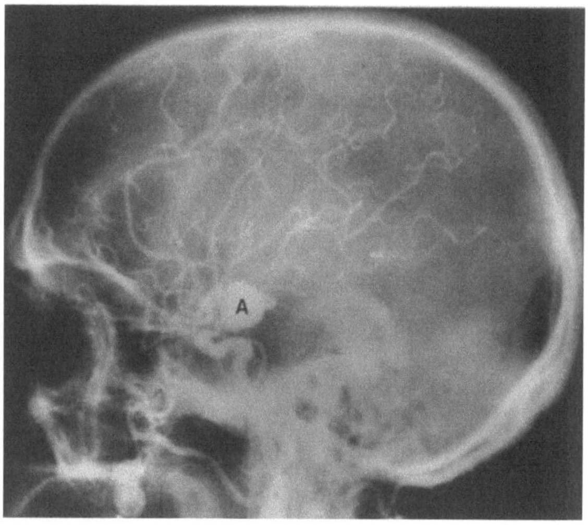

Fig. 301. Horizontal US. DRF 100, GPS probe, 5 MHz

CASE 66 (Figs. 302-306)

Internal carotid artery aneurysm in a 53-year-old man operated upon 2 days after subarachnoid hemorrhage via a left pterional approach.

The basal cisterns are filled with blood, hyperechoic on US. The aneurysm is seen as a globular area of relatively low signal intensity with a clearly demarcated hyperechoic wall. The neck of the aneurysm can be appreciated on Fig. 305. The lateral ventricles on the coronal US section (Fig. 306) are barely visible because they have been narrowed to slits by external ventricular drainage.

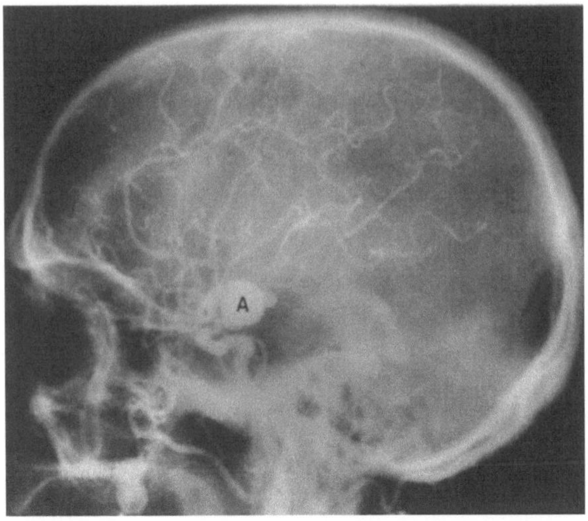

Fig. 302. Left internal carotid angiography: lateral view

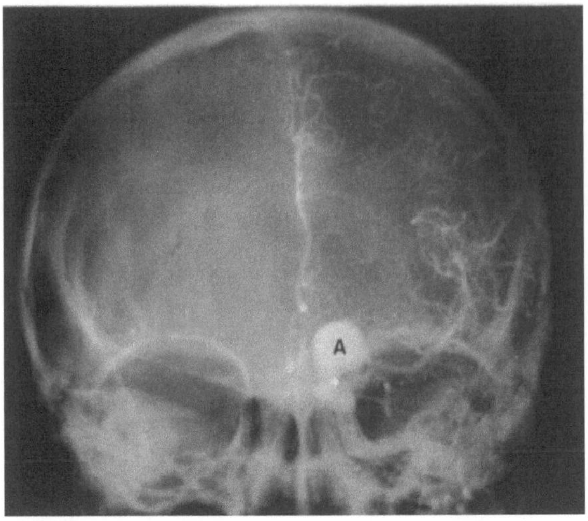

Fig. 303. Left internal carotid angiography: AP view

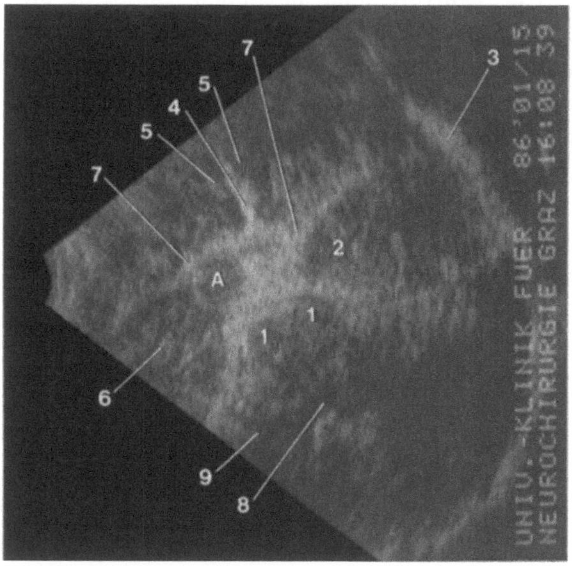

Fig. 304. Horizontal US. DRF 100, GPS probe, 5 MHz

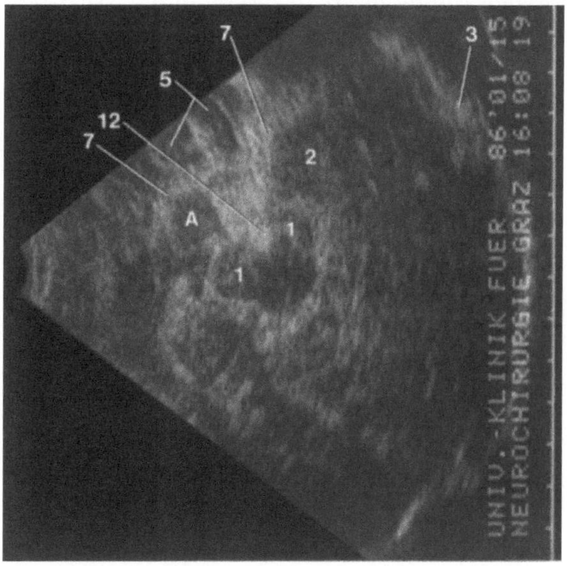

Fig. 305. Horizontal US. DRF 100, GPS probe, 5 MHz

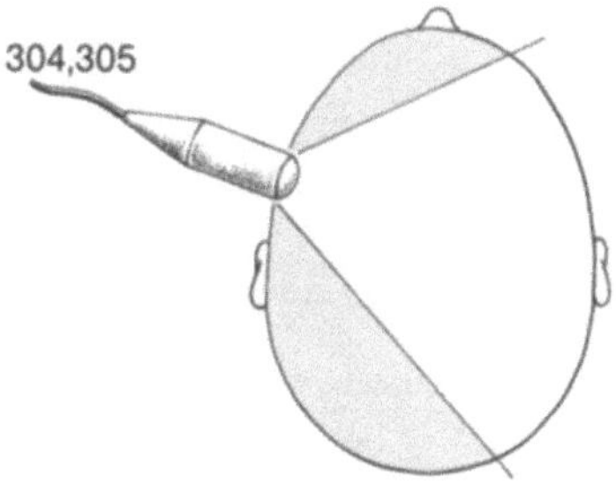

1 Crura cerebri
2 Right temporal lobe
3 Right temporal bone
4 Interhemispheric fissure
5 Gyrus rectus
6 Left temporal lobe
7 Sylvian cistern
8 Fourth ventricle
9 Cerebellum
10 Floor of middle cranial fossa
11 Slit-like lateral ventricles
12 Interpeduncular cistern
13 Corpus callosum
14 Third ventricle
A Aneurysm

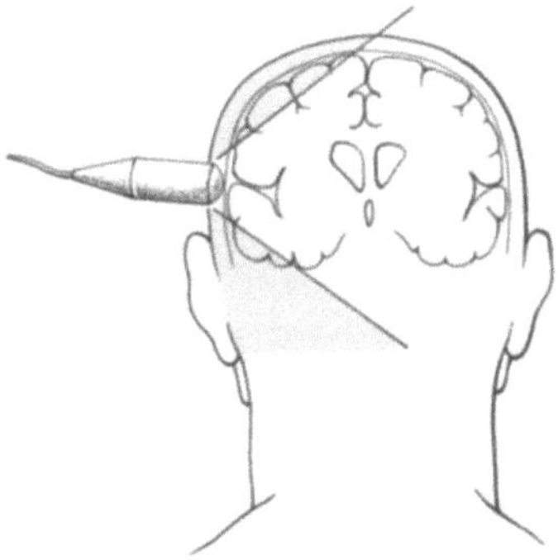

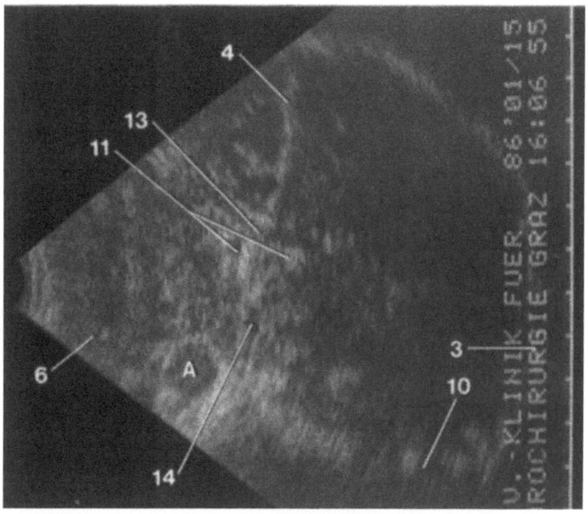

Fig. 306. Coronal US. DRF 100, GPS probe, 5 MHz

CASE 67 (Figs. 307–313)

Internal carotid artery aneurysm in a 72-year-old woman operated upon 1 day after subarachnoid hemorrhage via a left pterional approach.

The relatively small aneurysm cannot be unequivocally recognized on a single US image; however, during the imaging process, turbulence of the blood flow within the aneurysm allows clear diagnosis of the lesion. The basal cisterns are filled with blood, appearing hyperechoic.

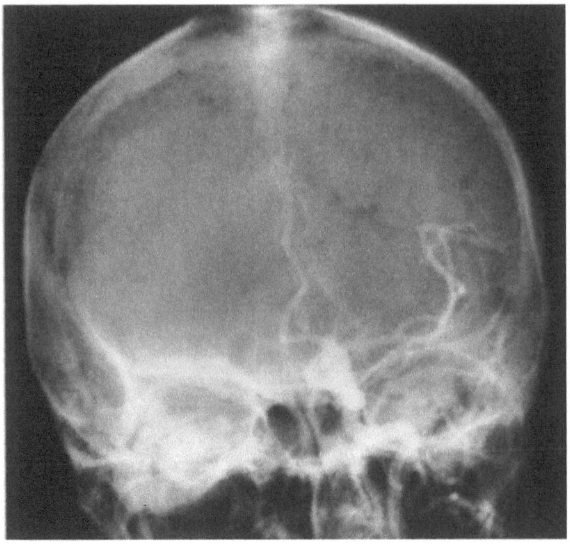

Fig. 307. Left internal carotid angiography: AP view

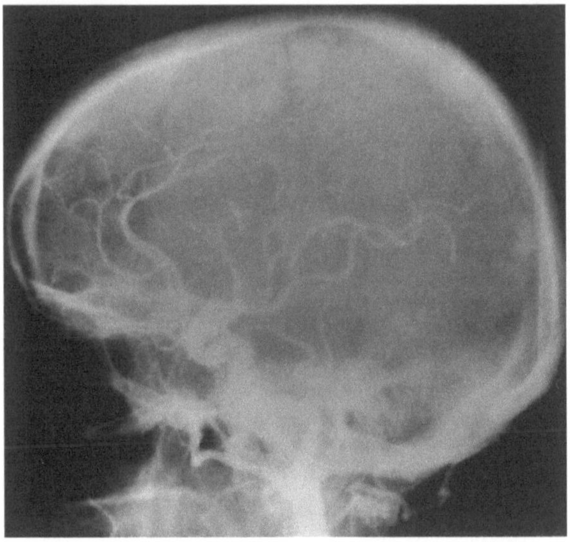

Fig. 308. Left internal carotid angiography: lateral view

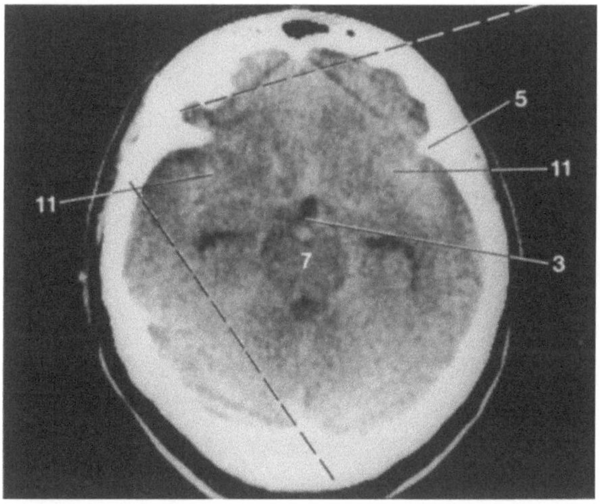

Fig. 309. Horizontal CT

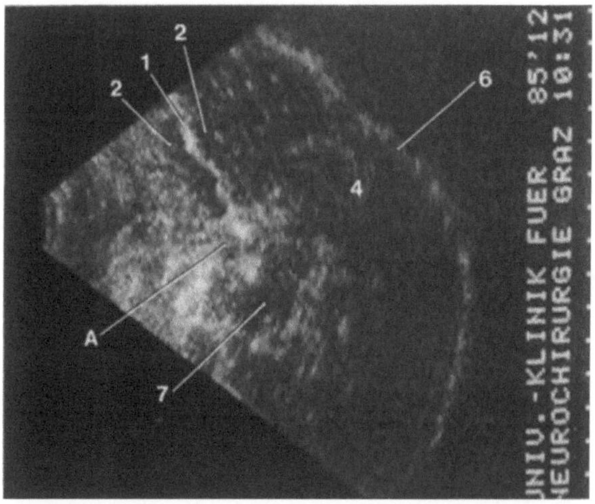

Fig. 310. Horizontal US. DRF 100, GPS probe, 5 MHz

1 Interhemispheric space
2 Gyrus rectus
3 Interpeduncular fossa
4 Right temporal fossa
5 Right sphenoid wing
6 Right temporal bone
7 Midbrain
8 Pons
9 Tentorium
10 Frontal horn
11 Sylvian fissure
A Aneurysm

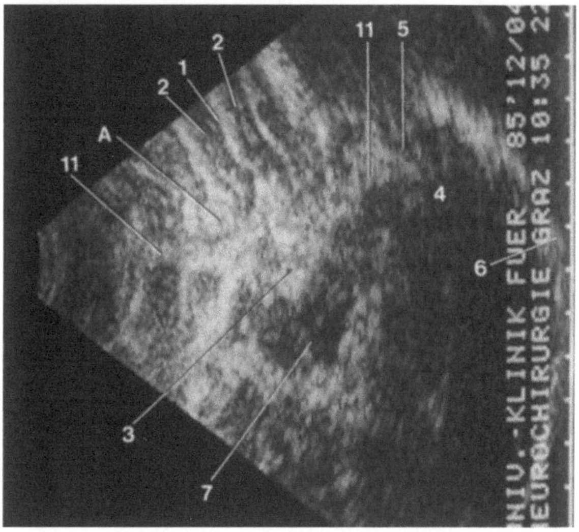

Fig. 311. Horizontal US. DRF 100, GPS probe, 5 MHz

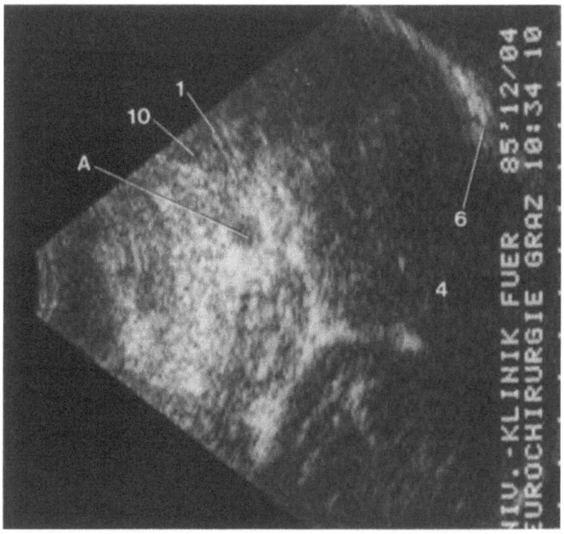

Fig. 313. Diagonal coronal US. DRF 100, GPS probe, 5 MHz

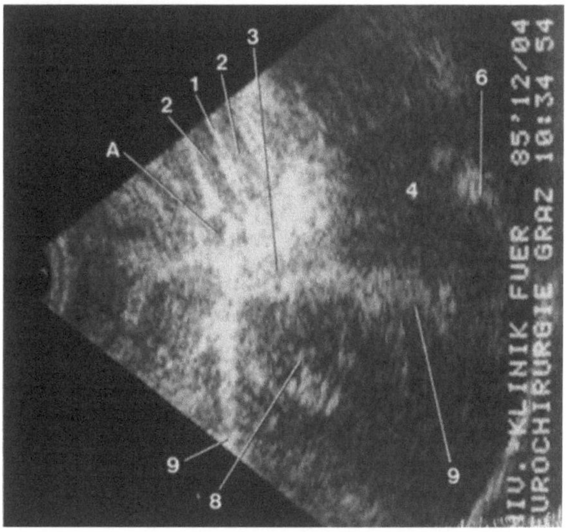

Fig. 312. Horizontal US. DRF 100, GPS probe, 5 MHz

CASE 68 (Figs. 314-320)

Ophthalmic artery aneurysm in a 30-year-old man operated upon via a left pterional approach.

The aneurysm is unruptured. The aneurysm's interior displays a low signal intensity, the wall is clearly hyperechoic. Figs. 317-320 show horizontal sections at different levels; in Fig. 319 the top of the dome of the aneurysm is sectioned tangentially. The horizontal CT plane of Fig. 317 corresponds to the horizontal US plane of Fig. 318. The coronal US section in Fig. 316 shows the parietobasal extension of the aneurysm as apparent on the angiograms (Figs. 314, 315).

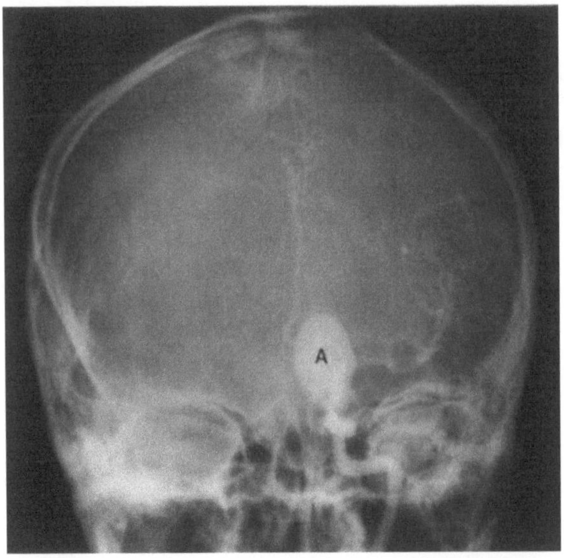

Fig. 314. Left internal carotid angiography: AP view

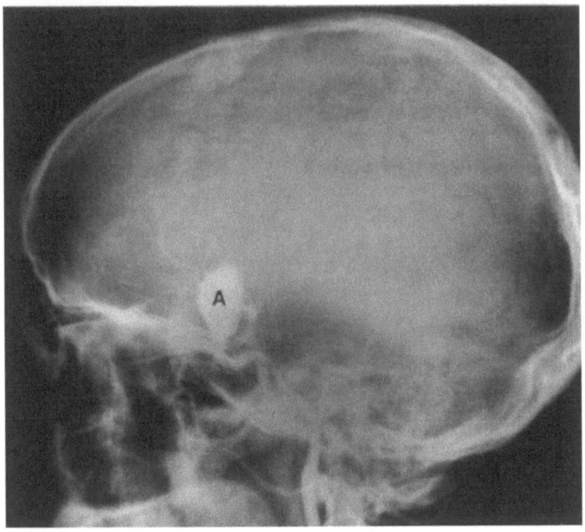

Fig. 315. Left internal carotid angiography: lateral view

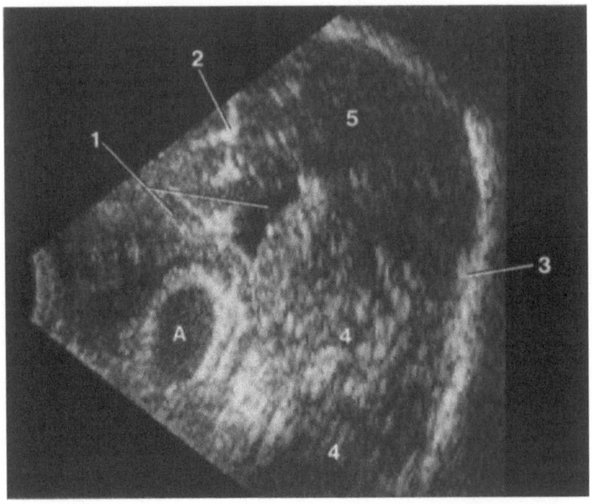

Fig. 316. Coronal US. DRF 100, GPS probe, 5 MHz

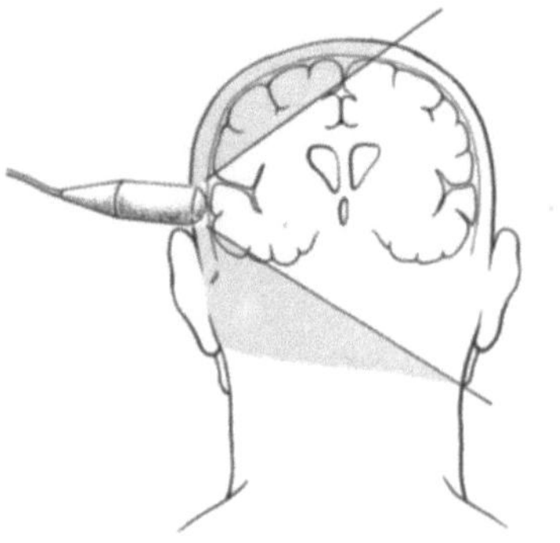

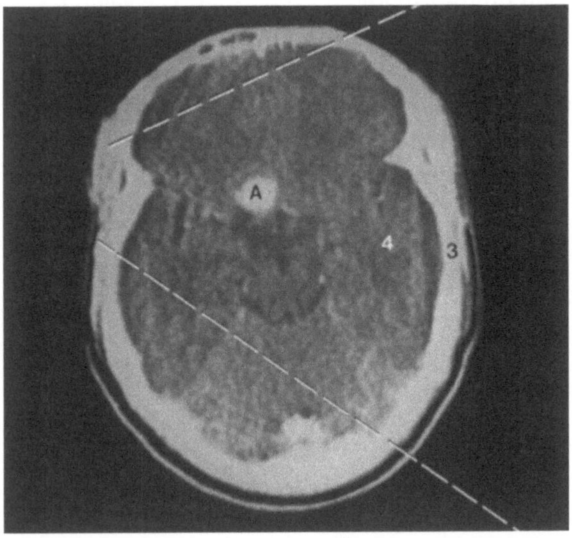

Fig. 317. Horizontal CT

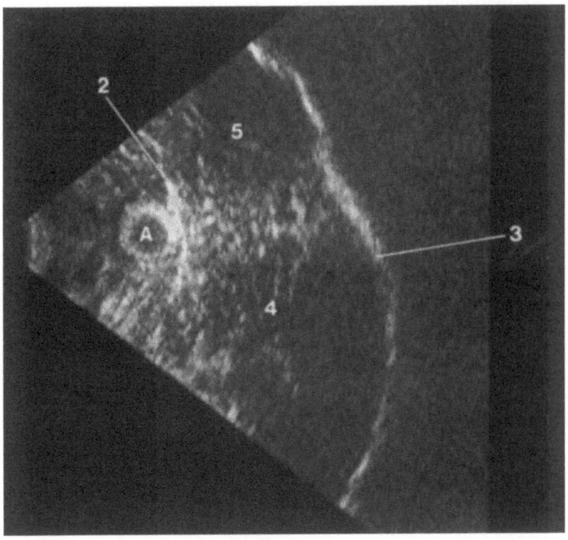

Fig. 318. Horizontal US. DRF 100, GPS probe, 5 MHz

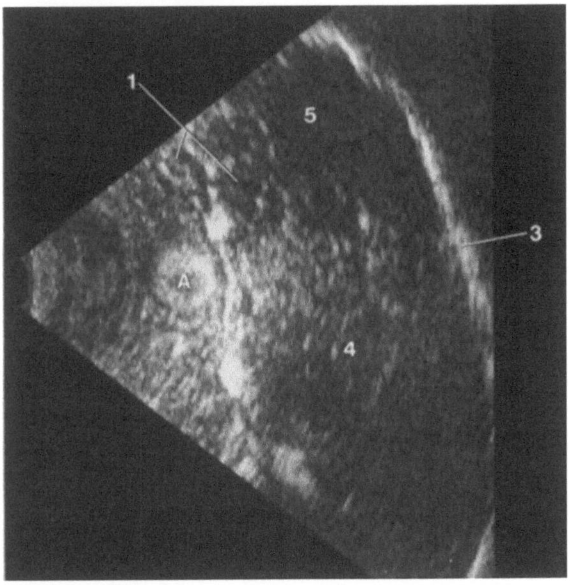

Fig. 319. Horizontal US. DRF 100, GPS probe, 5 MHz

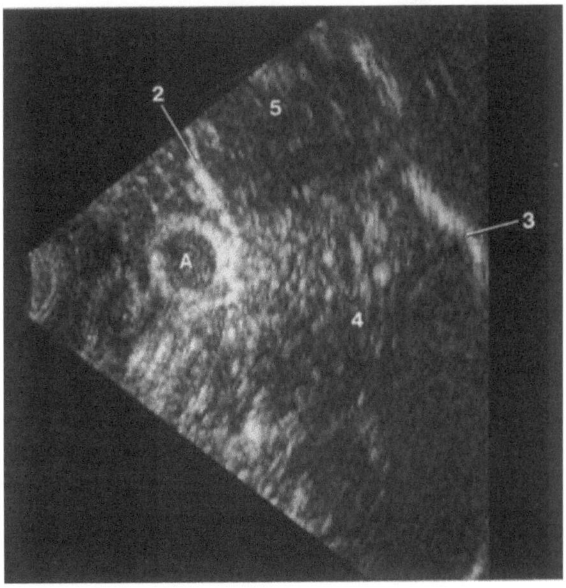

Fig. 320. Horizontal US. DRF 100, GPS probe, 5 MHz

1 Frontal horn
2 Interhemispheric space
3 Right temporal bone
4 Right temporal lobe
5 Right frontal lobe
A Aneurysm

CASE 69 (Figs. 321-326)

Thrombosed giant aneurysm of a pericallosal artery in a 65-year-old man operated upon via bifrontal craniotomy.

The CT scan (Fig. 321) shows the thrombosed part as a hyperdense tumor; the open left posterior part of the aneurysm is more markedly hyperdense and corresponds to the small aneurysm seen on the angiogram (Fig. 322). The sagittal US sections show the thrombosed part as rather homogeneously hyperechoic; the open part is distinctly hypoechoic with a signal intensity similar to that of the adjacent frontal horn's CSF. The wall of the aneurysm is seen as hyperechoic in Fig. 326, while the interior is almost isoechoic.

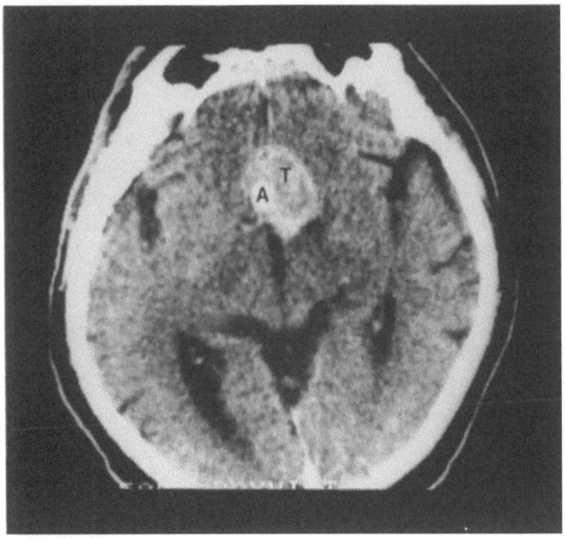

Fig. 321. Horizontal CT

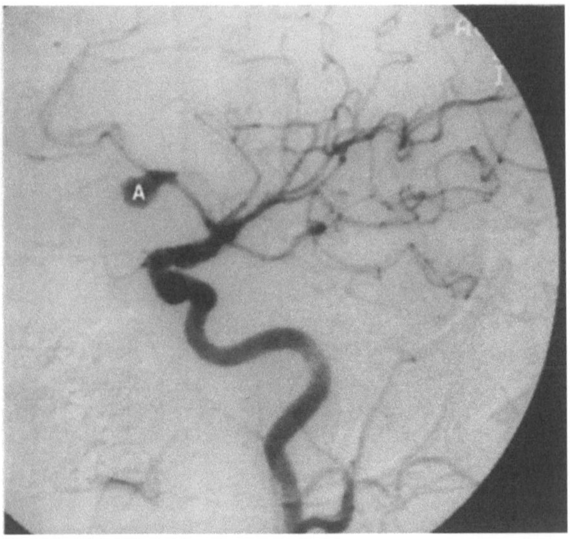

Fig. 322. Left internal carotid angiography: lateral view

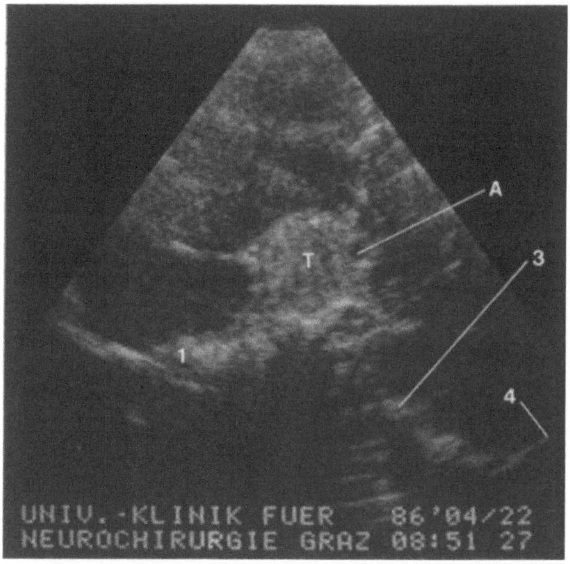

Fig. 323. Sagittal US. DRF 100, GPS probe, 5 MHz

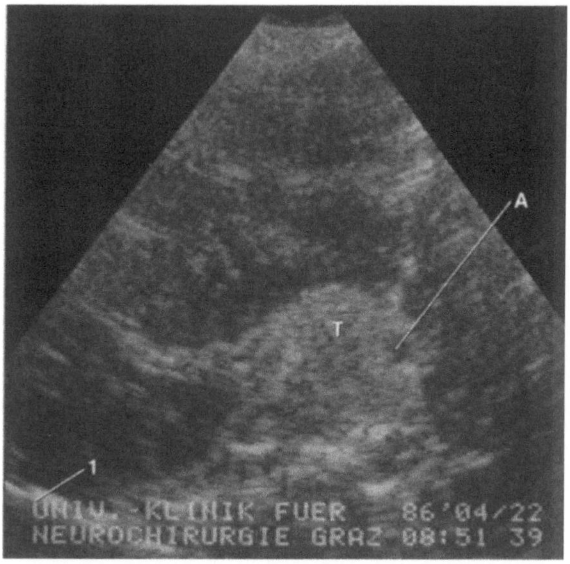

Fig. 324. Sagittal US. DRF 100, GPS probe, 5 MHz

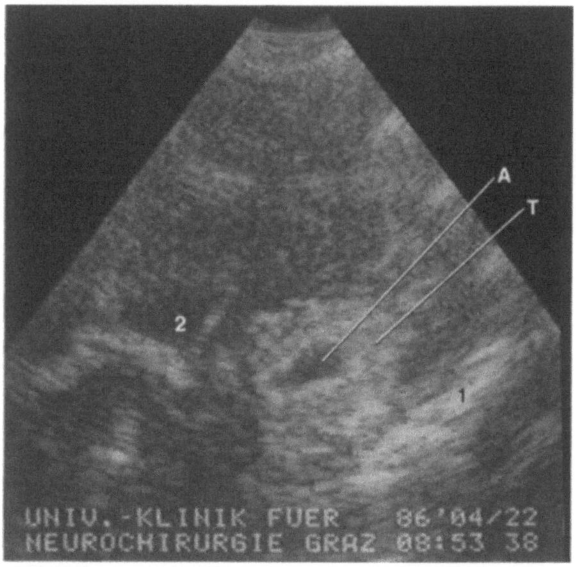

Fig. 325. Sagittal US. DRF 100, GPS probe, 5 MHz

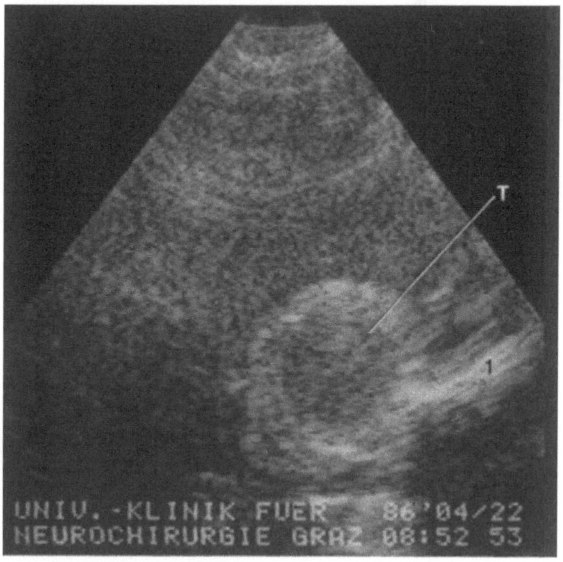

Fig. 326. Sagittal US. DRF 100, GPS probe, 5 MHz

1 Frontal bone
2 Frontal horn of the left lateral ventricle
3 Clivus
4 Occipital bone
A Open part of aneurysm
T Thrombosed part of aneurysm

CASE 70 (Figs. 327-334)

Left *trigonal AVM* in a 13-year-old girl operated upon via a parietooccipital approach.

The AVM is inhomogeneously hyperechoic; the choroid plexus displays clearly higher signal intensity and is tightly attached to the AVM. As shown by the angiograms, the AVM is fed mostly by the choroidal arteries. The blood clot in the ventricle, several days old, is isoechoic, as seen on the sagittal US sections.

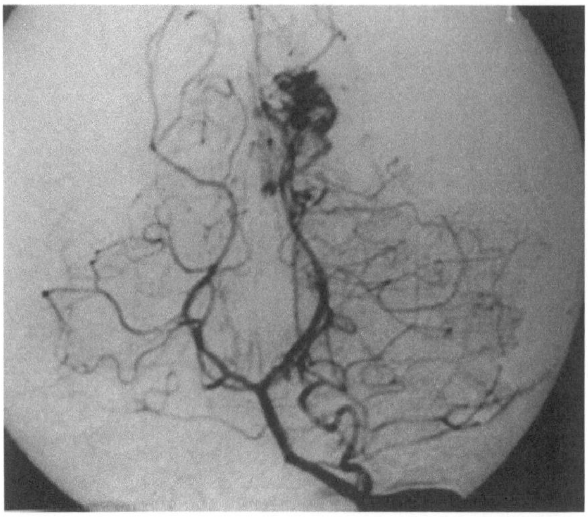

Fig. 327. Left vertebral angiography: AP view

1 Interhemispheric space
2 Lateral ventricle
3 Choroid plexus
4 Blood clot
5 Occipital lobe
6 Tentorium
7 Cerebellum
8 Fourth ventricle
T AVM nidus

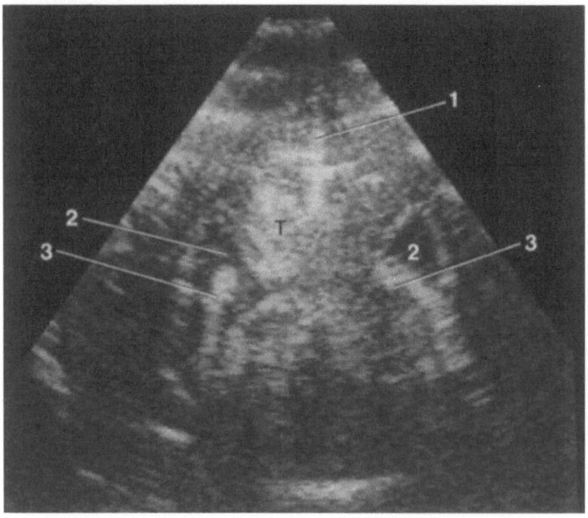

Fig. 328. Coronal US. DRF 100, GPS probe, 5 MHz

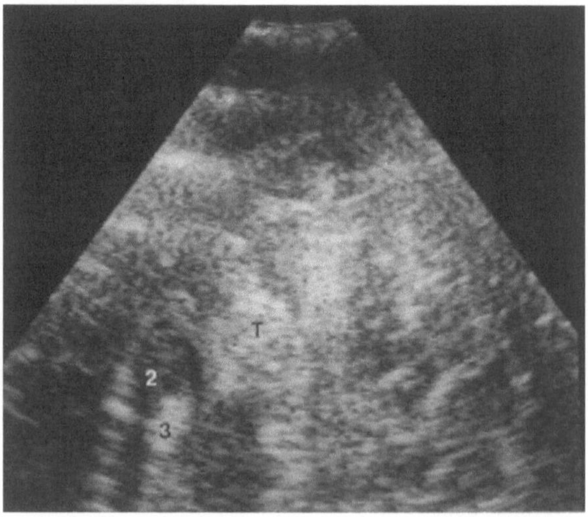

Fig. 329. Coronal US. DRF 100, GPS probe, 5 MHz

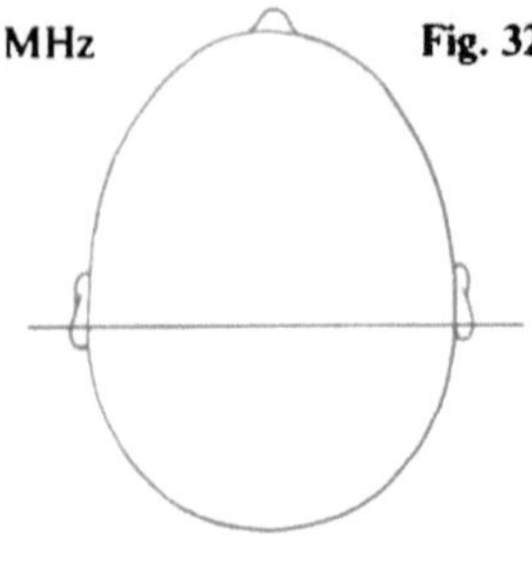

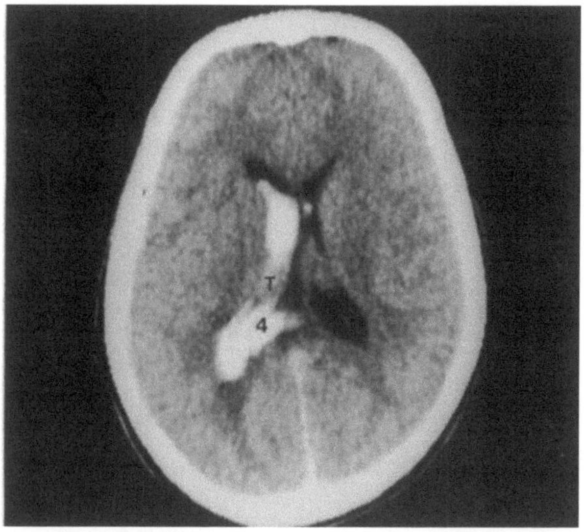

Fig. 330. Horizontal CT

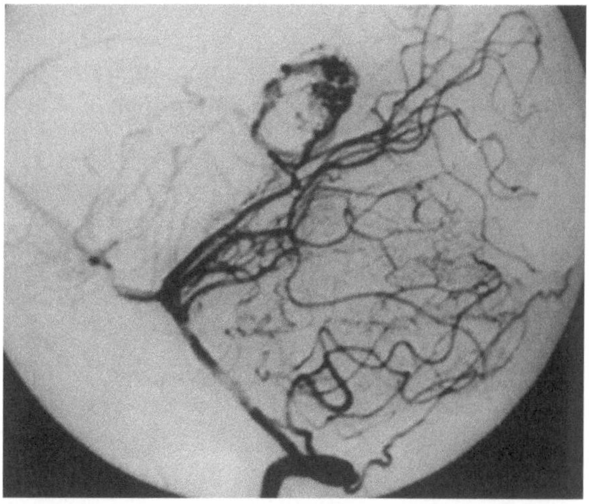

Fig. 331. Left vertebral angiography: lateral view

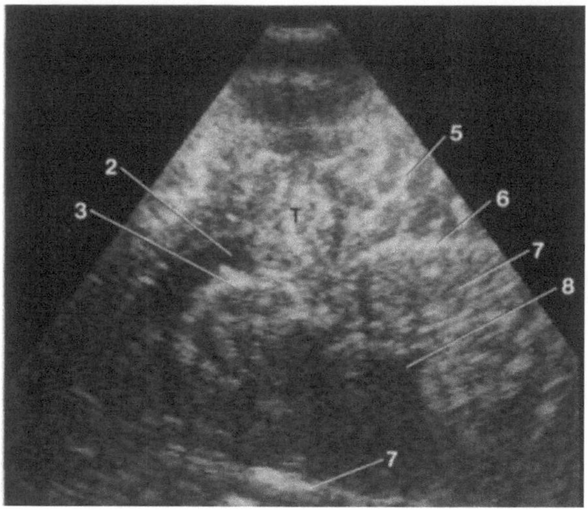

Fig. 332. Sagittal US. DRF 100, GPS probe, 5 MHz

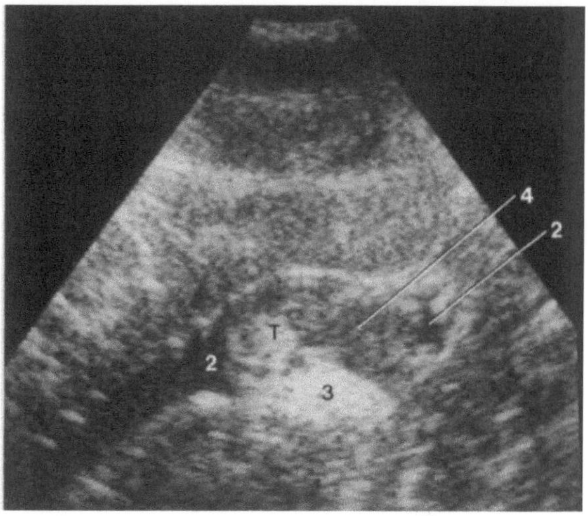

Fig. 333. Sagittal US. DRF 100, GPS probe, 5 MHz

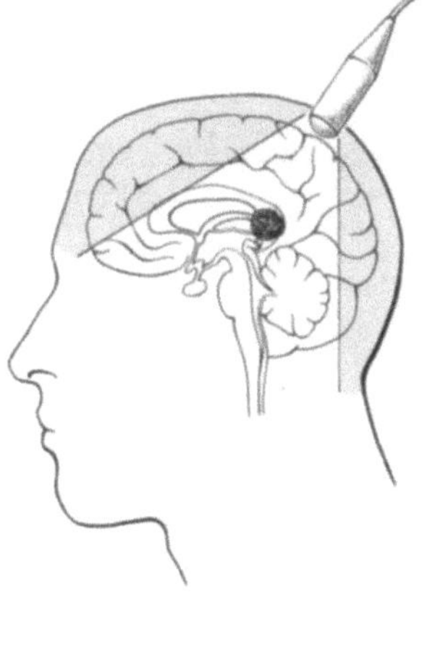

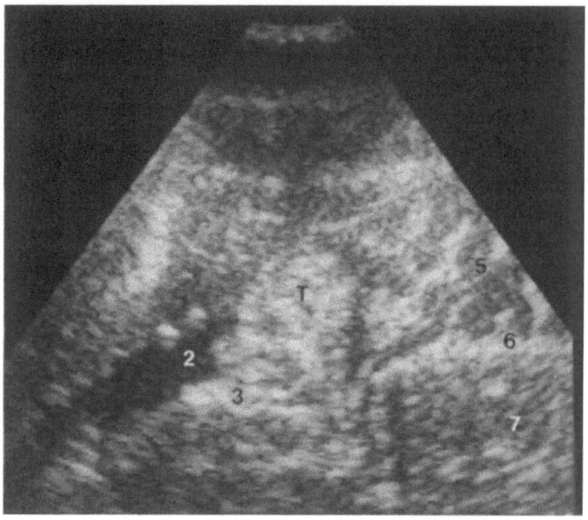

Fig. 334. Sagittal US. DRF 100, GPS probe, 5 MHz

CASE 71 (Figs. 335-341)

Occipital AVM in a 24-year-old man operated upon via left temporooccipital craniotomy.

Part of the lesion shows up on US as a hyperechoic mass like a tumor, in the other part vessels of various size are seen with hypoechoic lumina.

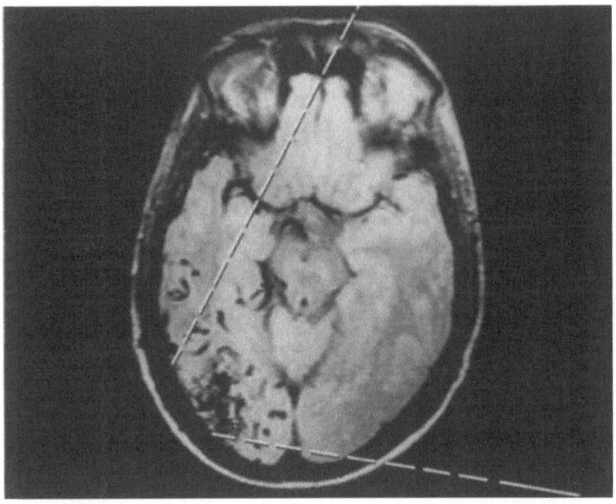

Fig. 335. Horizontal MRI. Stippled lines = sector lines for Figs. 337-339

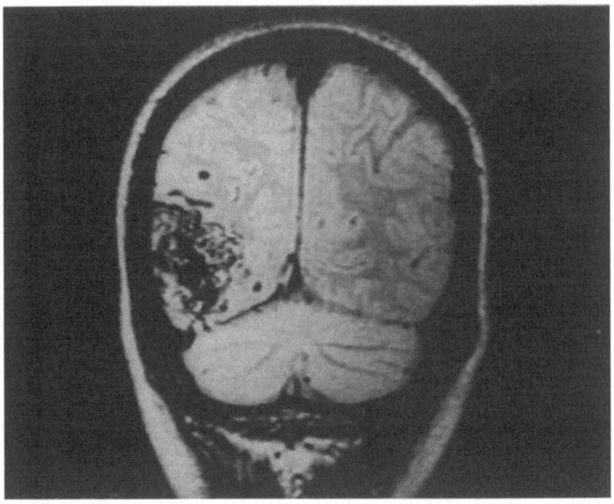

Fig. 336. Coronal MRI

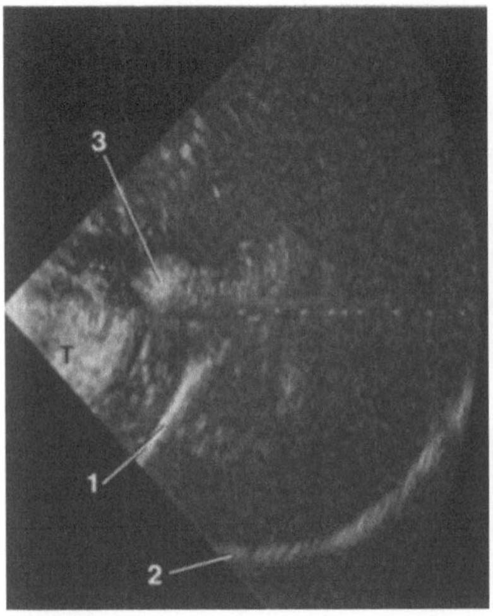

Fig. 337

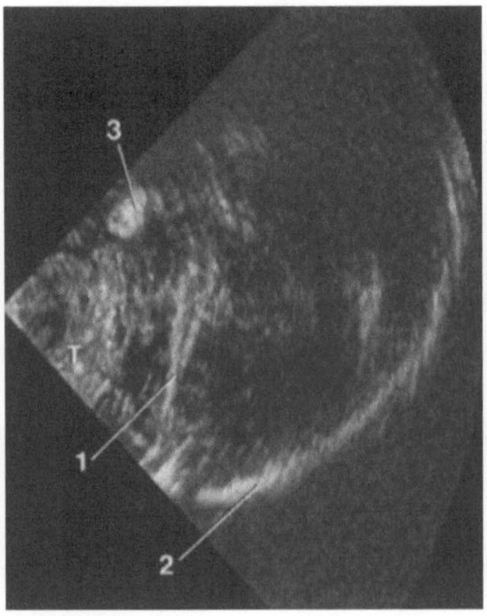

Fig. 338

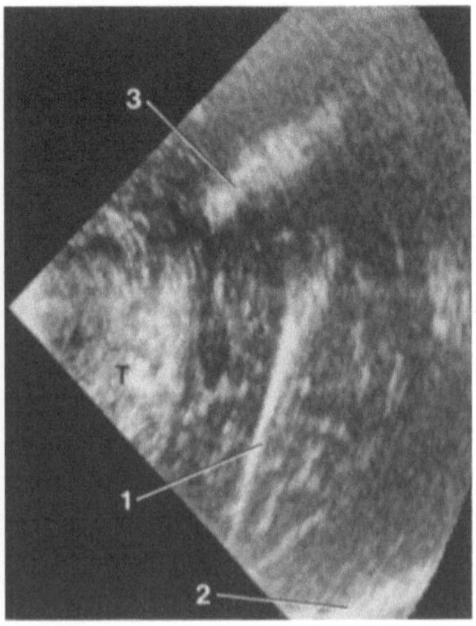

Fig. 339

Figs. 337-339. Horizontal US. SSA 100A, 5 MHz

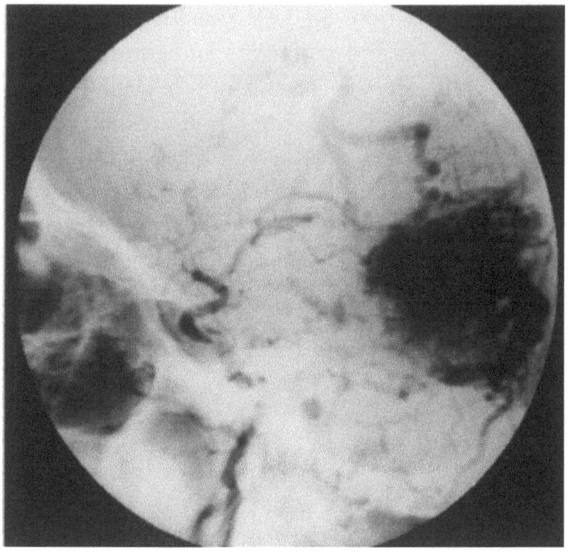

Fig. 340. Left internal carotid angiography: lateral view

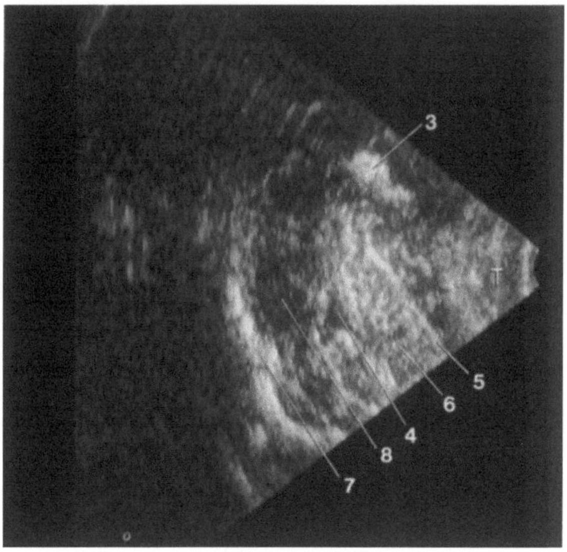

Fig. 341. Sagittal US. DRF 100, GPS probe, 5 MHz

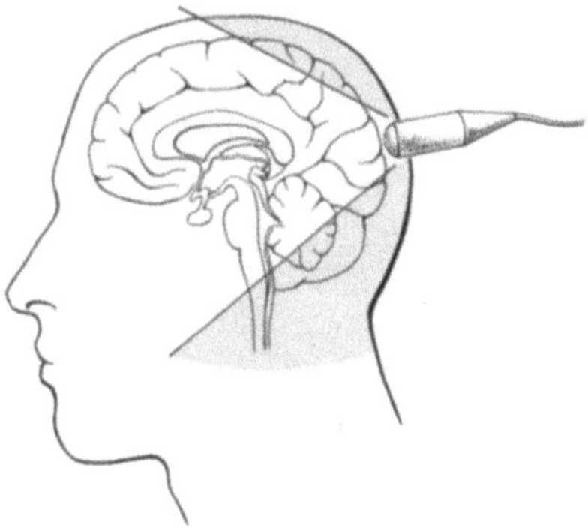

1 Falx
2 Contralateral occipital bone
3 Choroid plexus of left trigonum
4 Fourth ventricle
5 Tentorium
6 Cerebellum
7 Clivus
8 Pons
T AVM nidus

Intracerebral Hematomas

Acute intracerebral hematomas mostly display higher echo intensity than the normal brain; fluid compartments can, however, show up as isoechoic areas within the hematoma. With increasing time after the bleeding the signal intensity decreases, until the interior of the hematoma finally gives a mostly hypoechoic appearance [see also ref. 15]. The increasing zone of necrosis and edema around the hematoma, hypodense on CT, is hyperechoic on US. The following pages show a few examples of acute and chronic hematomas in different locations and their anatomical landmarks. Further examples are given in the chapter on the practical use of intraoperative US, where US-guided aspiration techniques are described (p. 156). Cerebellar hematomas are dealt with in the section on posterior fossa lesions (p. 91).

CASE 72 (Figs. 342-344)

Extensive *acute traumatic frontal hematoma* in a 42-year-old man operated upon by endoscopy via a right frontal burrhole.

The hematoma is markedly hyperechoic and ill defined at its border. The two horizontal US sections are taken with two different 5-MHz devices.

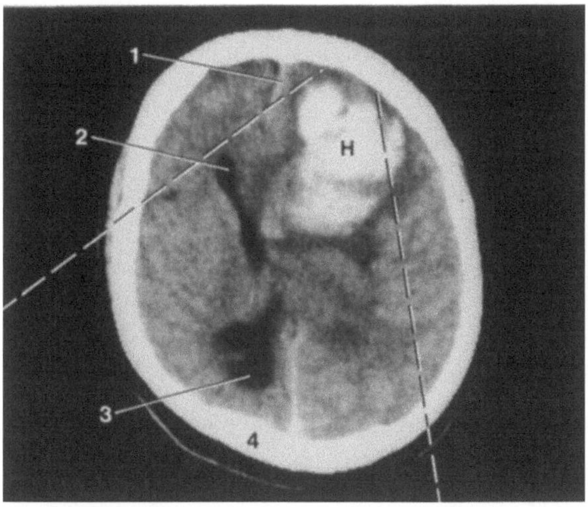

Fig. 342. Horizontal CT

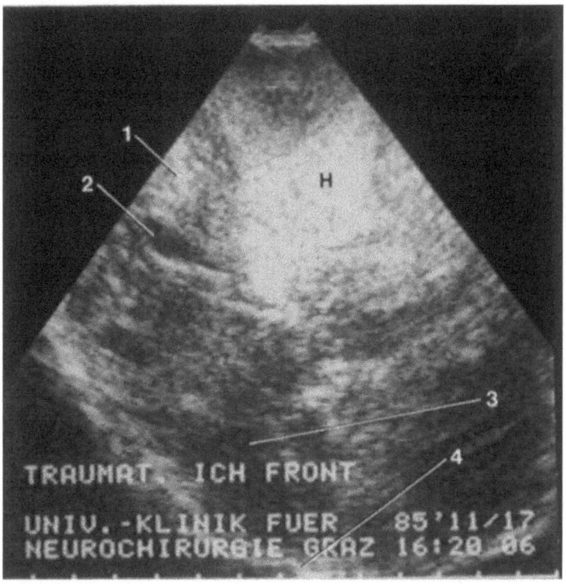

Fig. 343. Diagonal/horizontal US. DRF 100, GPS probe, 5 MHz

1 Falx
2 Left frontal horn
3 Left occipital horn
4 Occipital bone
H Hematoma

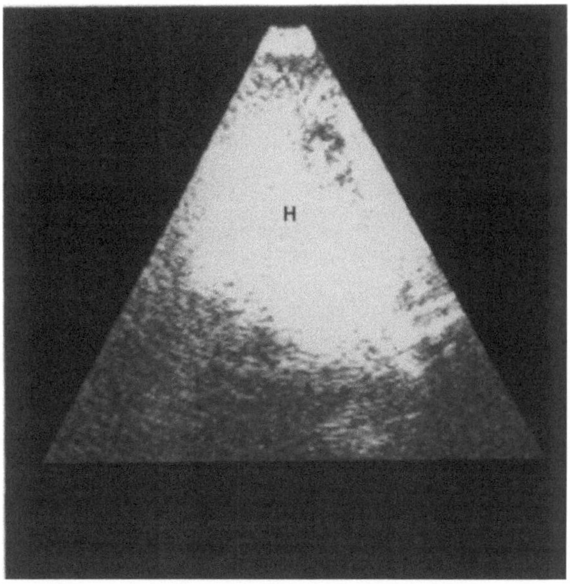

Fig. 344. Diagonal/horizontal US. DRF 100, IOP probe, 5 MHz

CASE 73 (Figs. 345, 346)

Temporoparietal acute intracerebral hematoma in a 66-year-old man operated upon by endoscopy via a burrhole.

The markedly hyperechoic hematoma is clearly demarcated, as on CT.

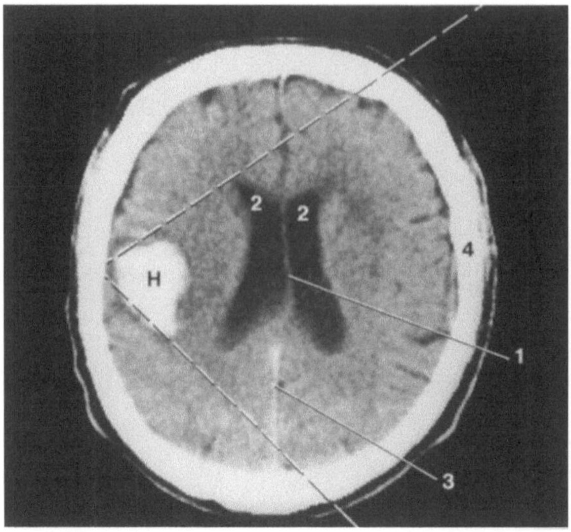

Fig. 345. Horizontal CT

1 Septum pellucidum
2 Lateral ventricle
3 Occipital falx
4 Right temporal bone
H Hematoma

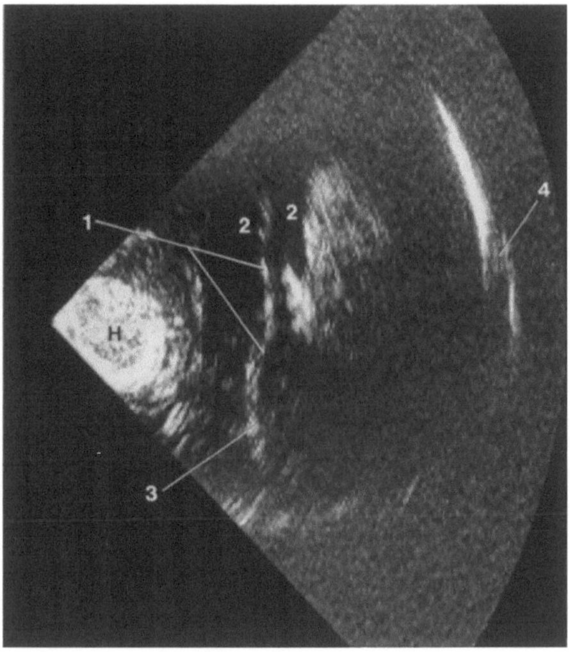

Fig. 346. Horizontal US. SSA 100A, 5 MHz

CASE 74 (Figs. 347-349)

Acute hypertensive basal ganglionic hemorrhage in a 69-year-old man operated upon by endoscopy via a left temporal burrhole.

The hematoma is hyperechoic with different signal intensities. The two horizontal sections were taken with the small intraoperative probe at 5 MHz with different levels of echo gain.

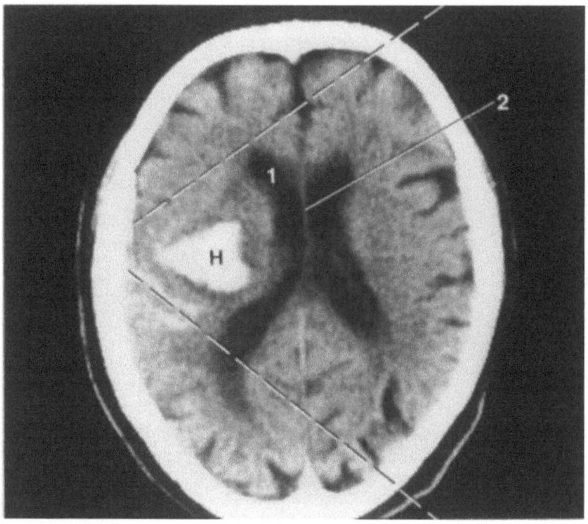

Fig. 347. Horizontal CT

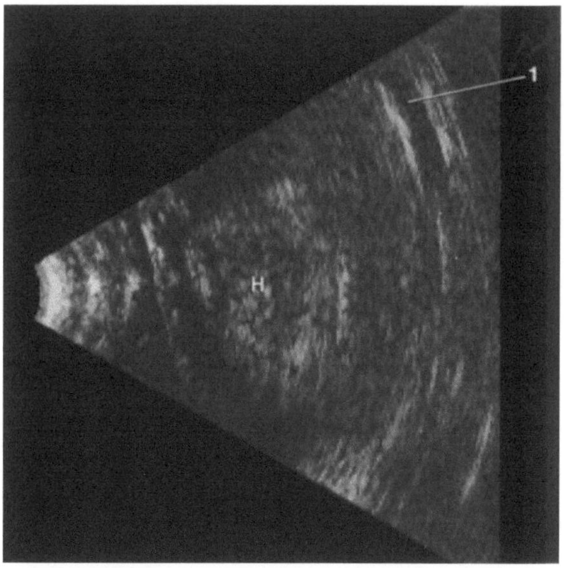

Fig. 348. Horizontal US. DRF 100, IOP probe, 5 MHz

1 Left lateral ventricle
2 Septum pellucidum
H Hematoma

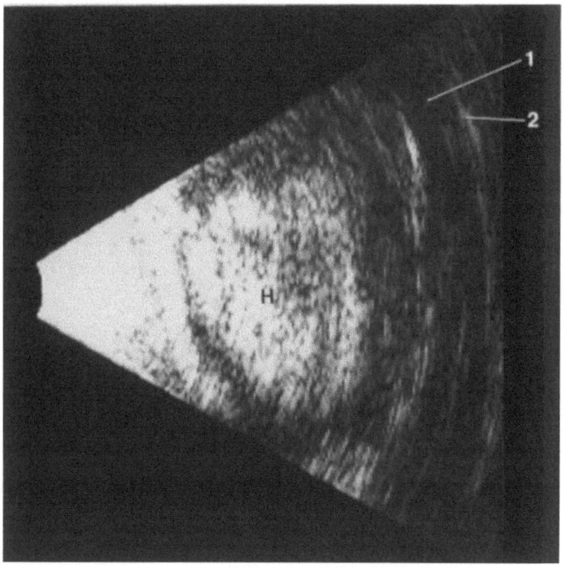

Fig. 349. Horizontal US. DRF 100, IOP probe, 5 MHz

CASE 75 (Figs. 350, 351)

Acute basal ganglionic hemorrhage in a 60-year-old patient operated upon by endoscopy via a right frontal burrhole.

The clot is hyperechoic but its border ill defined.

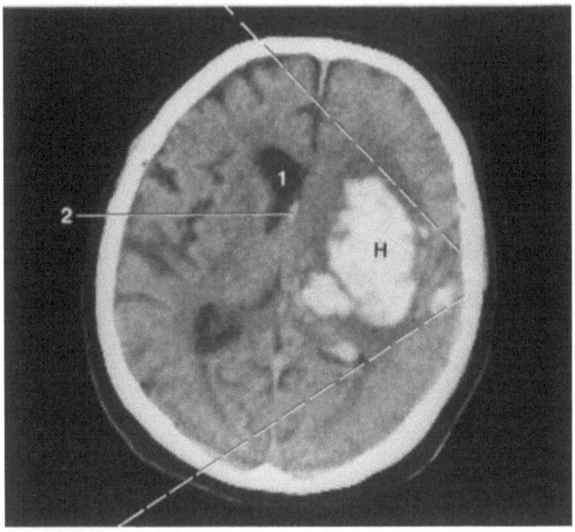

Fig. 350. Horizontal CT

1 Left lateral ventricle
2 Small clot in displaced and compressed right lateral ventricle
H Hematoma

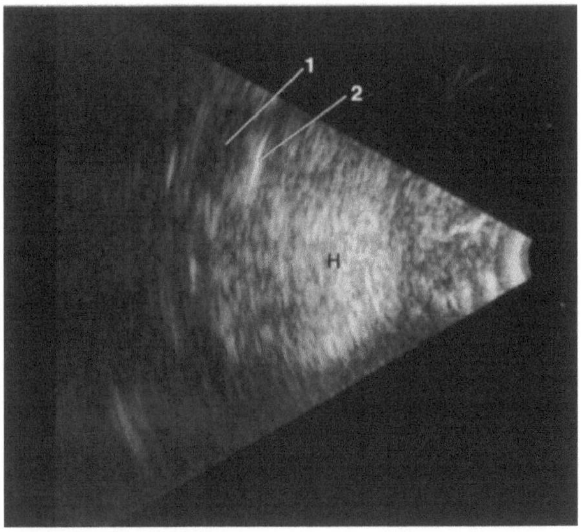

Fig. 351. Horizontal US. DRF 100, IOP probe, 5 MHz

CASE 76 (Figs. 352, 353)

Intraventricular hematoma located partly within the choroid plexus of a new-born baby.

US imaging through the fontanelle shows a clot of mixed echo intensity.

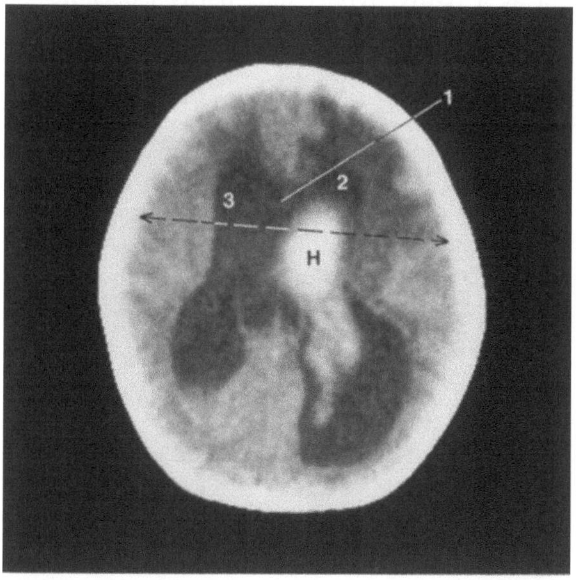

Fig. 352. Horizontal CT. Stippled line = sector plane for Fig. 353

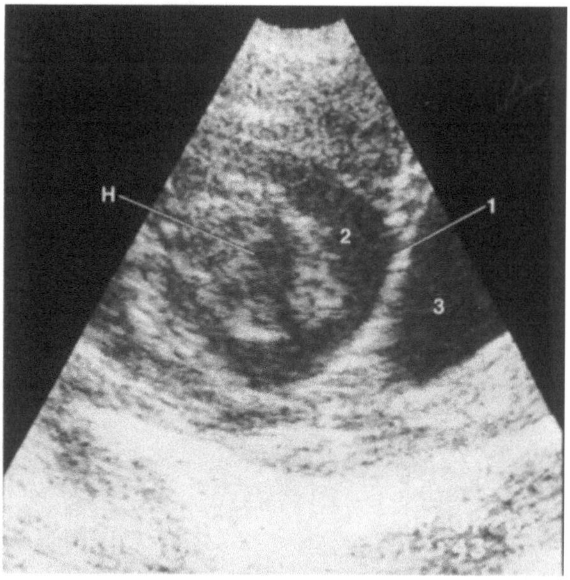

Fig. 353. Coronal US. DRF 100, IOP probe, 5 MHz

1 Septum pellucidum
2 Right lateral ventricle
3 Left lateral ventricle
H Hematoma of choroid plexus and ventricle

CASE 77 (Figs. 354–358)

Chronic spontaneous intracerebral hematoma in the left temporooccipital region in a 26-year-old woman operated upon by endoscopy via a burr-hole.

CT (Fig. 356) shows the hyperdense clot with a hypodense ring around. On MRI (Figs. 354, 355), the hematoma displays low signal intensity; the T2 image shows a high-signal ring around the hematoma. US (Figs. 357, 358) shows this hematoma as a partly hypoechoic, partly isoechoic lesion surrounded by a hyperechoic ring.

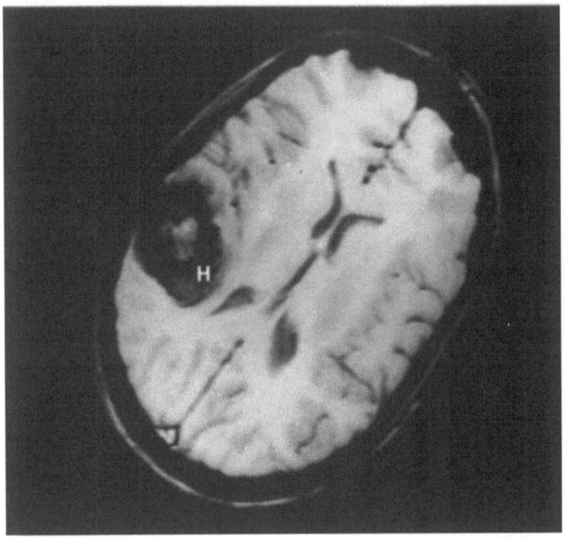

Fig. 354. Horizontal MRI

H Hematoma

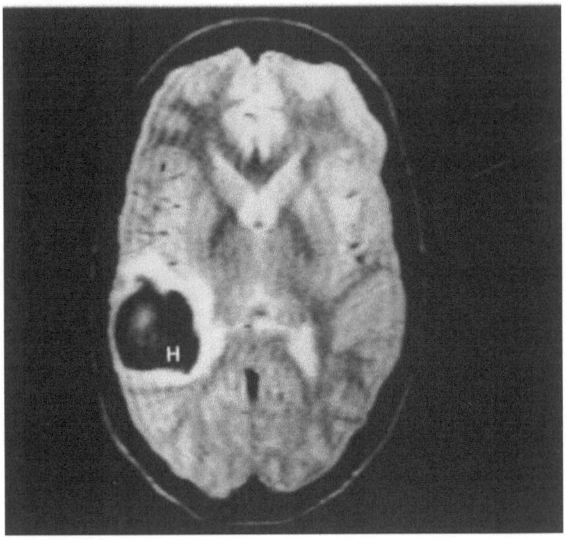

Fig. 355. Horizontal MRI

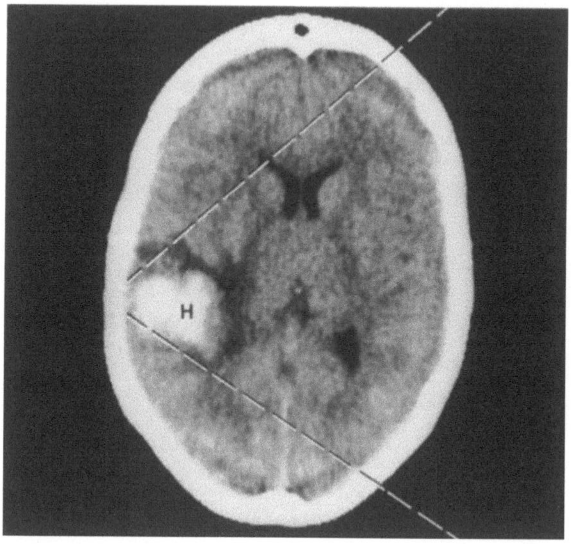

Fig. 356. Horizontal CT

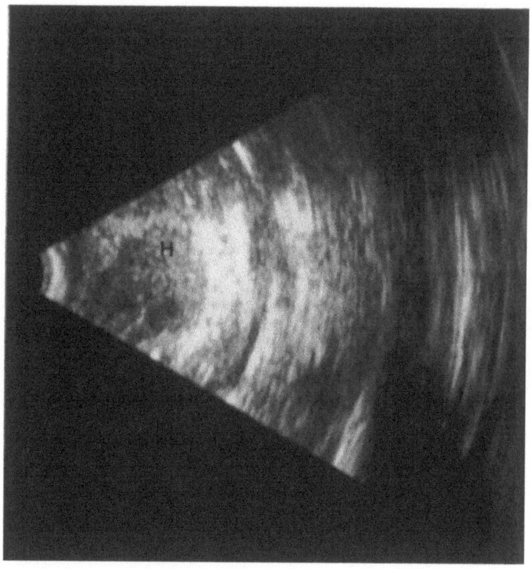

Fig. 357. Horizontal US. DRF 100, IOP probe, 5 MHz

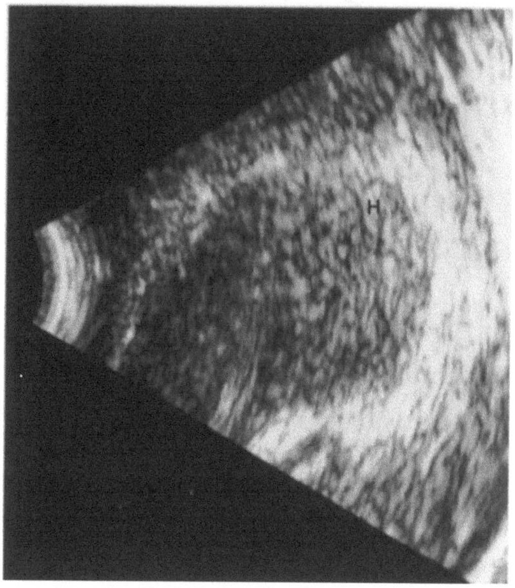

Fig. 358. Horizontal US. DRF 100, IOP probe, 5 MHz

CASE 78 (Figs. 359–361)

Chronic spontaneous intracerebral hematoma in a 64-year-old woman operated upon via craniotomy.

The hyperdense clot on CT is surrounded by a large hypodense area. On US, by contrast, the hematoma is hypoechoic whereas the surrounding zone is isoechoic to hyperechoic.

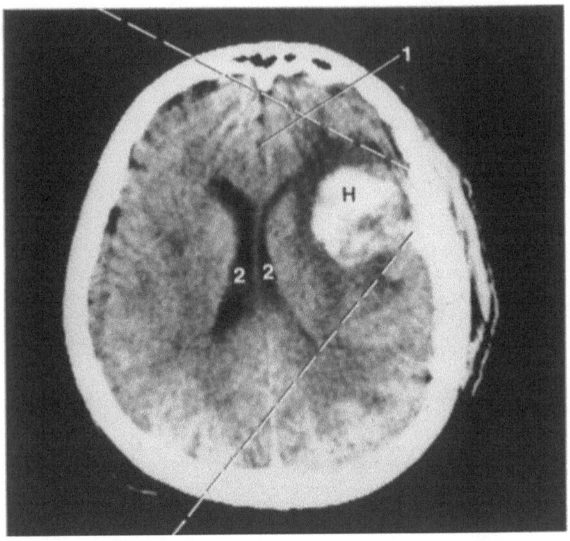

Fig. 359. Horizontal CT

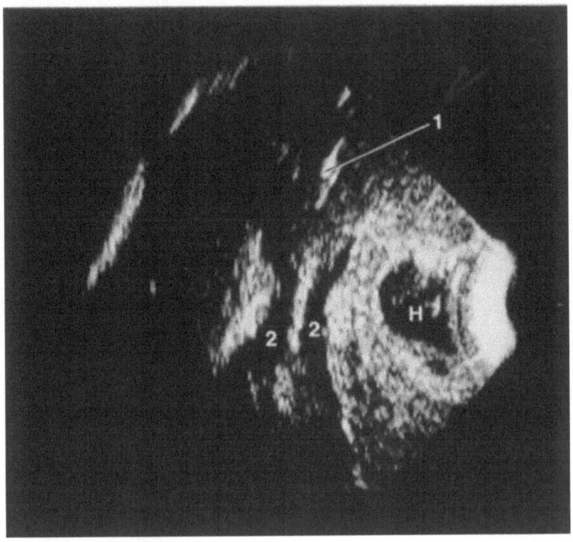

Fig. 360. Horizontal US. NS, 5 MHz

1 Falx
2 Lateral ventricle
H Hematoma

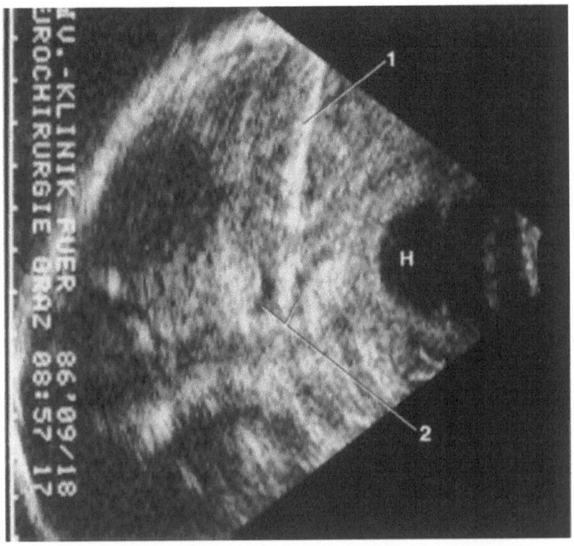

Fig. 361. Horizontal US. DRF 100, GPS probe, 5 MHz

Practical Application of Intraoperative Imaging

The practical applications of intraoperative US imaging can be divided into two categories: guidance for stereotactic interventions (see also p. 152), and anatomical orientation during conventional neurosurgical operations [6, 7, 11, 22, 24, 32, 33, 37, 43, 46, 52, 54, 55, 56, 57, 61, 67]. It may often be reassuring for the surgeon to confirm that the tumor is indeed in the expected location before the dura is opened; in some instances, it may then be possible to operate through a smaller dural opening than would otherwise have been necessary. Moreover, transdural imaging will help improve spatial orientation as it visualizes the underlying brain and enables the surgeon to imagine the lateral and central borders of lesions more clearly. Foreign bodies like wood, bone and metal can be visualized; especially metal can be expected to be seen more clearly on US than on CT [14].

At the end of a tumor operation, the surgeon may want to check radicality (see p. 147 for detailed description).

Intraoperative Anatomical Orientation

The use of US for intraoperative anatomical orientation is illustrated below for three groups of problems.

Localization of Circumscribed Intracerebral Lesions. Circumscribed subcortical or deep-seated lesions may be difficult to find during operation. Intraoperative US is the first direct method of brain imaging during surgery. Using the appropriate probe, even very small tumors can be visualized clearly and in their anatomical surroundings. Consequently, the operation can be planned more precisely, with a smaller approach through viable tissue. Sometimes it may be helpful to insert a Cushing needle, or similar, toward the tumor surface and observe this movement on the US monitor. The same goes for lesions located deep in the white matter.

Tumor Invasion of Venous Sinuses. With a 10-MHz probe the lumen of venous sinuses can be inspected in the case of suspected tumor invasion; this may be especially helpful in falx meningiomas, where imaging can be done at the beginning of the operation, before opening the dura, or later on, when the bulk of the tumor has been removed and invasion or compression of a sinus region is suspected on angiography.

Placement of Ventricular Shunt Catheters. As already mentioned (p. 99), US imaging for hydrocephalus may also be a practical intraoperative procedure in children with open fontanelles; the ventricular shunt catheter is introduced with US monitoring, in a sagittal or coronal plane, of the position of the catheter tip in relation to the choroid plexus [60].

CASE 79 (Figs. 362, 363)

Metastasis from bronchial carcinoma in a 56-year-old man operated upon via left parietooccipital craniotomy.

US at 5 MHz shows the tumor, 2 cm in diameter, only faintly as a hypoechoic lesion surrounded by edematous tissue of the precentral and postcentral gyri which is hyperechoic compared to the same areas in the right hemisphere.

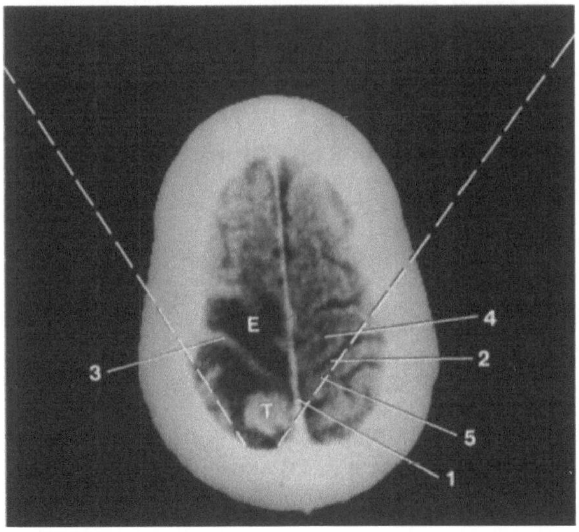

Fig. 362. Horizontal CT

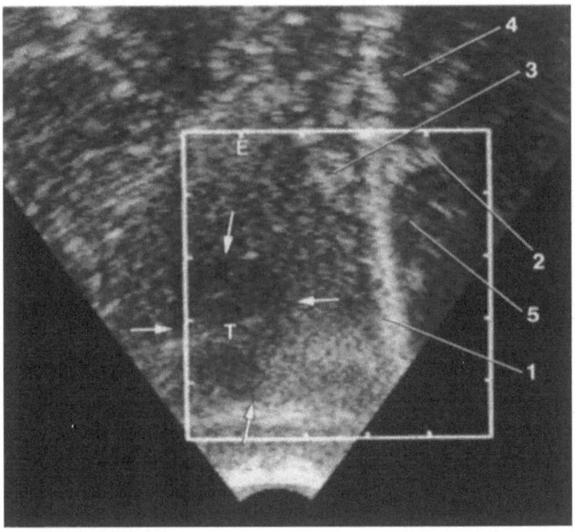

Fig. 363. Horizontal US. DRF 100, GPS probe, 5 MHz

1 Falx
2 Right rolandic fissure
3 Left rolandic fissure
4 Right precentral gyrus
5 Right postcentral gyrus
E Edema
T Tumor
→ Border of tumor

CASE 80 (Figs. 364, 365)

Metastasis from bronchial carcinoma in a 59-year-old man operated upon via left frontal craniotomy.

The 5-MHz US investigation reveals a slightly hyperechoic tumor with a markedly hyperechoic, rather well demarcated capsule. The edematous tissue from a distance of 1-2 cm from the capsule outward is hyperechoic, as in the other metastases investigated; the hypoechoic zone immediately surrounding the capsule seems to be the result of a technical artifact which also gives the metastasis itself a less hyperechoic appearance.

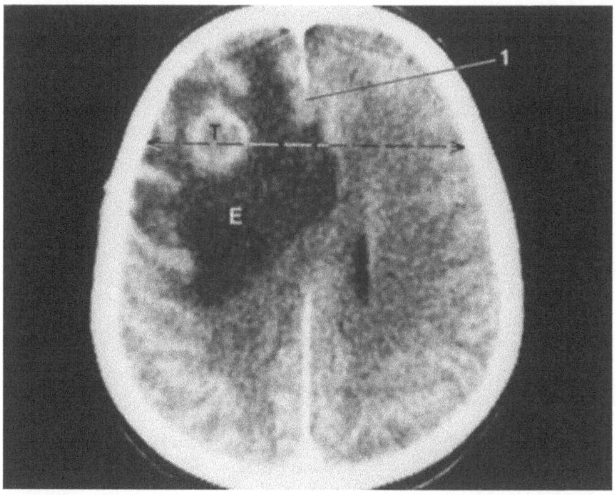

Fig. 364. Horizontal CT. Stippled line = sector plane for Fig. 365

1 Interhemispheric space
A Artifact
E Edema
T Tumor
→ Border of tumor

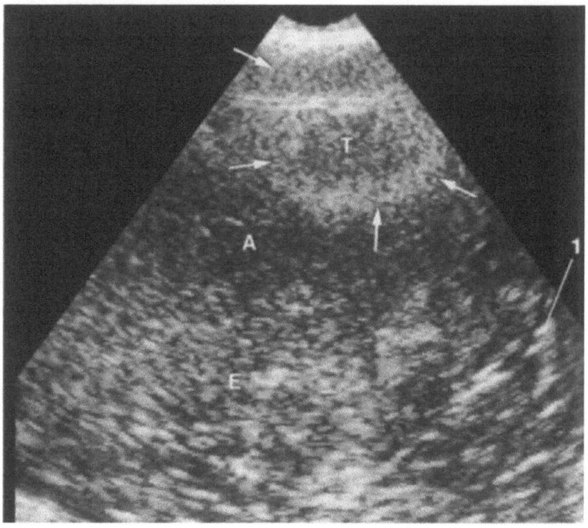

Fig. 365. Coronal US. DRF 100, GPS probe, 5 MHz

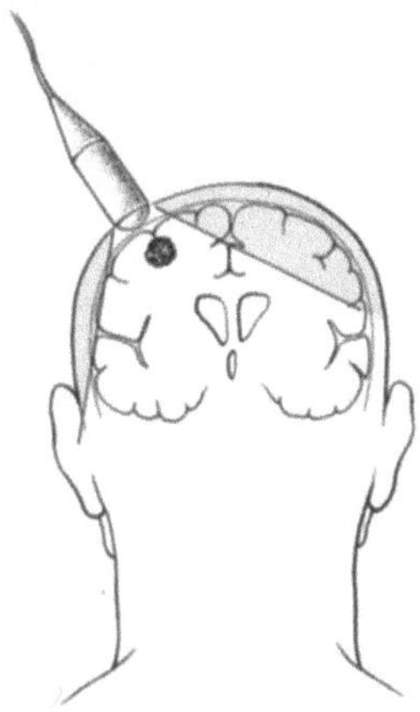

CASE 81 (Figs. 366, 367)

Metastasis from pulmonary carcinoma in a 55-year-old woman operated upon via right parietal craniotomy.

The tumor, almost 2 cm in diameter, is detected by 5-MHz imaging; however, the exact outline of the border cannot be clearly distinguished. The superficial location of the lesion would warrant the use of a 7.5-MHz or 10-MHz probe.

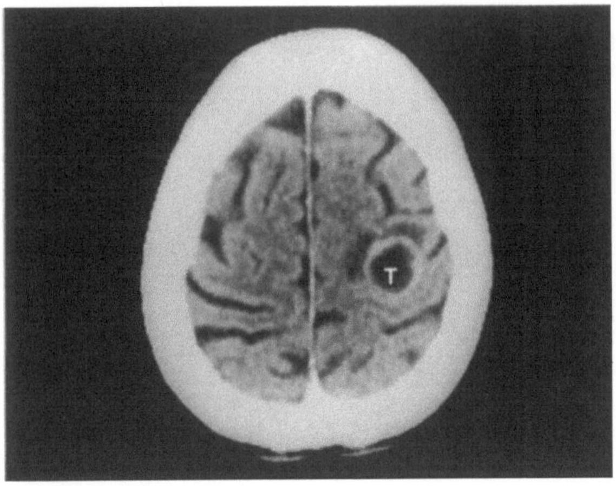

Fig. 366. Horizontal CT

1 Falx
2 Left lateral ventricle
3 Right lateral ventricle
4 Choroid plexus
T Tumor
→ Tumor capsule

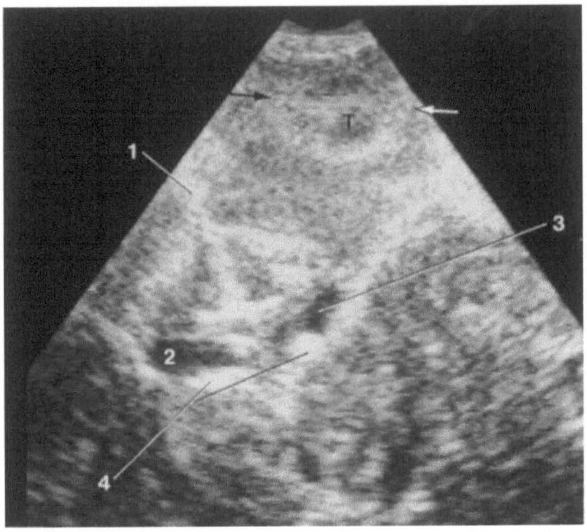

Fig. 367. Coronal US. DRF 100, GPS probe, 5 MHz

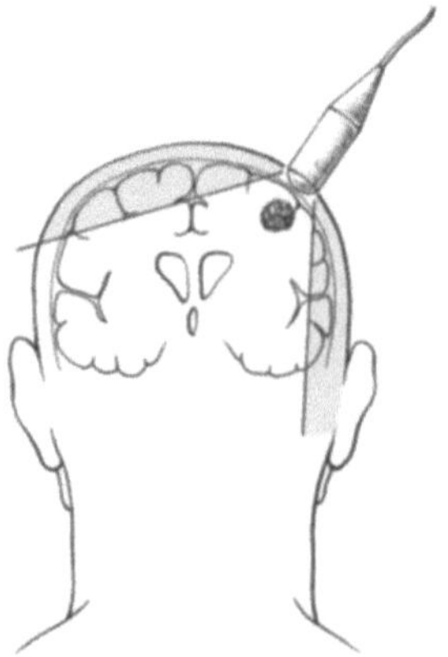

CASE 82 (Figs. 368–371)

Metastasis from renal cell carcinoma in a 55-year-old man operated upon via right frontal craniotomy.

The 7-mm lesion is undetectable on 5-MHz imaging (Fig. 369), whereas with the 7.5-MHz probe it appears clearly as a markedly hyperechoic globule (Figs. 370, 371). The surrounding white matter edema is hyperechoic and thus demarcated from the adjacent cortical regions with their markedly lower signal intensity.

1 Falx
2 Cortex of superior frontal lobule
3 Lateral ventricles
4 Cingulate sulcus
5 Paracentral sulcus
E Edema
T Tumor

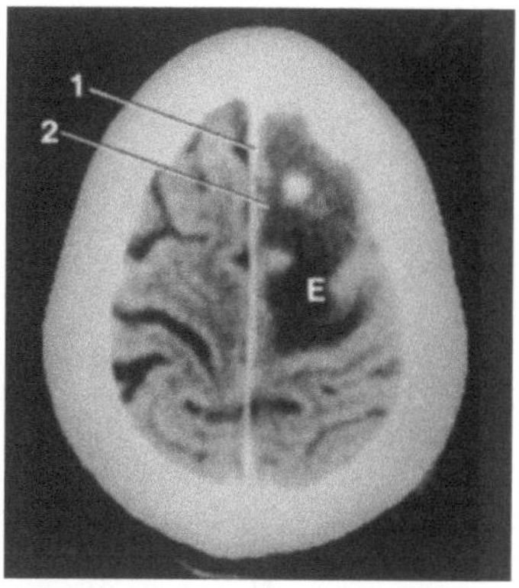

Fig. 368. Horizontal CT

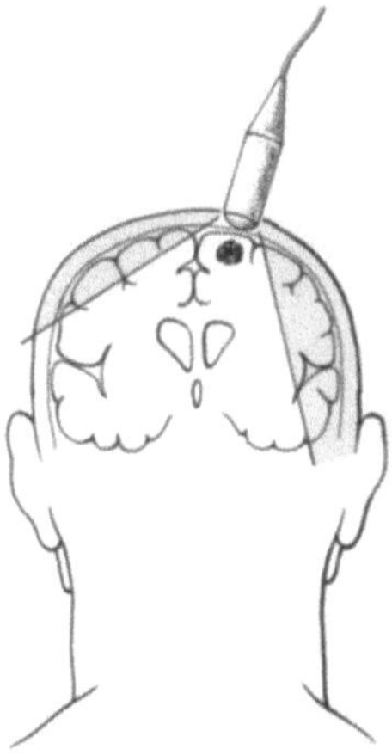

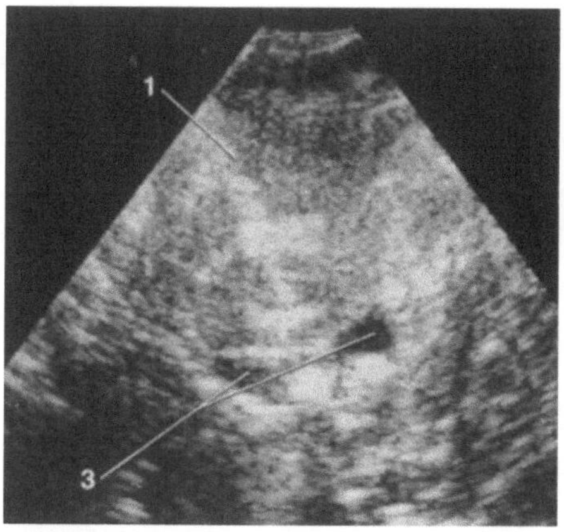

Fig. 369. Coronal US. DRF 100, GPS probe, 5 MHz

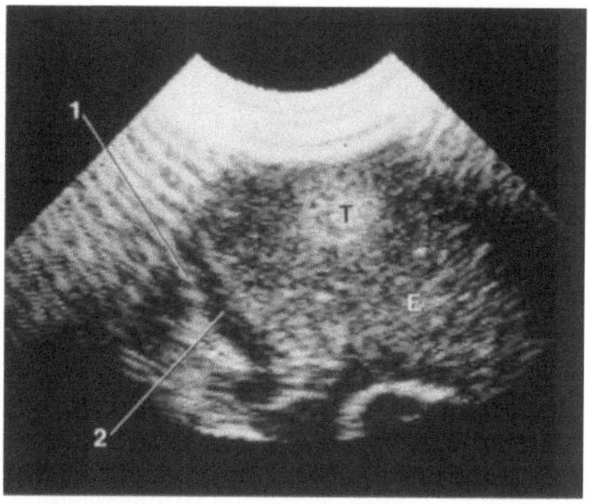

Fig. 370. Coronal US. NS, 7.5 MHz

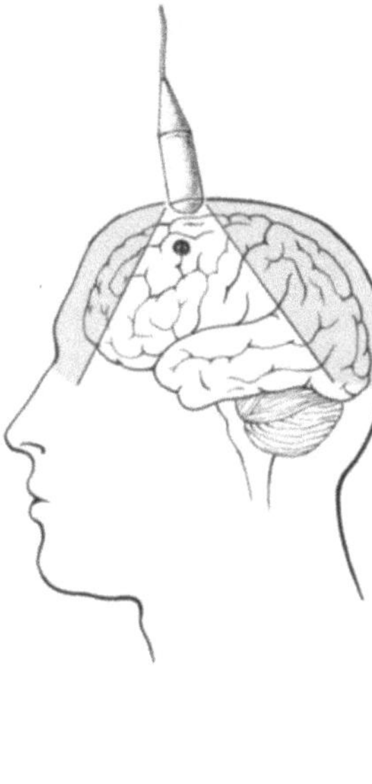

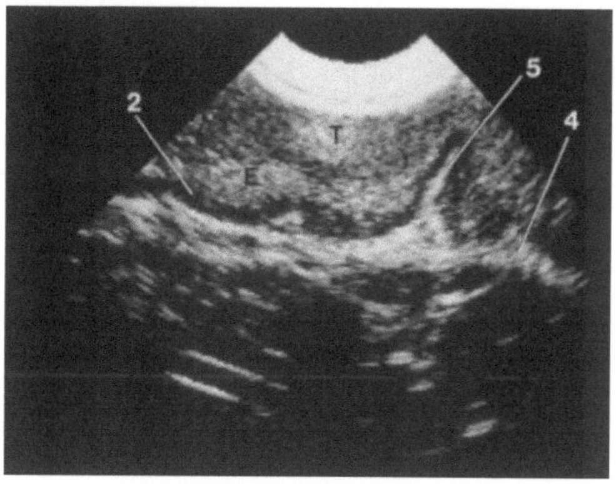

Fig. 371. Sagittal US. NS, 7.5 MHz

CASE 83 (Figs. 372-374)

Grade 2 astrocytoma in a 15-year-old boy with epileptic fits, operated upon via parietal craniotomy.

US at 5 MHz does not clearly visualize the lesion in the paracentral lobule (Fig. 374). At 7.5 MHz, however, the very well demarcated tumor appears with clear anatomical delineation (Fig. 373).

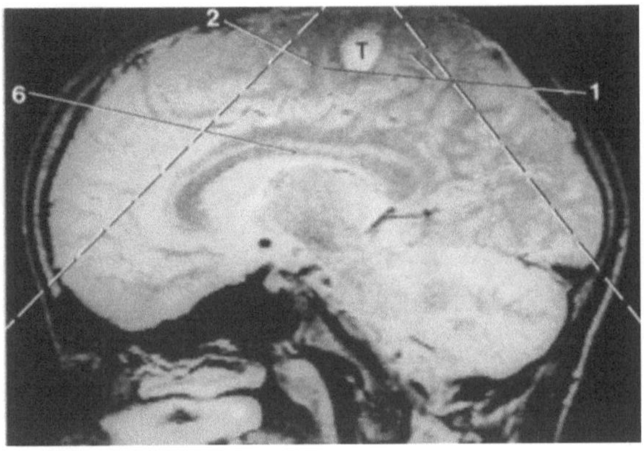

Fig. 372. Sagittal MRI

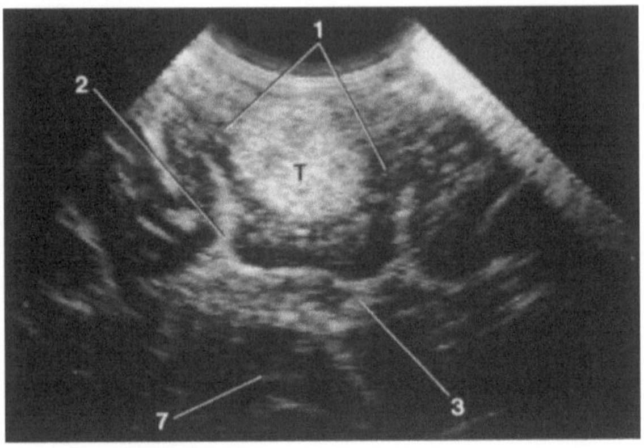

Fig. 373. Sagittal US. NS, 7.5 MHz

1 Cortex of paracentral lobule
2 Paracentral sulcus
3 Cingulate sulcus
4 Falx
5 Left temporal bone
6 Corups callosum
7 Cingulate gyrus
T Tumor

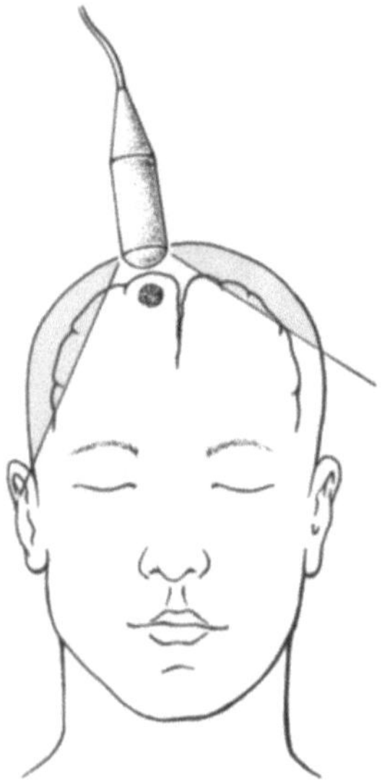

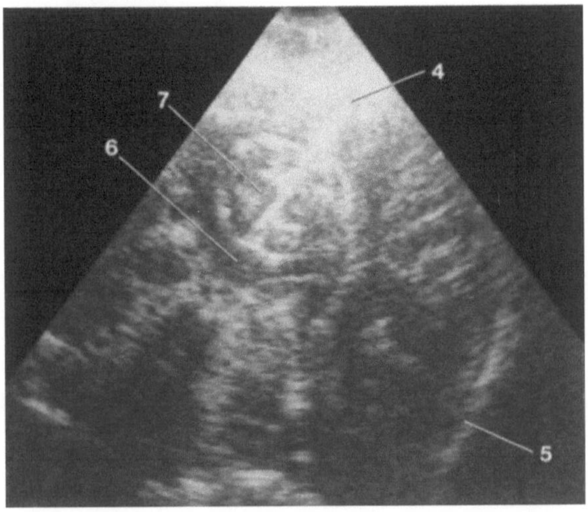

Fig. 374. Coronal US. DRF 100, GPS probe, 5 MHz

CASE 84 (Figs. 375-377)

Metastasis from colon carcinoma in the right cerebellar hemisphere of a 62-year-old woman operated upon via occipital craniotomy.

At 10 MHz, US imaging provides excellent delineation and anatomical correlation of the 6-mm tumor, which appears isoechoic to the cerebellar tissue.

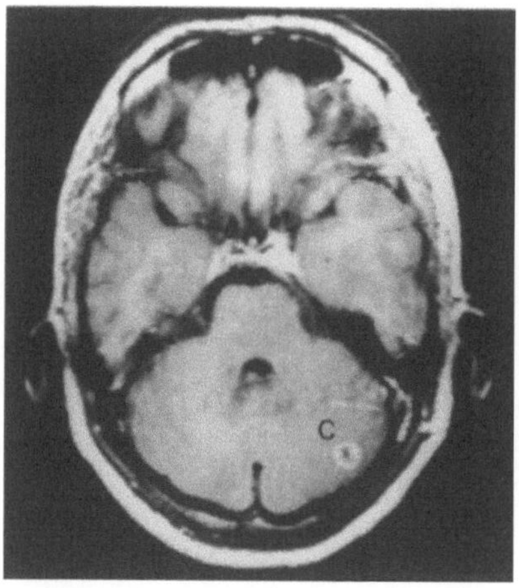

Fig. 375. Horizontal MRI

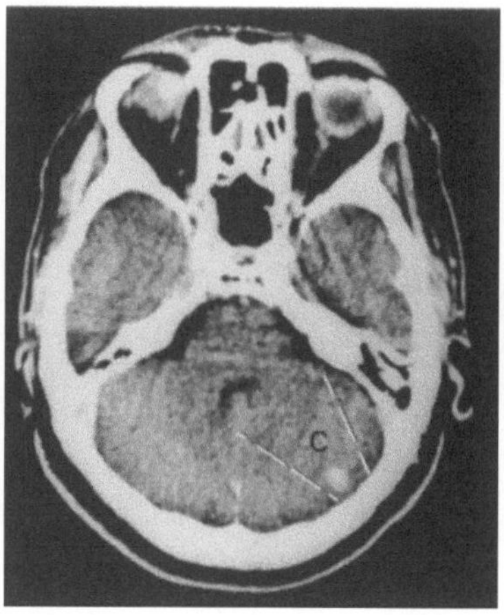

Fig. 376. Horizontal CT

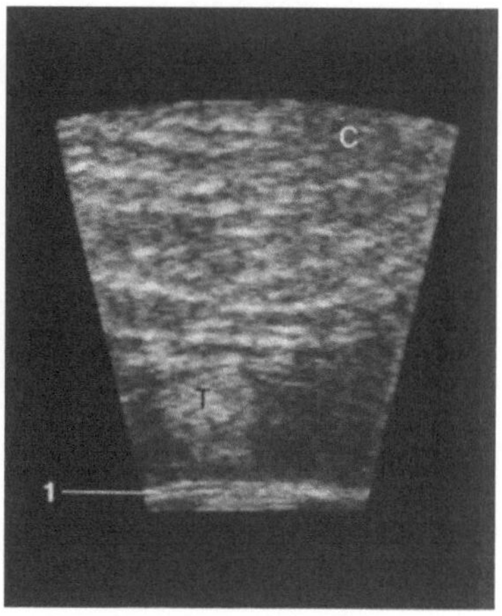

Fig. 377. Horizontal US. DRF 100, NF probe, 10 MHz

1 Dura
C Cerebellar hemisphere with structure of lobuli
T Tumor

CASE 85 (Figs. 378–382)

Metastasis 1 cm in diameter *from renal cell carcinoma* at the lateral base of the left cerebellar hemisphere in a 56-year-old man operated upon via lateral occipital craniotomy.

At 10 MHz in horizontal and sagittal projections, the tumor is shown as a hyperechoic, well-demarcated lesion with excellent demarcation from the surrounding cerebellar tissue.

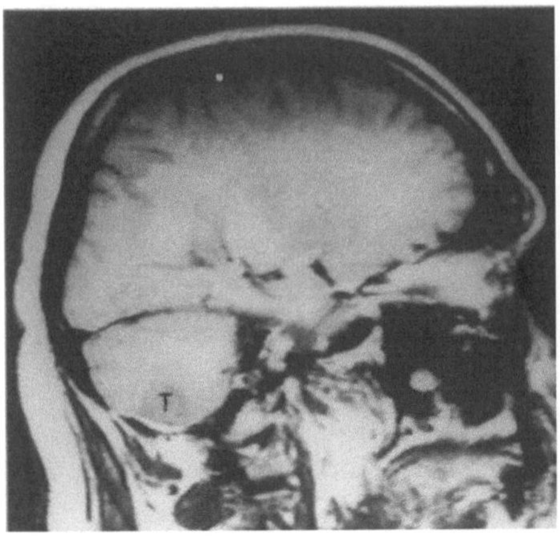

Fig. 378. Sagittal MRI

1 Cut edge of occipital bone
2 Dura
3 Cerebellar hemisphere
T Tumor

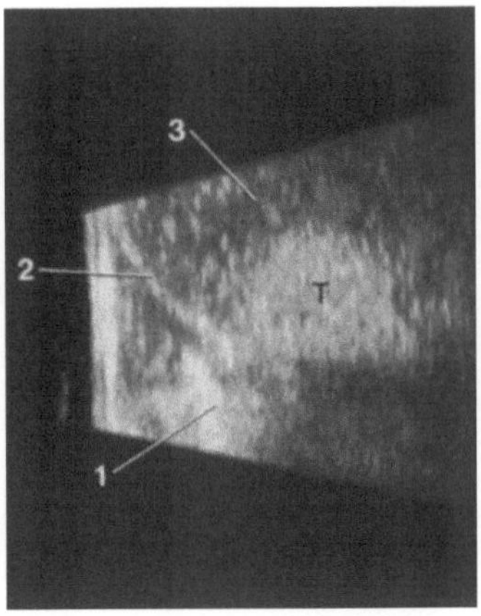

Fig. 379. Sagittal US. DRF 100, NF probe, 10 MHz

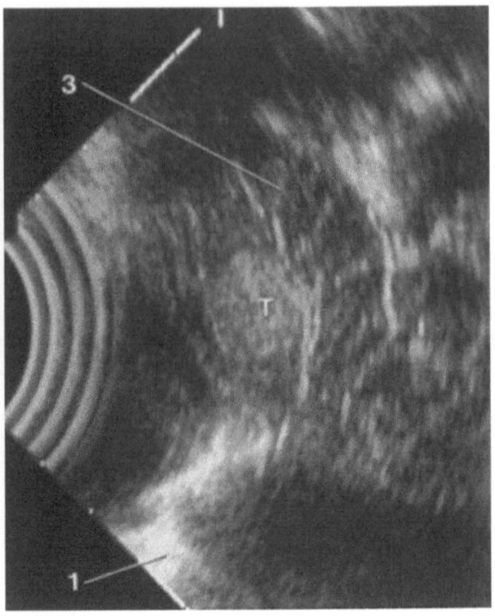

Fig. 380. Sagittal US. UM 8, annular array probe, 7.5 MHz

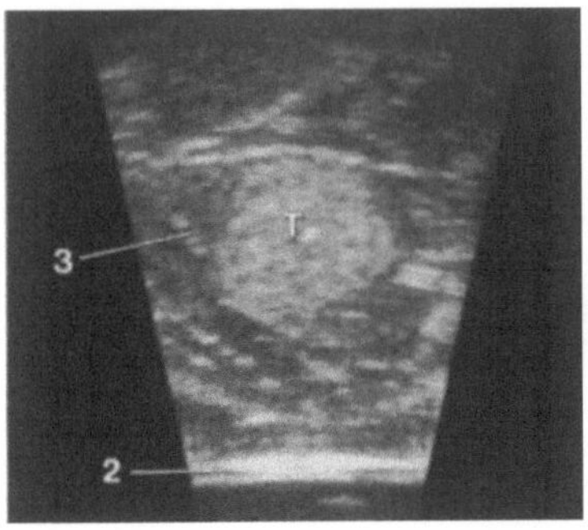

Fig. 381. Horizontal US. DRF 100, NF probe, 10 MHz

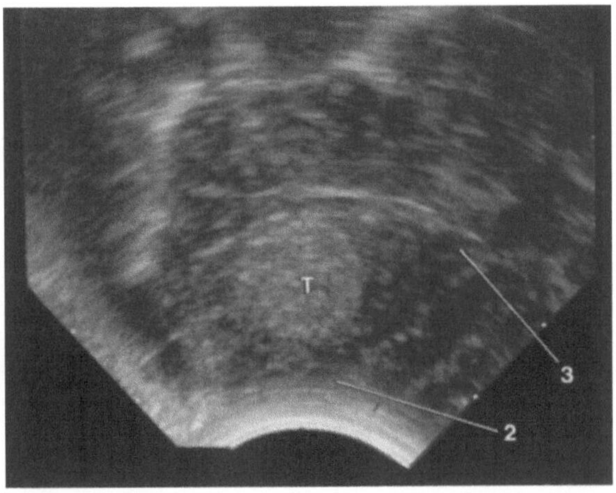

Fig. 382. Horizontal US. UM 8, annular array probe, 10 MHz

CASE 86 (Figs. 383-391)

Falx meningioma in a 52-year-old man operated upon via left parietooccipital craniotomy.

On CT, the hyperdense tumor shows a hypodense center, probably because of necrosis. The tumor grows through the fenestrated falx.

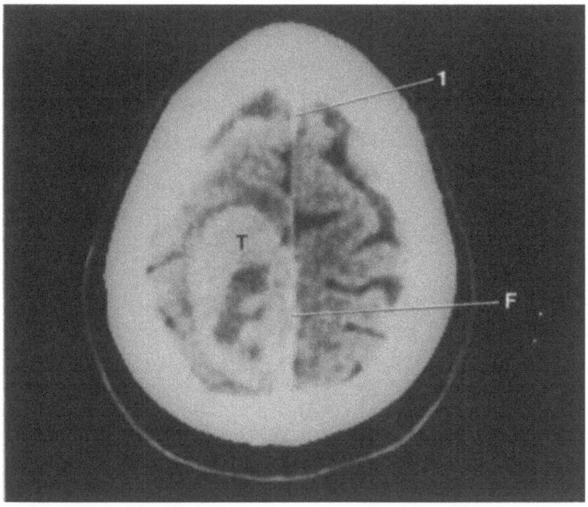

Fig. 383. Horizontal CT

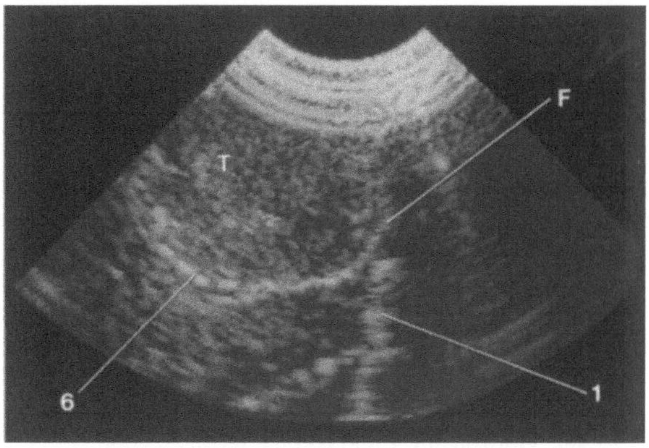

Fig. 384. Coronal US. NS, 7.5 MHz

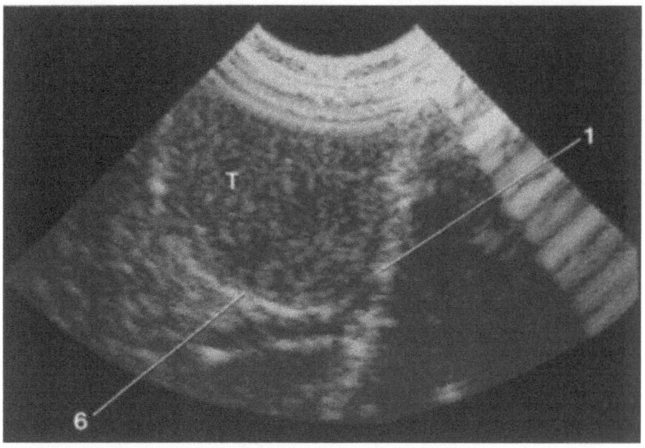

Fig. 385. Coronal US. NS, 7.5 MHz

1 Falx
6 Hyperechoic tumor capsule
F Fenestration of falx by tumor
T Tumor

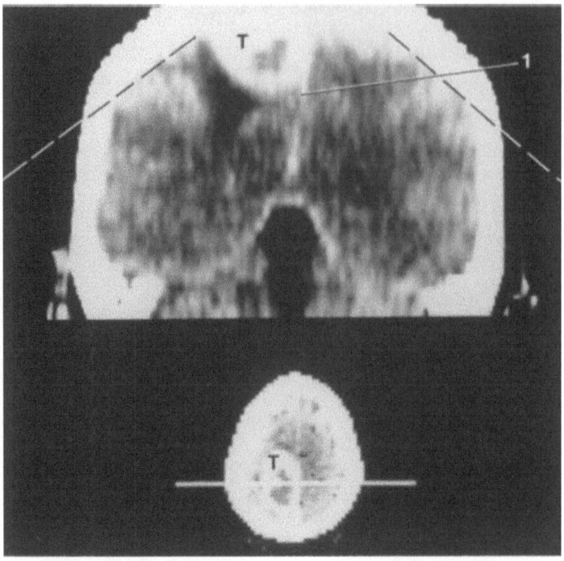

1 Falx
2 Choroid plexus
3 Tentorium
4 Occipital bone
5 Pyramidal bone
6 Hyperechoic tumor capsule
7 Cerebellar hemisphere
8 Splenium of corpus callosum
9 Lateral ventricle
10 Temporal cranial fossa
F Fenestration of falx by tumor
L Narrowed lumen of sagittal sinus
T Tumor
→ Tumor invasion of side wall of sagittal sinus

Fig. 386. Horizontal CT and coronal reconstruction

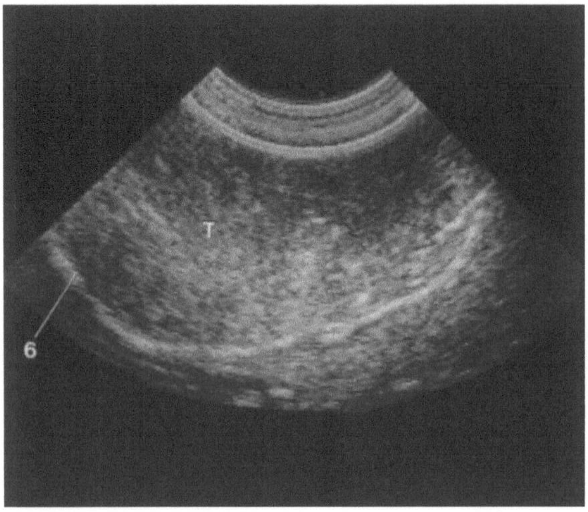

Fig. 387. US at 7.5 MHz. NS

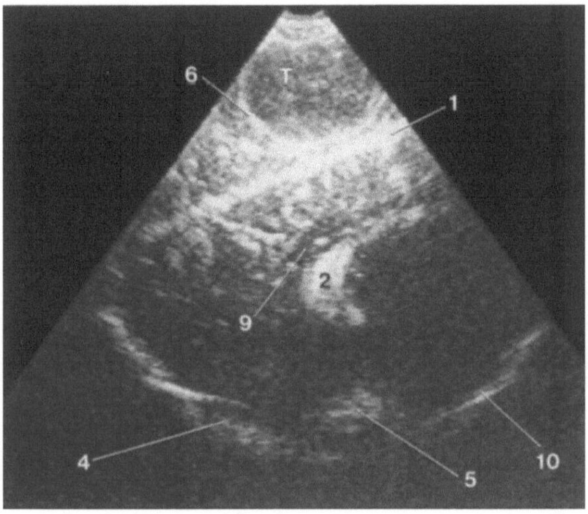

Fig. 388. Diagonal sagittal US. DRF 100, GPS probe, 5 MHz

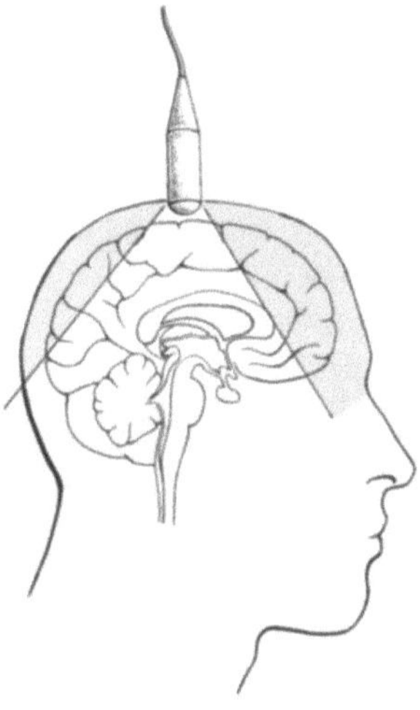

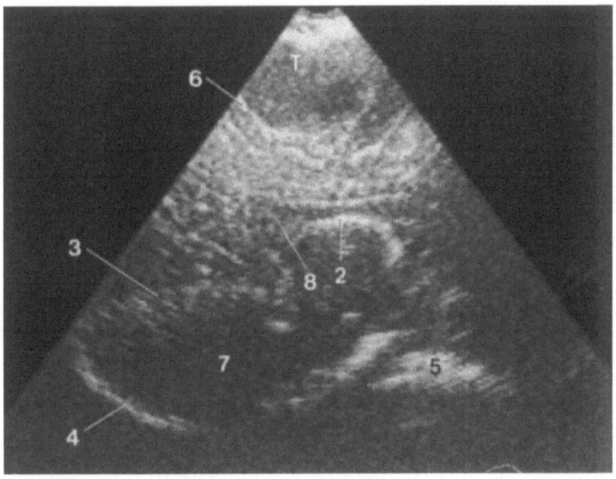

Fig. 389. Sagittal US. DRF 100, GPS probe, 5 MHz

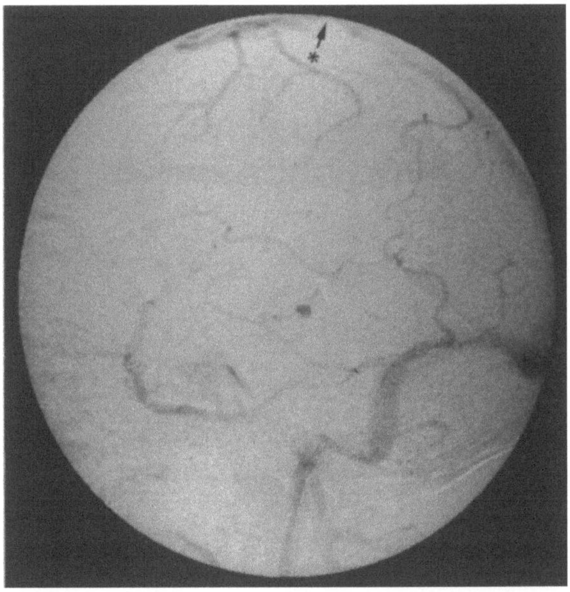

Fig. 390. Left internal carotid angiography: lateral view, venous phase

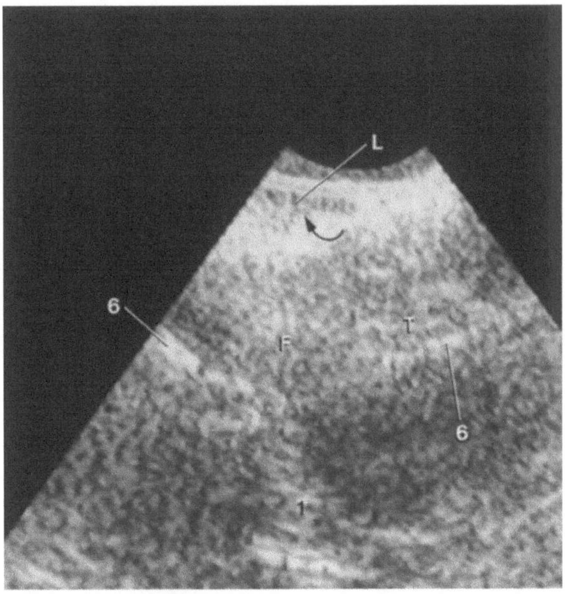

Fig. 391. Coronal US. DRF 100, GPS probe, 5 MHz

The venous angiogram (Fig. 390) shows poor filling of the superior sagittal sinus as well as an area where invading tumor seems to occlude the lumen (*). Obviously, US at 5 MHz does not provide excellent visualization of the immediately underlying sagittal sinus; however, as shown in Fig. 391, the sinus can be demonstrated as partly open and invaded by tumor. The tumor fenestrates the falx and grows to the contralateral side; however, the contralateral sinusal side wall remains intact. Surgical exposure verified this. The invaded sinusal side wall was excised and reconstructed, and the intrasinusal tumor was removed. The tumor is isoechoic or even slightly hypoechoic with a markedly hyperechoic capsule; the distinct differences of density seen on CT do not appear on US.

CASE 87 (Figs. 392–395)

Frontoparietal falx meningioma in a 62-year-old woman.

After removal of the tumor bulk, a 10-MHz probe was placed in the midline over the sagittal sinus for imaging in the coronal plane. Figure 394, in agreement with the venous angiogram (Fig. 393), shows the posterior end of the sinus lumen subtotally occluded by tumor invasion. Figure 395, taken in a slightly more posterior coronal plane, shows the beginning of the open sinus, as also demonstrated on the angiogram (Fig. 393).

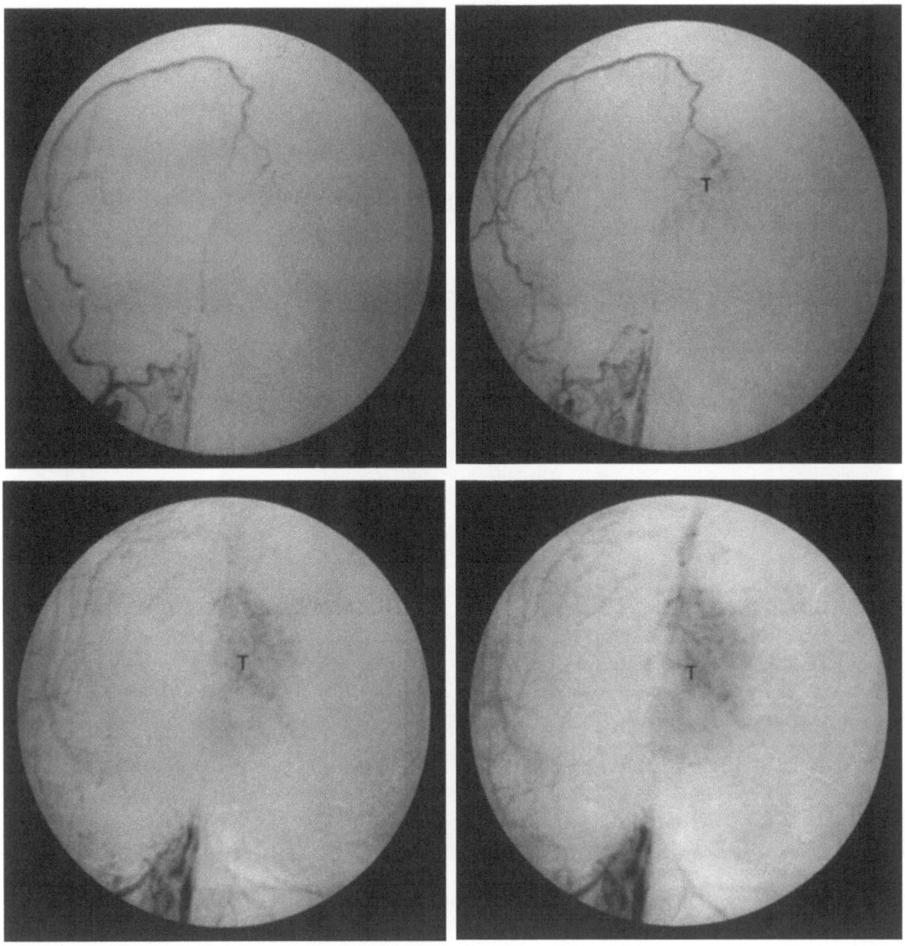

Fig. 392. Right external carotid angiography: AP view

1 Dural roof of sagittal sinus
2 Dural side wall of sinus
3 Lumen of sinus
T Tumor
→ Subtotally occluded part of sagittal sinus invaded by tumor
➧ Open sagittal sinus at posterior end of lumen

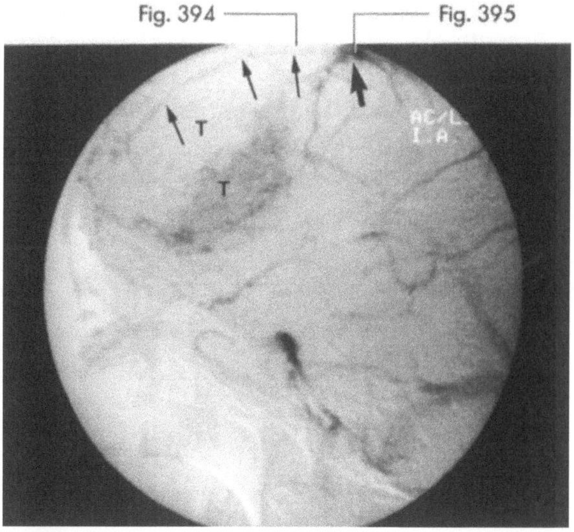

Fig. 393. Left internal carotid angiography: lateral view, venous phase

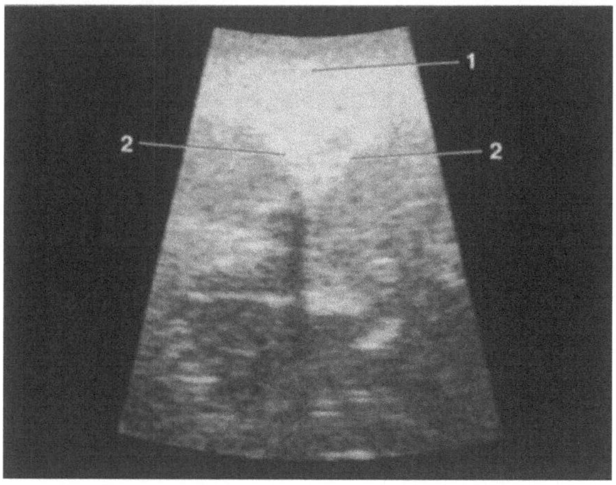

Fig. 394. Coronal US. DRF 100, NF probe, 10 MHz

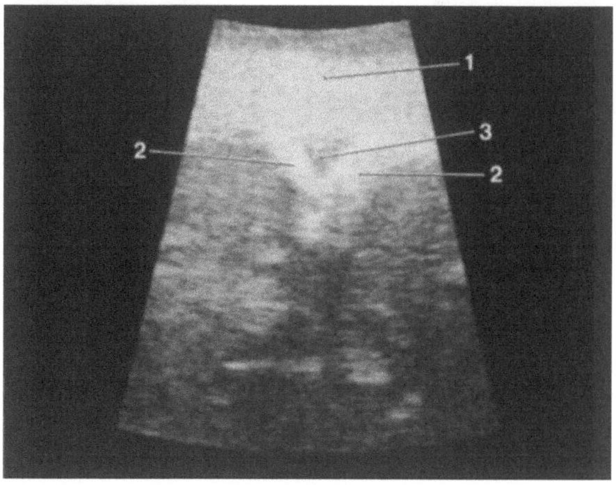

Fig. 395. Coronal US. DRF 100, NF probe, 10 MHz

CASE 88 (Figs. 396, 397)

Shunt implantation via the right occipital horn in a 2-month-old baby with *posthemorrhagic hydrocephalus*.

The hemorrhage had occurred shortly after birth (in the 33rd week of gestation). The two coronal US sections taken through the frontal fontanelle show the enlarged ventricular system before (Fig. 396) and during (Fig. 397) introduction of the ventricular catheter.

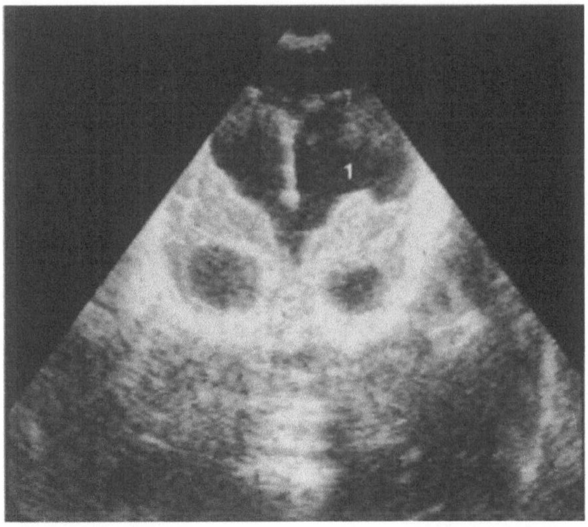

Fig. 396

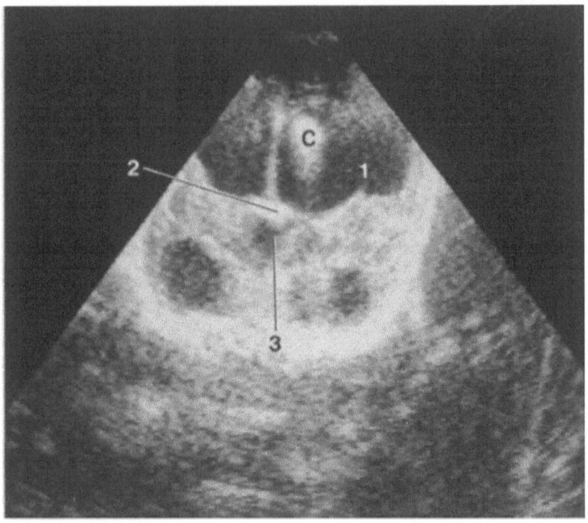

Fig. 397

Figs. 396, 397. Coronal US. DRF 100, GPS probe, 5 MHz

1 Lateral ventricle
2 Choroid plexus
3 Third ventricle
C Ventricular catheter

CASE 89 (Figs. 398-401)

Hydrocephalus in a 1-year-old child.

The parasagittal US sections show the enlarged right lateral ventricle through the frontal fontanelle before (Fig. 400) and during (Fig. 401) insertion of the ventricular catheter.

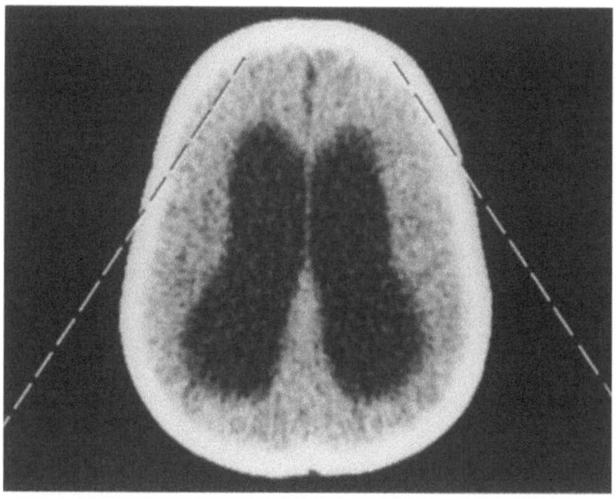

Fig. 398. Horizontal CT

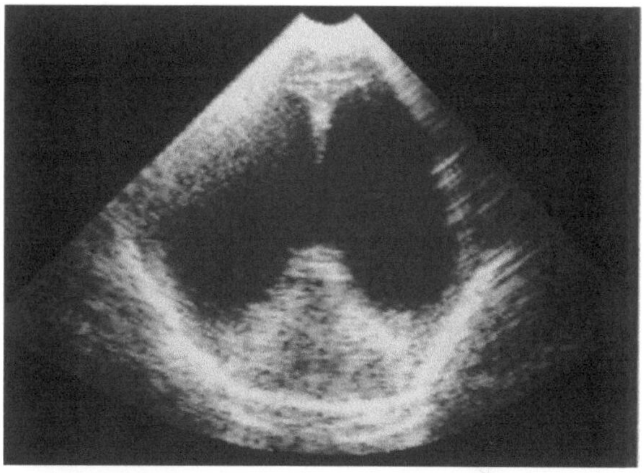

Fig. 399. Horizontal US. NS, 5 MHz

Figs. 400, 401. Sagittal US. NS, 5 MHz (see schema) ▷

1 Choroid plexus
2 Frontal horn of lateral ventricle
3 Temporal horn of lateral ventricle
4 Occipital horn of lateral ventricle
C Ventricular catheter

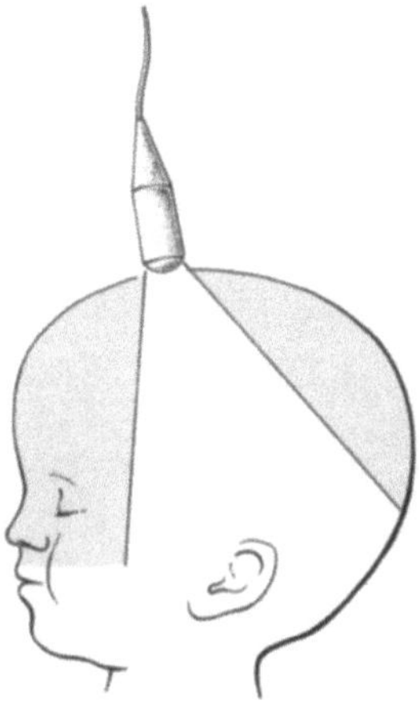

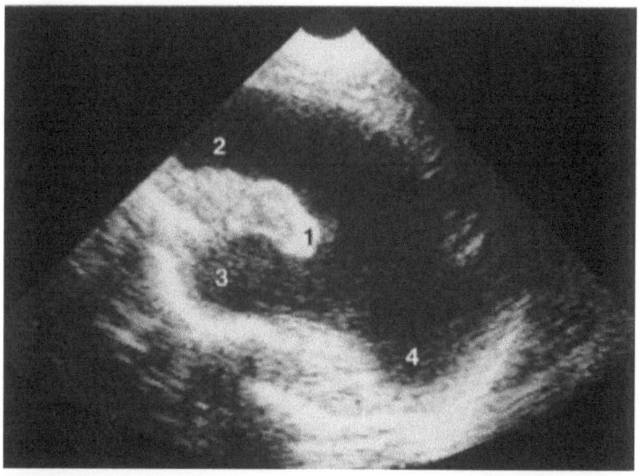

Fig. 400

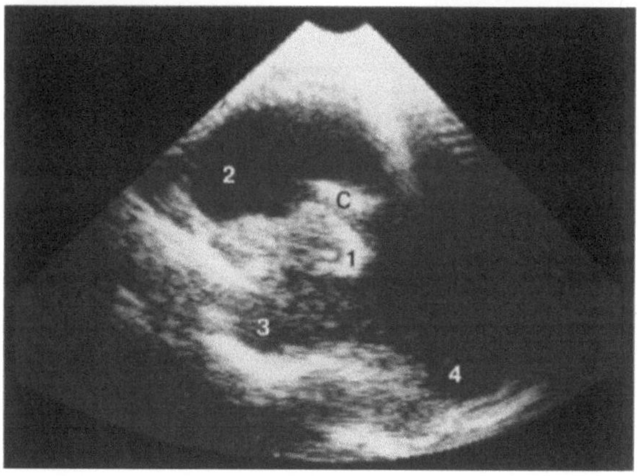

Fig. 401

Intraoperative Control After Tumor Removal

One of the expected practical applications of intraoperative US imaging in daily clinical neurosurgery was the control of radical removal of difficult tumors, especially of glimoas, which are ill-defined on CT and MRI and even more so during operation, there being no clear cleavage plane between the tumor and the surrounding edema. This expectation has not been fulfilled for the vast majority of circumstances, for the following reason: it has already been shown in earlier chapters that the outer border of tumors in the brain is hyperechoic, with very few exceptions. The edema surrounding gliomas and metastases is also hyperechoic, though less markedly so than the tumor. As soon as the tumor has been removed, small clots of blood in the wall of the cavity will show up as hyperechoic areas which often even cast a shadow behind them and thus hinder imaging of the tissue beyond. This makes it difficult to differentiate between hyperechoicity of the wall itself and hyperechoicity from residual tumor. The following examples are provided in order to illustrate the fact that one generally cannot rely on an intraoperative control image to make this distinction. In exceptional cases, however, it may be possible (61), as shown by the first example (Fig. 402).

CASE 90 (Fig. 402)

In this case the surgeon was of the opinion that it would be easy to go for this small, *subcortically located tumor.*

When it became apparent that the chosen approach to the lesion did not allow clear exposure and removal as expected, US imaging was performed with a 10-MHz probe after filling the defect created by the approach with Ringer solution: the image shows that the tumor was very slightly missed in the lateral floor of the approach. The operation could be uneventfully continued and completed with radical removal of the tumor.

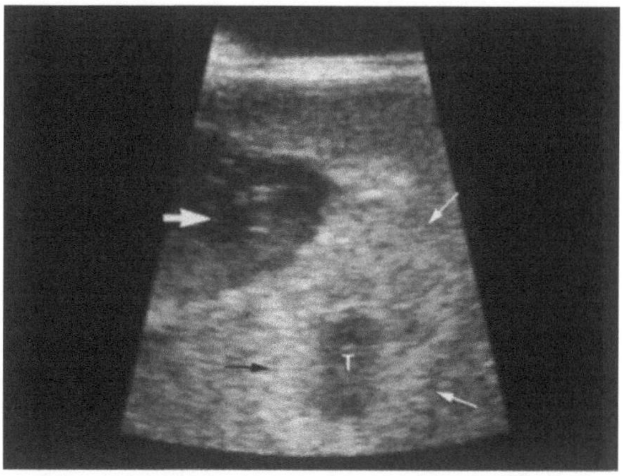

Fig. 402. US at 10 MHz. DRF 100, NF probe

T Tumor
→ Surface of tumor
➡ Surgical approach

CASE 91 (Figs. 403-408)

In this case, an *occipital metastasis* was removed via left occipital craniotomy.

The hyperechoic, well-demarcated tumor can be seen on the preoperative US images (Figs. 403, 405, 407). After removal of the tumor, a piece of Gelfoam was placed at the posterior end of the choroid plexus in the trigonum, where the tumor had been tightly adherent. From the control images (Figs. 404, 406, 408, corresponding respectively to Figs. 403, 405, 407) it is not unequivocally apparant whether complete removal of the tumor has been achieved, because the hyperechoic appearance of the Gelfoam resembles that of the tumor before it.

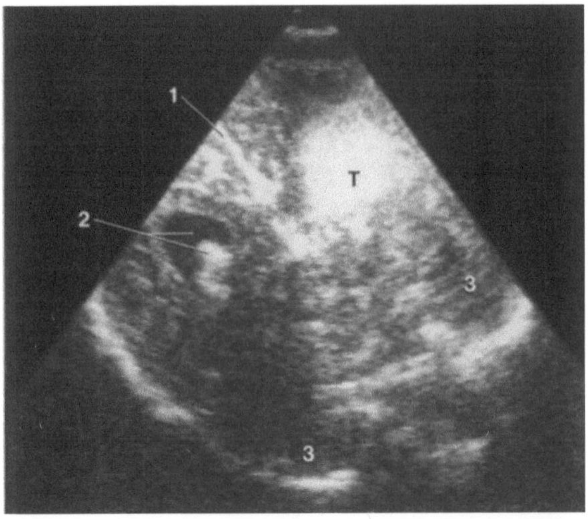

Fig. 403. Preoperative horizontal US. DRF 100, GPS probe, 5 MHz

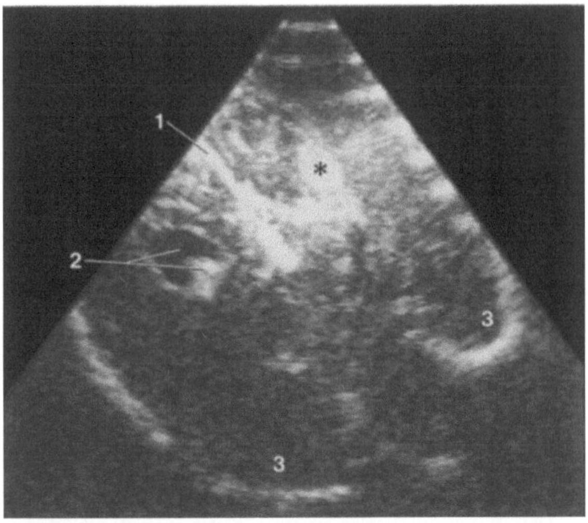

Fig. 404. Postoperative horizontal US corresponding to Fig. 403. DRF 100, GPS probe, 5 MHz

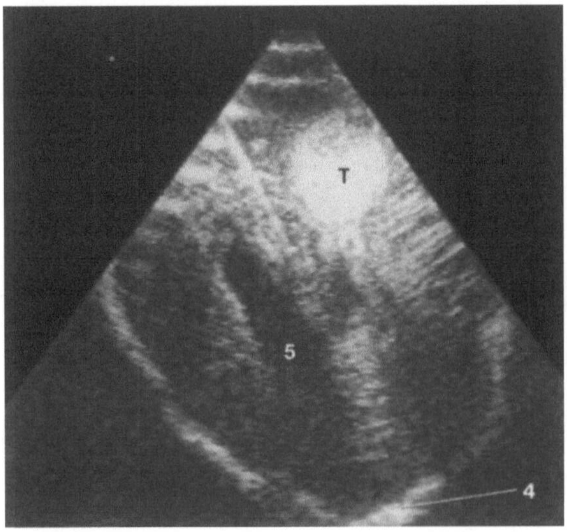

Fig. 405. Preoperative horizontal US. DRF 100, GPS probe, 5 MHz

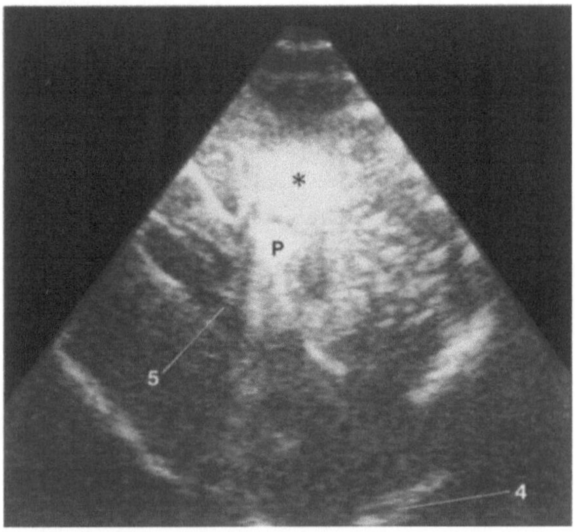

Fig. 406. Postoperative horizontal US corresponding to Fig. 405. DRF 100, GPS probe, 5 MHz

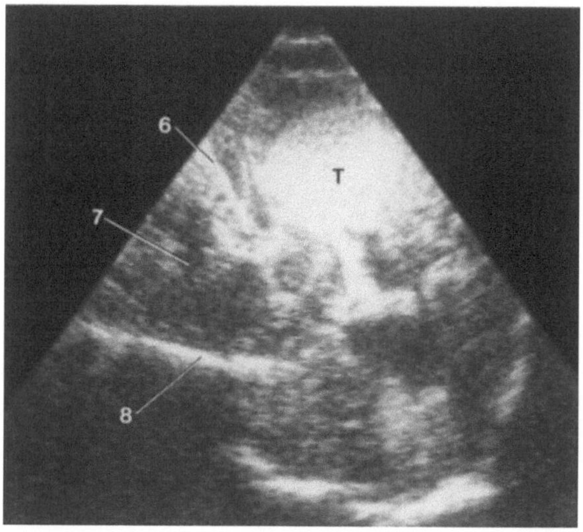

Fig. 407. Preoperative sagittal US. DRF 100, GPS probe, 5 MHz

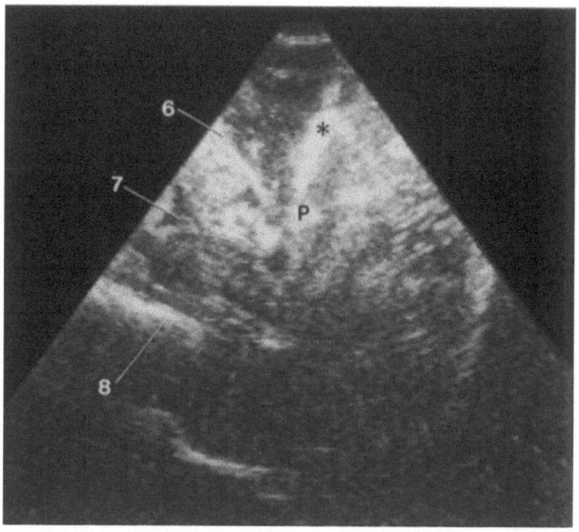

Fig. 408. Postoperative sagittal US corresponding to Fig. 407. DRF 100. GPS probe, 5 MHz

1 Occipital falx
2 Trigonal ventricle with choroid plexus
3 Middle fossa
4 Frontal bone
5 Lateral ventricle
6 Tentorium
7 Fourth ventricle
8 Clivus
P Choroid plexus
T Tumor
* Gelfoam

CASE 92 (Figs. 409–411)

In this patient, a small *occipital metastatis* was operated upon via right occipital craniotomy.

The hypoechoic interior is surrounded by a hyperechoic capsule. The surrounding edema is also hyperechoic and veils the border of the tumor (Fig. 409). After removal of the tumor, the somewhat collapsed cavity can be demonstrated on a control image (Figs. 410, 411); however, no clear-cut information is yielded as to whether complete removal has been achieved, since the tumor bed is as hyperechoic as was, or is, the tumor capsule.

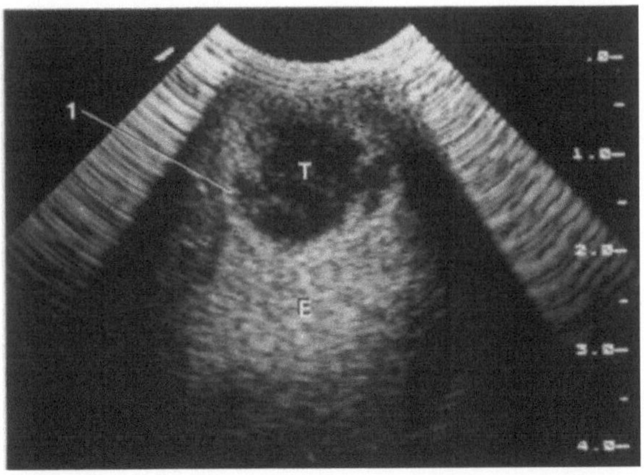

Fig. 409. Horizontal US. UM 8, annular array probe, 10 MHz

1 Tumor capsule
2 Wall of tumor cavity
C Tumor cavity
E Edema
T Tumor

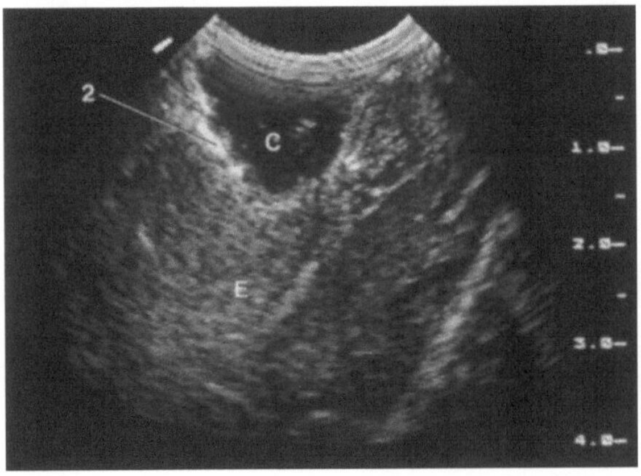

Fig. 410. Horizontal US. UM 8, annular array probe, 10 MHz

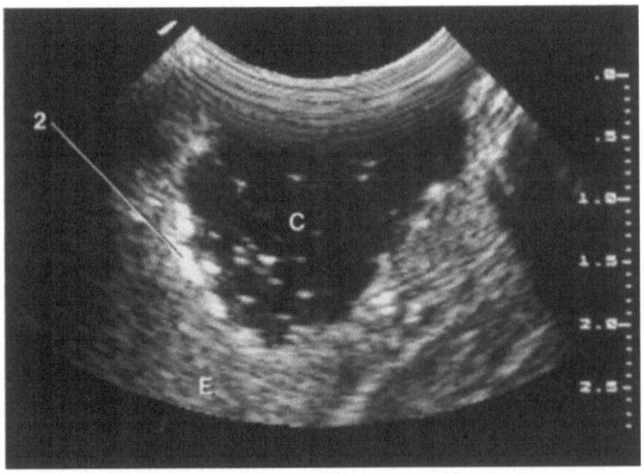

Fig. 411. Horizontal US. UM 8, annular array probe, 10 MHz

CASE 93 (Figs. 412-416)

Metastasis in the white matter of the parietal lobe operated upon via parietal craniotomy.

The 10-MHz probe clearly outlines the anatomical details of the tumor and the surrounding structures; thus, a sulcus can be detected which leads exactly to the surface of the metastasis. The tumor was approached with the aid of the operating microscope and enucleated in toto; Fig. 416 shows the 10-MHz control image which demonstrates the tumor bed and the narrow channel of approach. However, from the US image alone it cannot be unequivocally stated that the tumor has been radically removed. In particular, the bottom of the tumor bed displays hyperechoicity similar to that of the previously present capsule of the tumor.

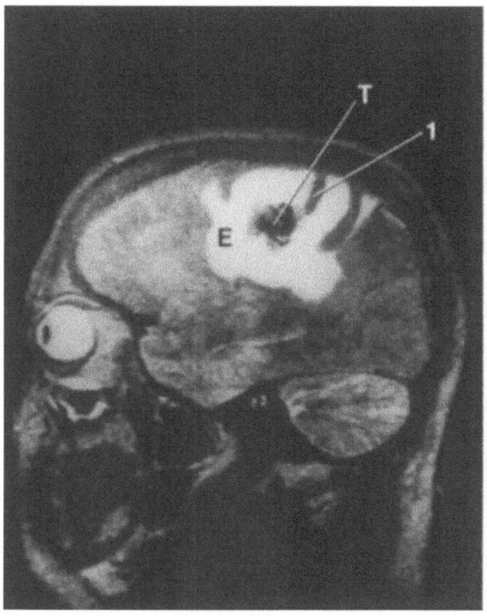

Fig. 412. Sagittal MRI

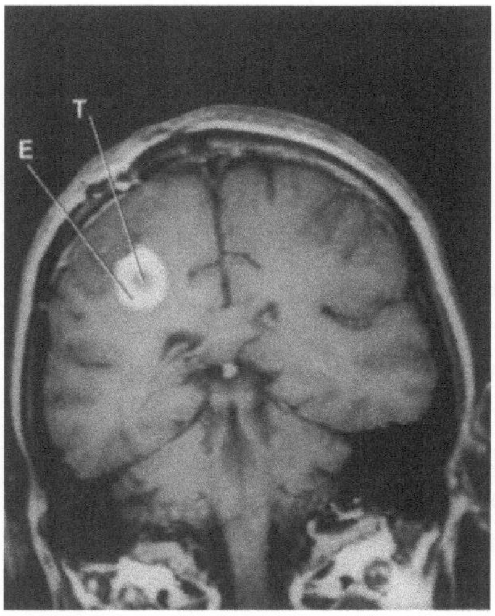

Fig. 413. Coronal MRI

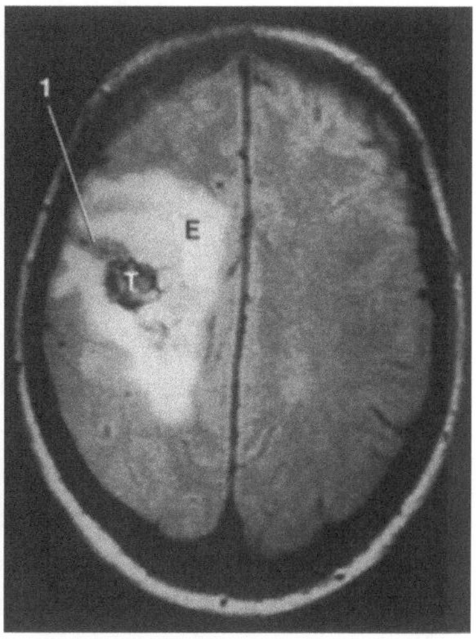

Fig. 414. Horizontal MRI

1 Sulcus
2 Channel of surgical approach
C Tumor cavity
E Edema
T Tumor

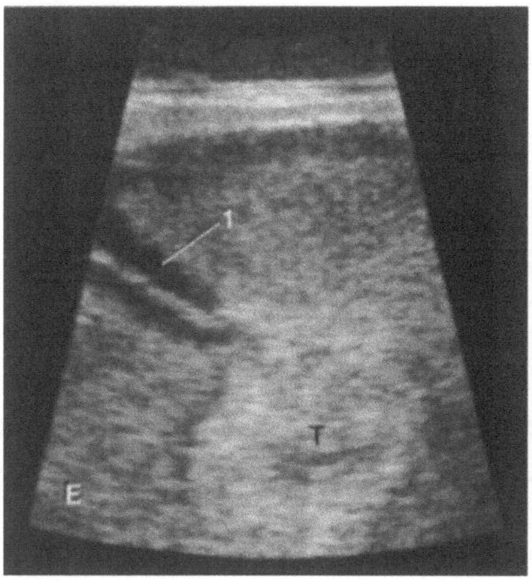

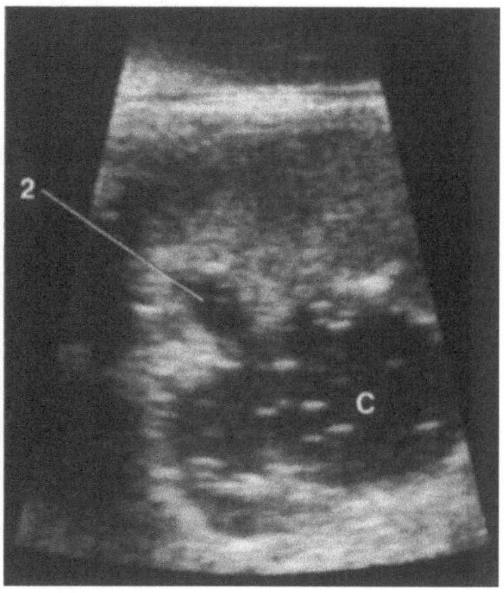

Figs. 415, 416. US at 10 MHz. DRF 100, NF probe

Ultrasound-Guided Stereotaxy

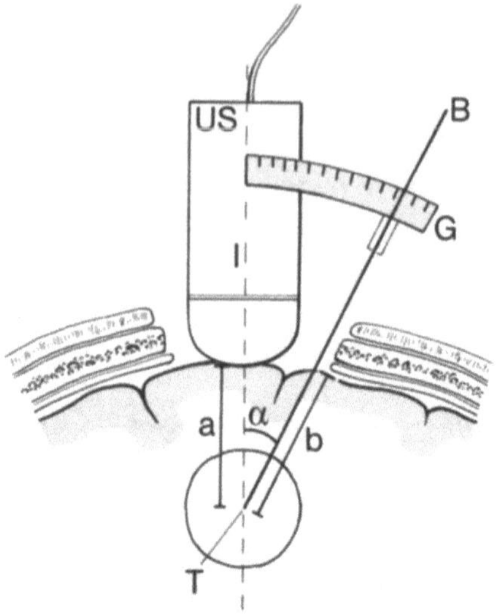

Fig. 417. Simultaneous US-guided stereotaxy

a Distance from brain surface to target point along line *l*
α Angle between *l* and *B*
b Distance from brain surface to target point along line *B*
B Biopsy needle
G Instrument guide with scale for angle *α*
l US centerline
T Target point
US Ultrasound probe

Stereotactic techniques, i.e. methods for orientation in the intracranial space, have been used in a variety of diagnostic and therapeutic neurosurgical procedures. These techniques use either indirect intraoperative imaging of an intracranial target area (e.g., ventriculography or angiography to show the immediate surroundings of a target), or direct preoperative imaging of the brain (e.g., CT). The former has the disadvantage of being too imprecise for certain targets, while the latter is often time-consuming and logistically complicated. CT is indispensable in some cases but unnecessary in others, for example large supratentorial lesions.

Intraoperative US is the first direct and real-time imaging method to show intracranial lesions. Besides providing pictures of the lesion in question and the surrounding brain structures, it allows the directing of an instrument such as a biopsy needle, an aspiration cannula or an endoscope to a target point in the real-time image. The distance from the surface to the target can be calculated with the aid of the computer systems which are built into all commercially available instruments of the last generation. There are basically two ways of reaching a predefined target point.

Simultaneous US-Guided Stereotaxy. The first way of reaching the target point involves mounting an instrument holder on the US probe (Fig. 417) and introducing the instrument alongside the transducer: the angle *(α)* between the longitudinal axis of the probe and the intrument guide *(G)* will then be a measure for the depth at which the instrument will meet the US centerline *(l)* and thereby the target point *(T)*. The distance from the probe surface to the target *(a)* can be used as the surface-target distance for the surgical instrument *(b)*, because the distance between instrument and probe is small enough to allow the assumption that the brain surface is a globe. As one major advance over all other stereotactic techniques, US guidance provides direct visual verification that the instrument has arrived in the target area. All further procedures can be performed under this direct visual control on the video monitor of the US apparatus. On disadvantage of this method is that it requires a small craniotomy to allow access for the probe and the surgical instrument (see case 102).

Consecutive US-Guided Stereotaxy. The second method of US-guided stereotaxy is the consecutive insertion of US probe and surgical instrument through the same fixation device via a burrhole: one such holder was designed by M. Berger [4] and is shown in Figs. 418–421. The holding device *(H)* for the probe is fixed thightly to the skull in a 2-cm burrhole; it includes a ball joint *(B)* for free movement of the probe until the target point *(T)* has been defined on the US image and the distance to it has been calculated (Fig. 418b). Thereafter, the ball joint is fixed in this position by means of the fixation ring *(R)*, so that it is now in the centerline (l) of the holding device, which points exactly to the target point. The probe itself is now removed and replaced by a plastic model *(P)* of the probe (Figs. 419–421). This model has a central channel of exactly the

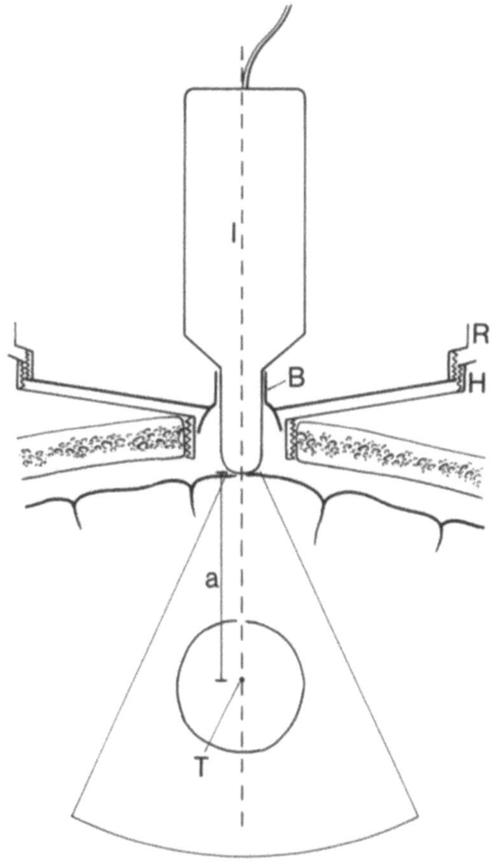

Fig. 418a. Consecutive US-guided stereotaxy

a Distance to target
B Ball joint
H Fixation for US probe and biopsy instrument
I US centerline
R Fixation ring
T Target point

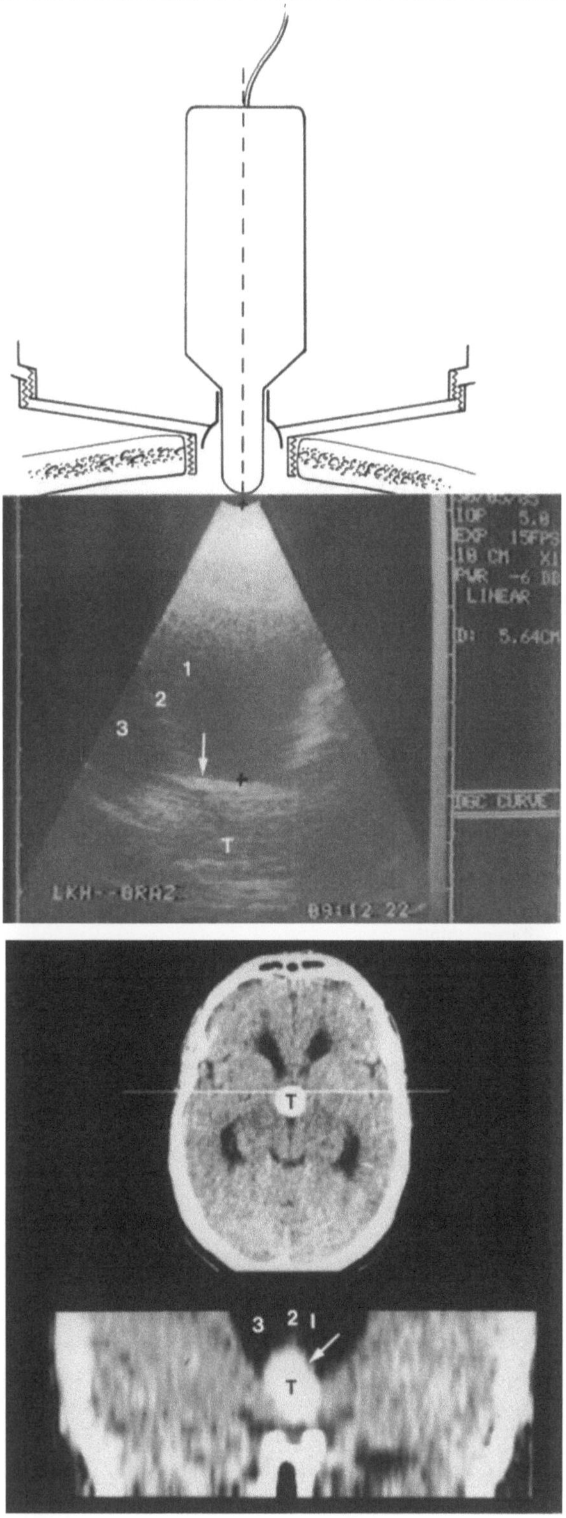

▷
Fig. 418b. Calculation of distance *a* by inbuilt computer as the distance between the two crosses in the US image. In this case of a third ventricular tumor, this distance was 5.64 cm. IOP, 5 MHz

1 Right lateral ventricle
2 Septum pellucidum
3 Left lateral ventricle
T Tumor
↓ Tumor bulging through enlarged foramen of Monro

diameter of the surgical instrument *(S)*. The latter is introduced through this channel in the model to the predefined depth. In the same way, an endoscope can be introduced (Fig. 420).

The advantage over the simultaneous technique is that it can be used via a burrhole; the disadvantage is that imaging is not available while the surgical instrument is in place. This dis-

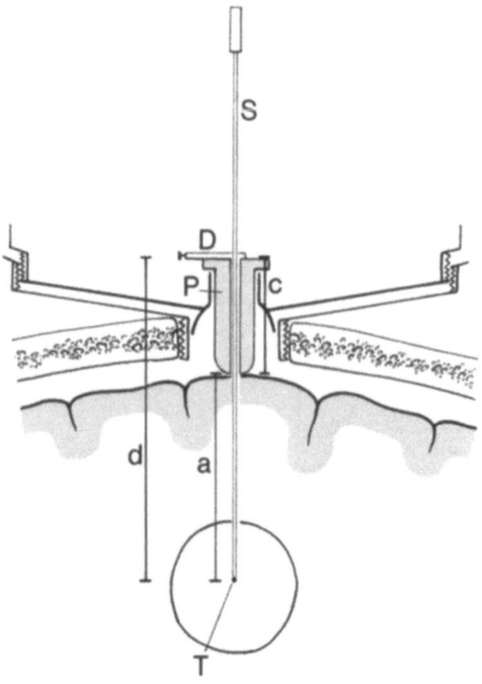

Fig. 419. Consecutive US-guided burrhole biopsy

a Distance to target minus length of *P*
c Length of *P*
d Distance to target for biopsy needle (*a*+ *c*)
D Holder for biopsy needle with fixation screw
P Plastic model of probe
S Biopsy needle
T Target point

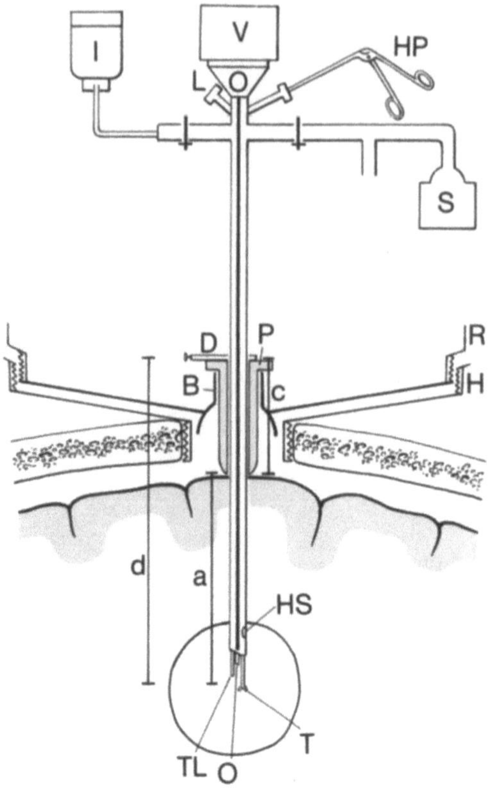

Fig. 420. US-guided endoscopy

a Distance to target minus length of *P*
c Length of *P*
d Distance to target for biopsy needle (*a*+ *c*)
B Ball joint
D Holder for biopsy needle with fixation screw
H Fixation for US probe and biopsy instrument
I Infusion system for irrigation
L Connector for Nd-YAG laser
O Optic system
P Plastic model of probe
R Fixation ring
S Suction
T Tip of biopsy forceps
V Video camera
HP Handpiece of biopsy forceps
HS Side hole for suction
TL Fiberoptic tip for laser

advantage can partly be compensated by alternating insertion of probe and instrument. Moreover, endoscopic biopsy can take over the visual control after the endoscope has been introduced to the target area.

Both techniques have the advantage over other stereotactic methods that the "operating field", i.e., the target area, can be controlled in the operating room, when the actual procedure is finished. Thus, any bleeding can be readily detected and treated if necessary.

The accuracy of these methods of US-guided stereotaxy is sufficient for the majority of supratentorial lesions, and they can be safely used for the burrhole evacuation of hematomas by means of simple needle aspiration, an Archimedes screw or an endoscope. They can also be used for biopsy of solid and cystic tumors in the hemispheres, the deep nuclei or the ventricular system, including the third ventricle. Numerous recent publications describe the procedure as fast and safe [refs. 13, 18, 19, 35, 57, 62, 65].

In cases of large, especially cystic, lesions it is no problem to perform puncture without needle guide, using the simultaneous technique, i.e., watching the movement of the needle on the US video monitor [53].

It is important, especially with thin-walled cysts, to take the biopsy specimen from the cyst wall before evacuating the cyst, because the collapsed wall may be difficult to find and biopsy. This problem does not exist when endoscopic biopsy is performed: as a first step, some of the cyst fluid is tapped using a Cushing needle for cytological investigation. Next, the remaining cyst fluid is washed out and replaced by artificial CSF or Ringer solution to prevent collapse of the cyst. Biopsies of the cyst wall can then be taken under direct visual control.

However, the precision is certainly insufficient to reach target points in the posterior fossa via a supratentorial approach; lesions of the cerebellum can be reached under US guidance via a suboccipital approach (burrhole) [8] with adequate accuracy. The visualization of the pons is often inadequate for precise target definition; the authors have personal experience with only one case of endoscopic evacuation of brainstem hemorrhage and there US-guided evacuation was successful.

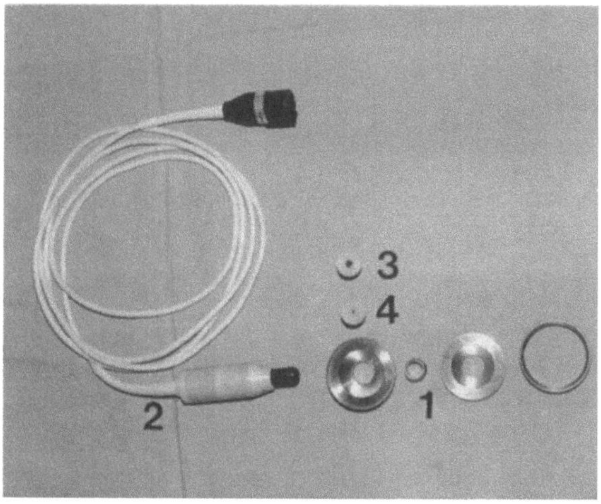

Fig. 421. Modified Berger set (Diasonics) for fixation of IOP US probe (Diasonics) through a 2-cm burrhole

1 Holding device, ball joint, fixation ring
2 US probe
3 Plastic model for endoscope
4 Plastic model for surgical instrument

Placement of Burrhole for US-Guided Stereotaxy. For hemispheric lesion, the approach via the shortest transcortical distance to target or through the least eloquent cortical area is usually defined with the aid of CT and/or MRI parameters, using different planes of imaging. Lesions in the lateral ventricles are reached through a classical frontal or occipital burrhole; trigonal lesions are conveniently approached through a parietooccipital burrhole through Brodmann's area 7a or 7b. If highly vascular lesions are situated along the track to the target, US-guided procedures should not be performed, because direct and sufficiently precise correlation with angiographic data is not possible. The anterior third ventricle is also reached safely through a classical frontal burrhole.

On the following pages examples will be given of the use of US-guided stereotaxy for endoscopic evacuation of hematoma, endoscopic biopsy of cystic hemispheric tumors, endoscopic biopsy of central tumors via the ventricular system, needle biopsy of brain tumors and drainage of brain abscesses.

Endoscopic Evacuation of Intracerebral Hematomas

CASE 94 (Figs. 422–425)

Spontaneous temporooccipital hematoma in a 73-year-old man. US-guided endoscopic evacuation (consecutive technique) was performed through a burrhole over the hematoma.

On US, the hematoma is partly hyperechoic and partly isoechoic (Fig. 423); during operation it turned out to be partly fluid and partly solid. At the end of the operation US control through the burrhole verified complete evacuation (Fig. 424). Postoperative CT shows the small defect and a catheter in the mostly collapsed cavity (Fig. 425).

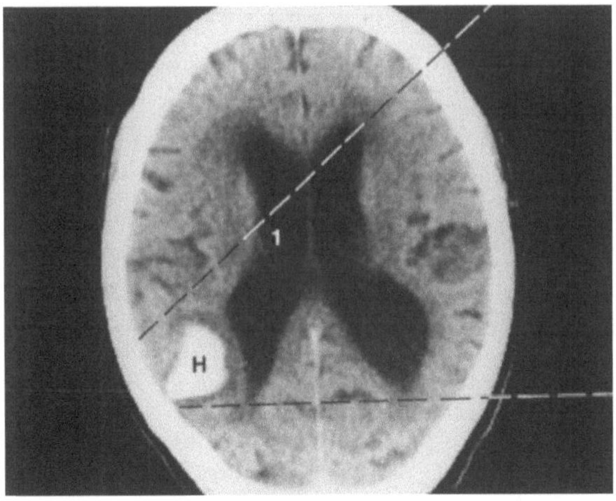

Fig. 422. Preoperative horizontal CT

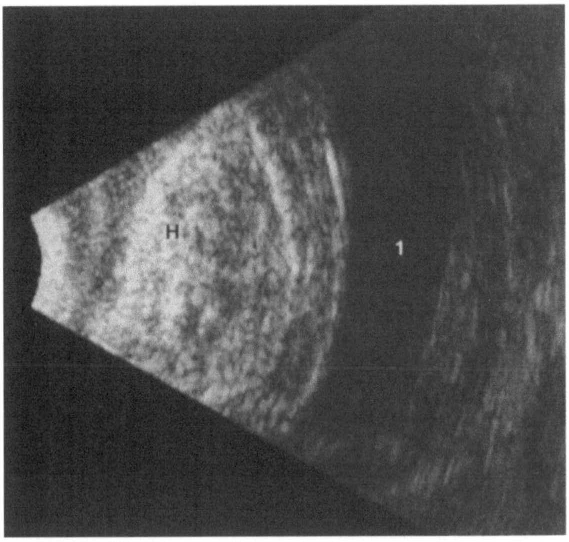

Fig. 423. Preoperative horizontal US. DRF 100, IOP probe, 7.5 MHz

1 Left lateral ventricle
2 Catheter in hematoma cavity
C Empty hematoma cavity
H Hematoma

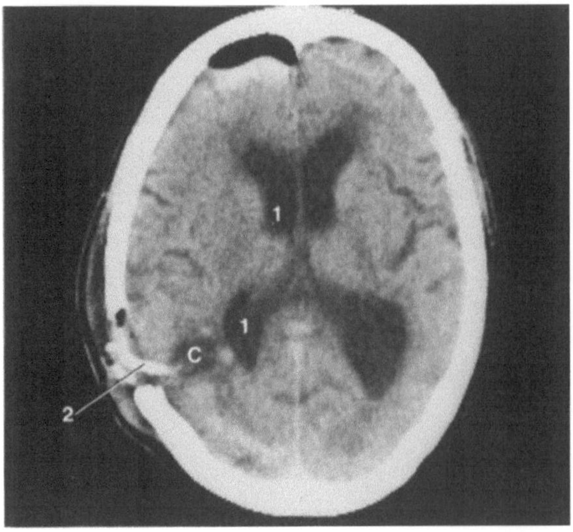

Fig. 424. Postoperative horizontal CT

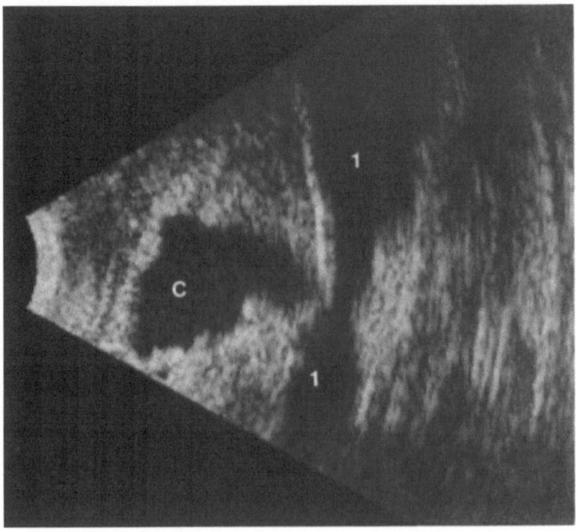

Fig. 425. Postoperative horizontal US. DRF 100, IOP probe, 7.5 MHz

CASE 95 (Figs. 426-428)

Hypertensive left frontotemporal hemorrhage in a 77-year-old man. US-guided endoscopic evacuation (consecutive technique) was done through a left frontal burrhole.

Fig. 427 shows the mostly hyperechoic mass before the start of evacuation. By removing the endoscope after partial evacuation, and inserting the small intraoperative US probe into the burrhole, the partly empty cavity can be visualized together with the remaining clot.

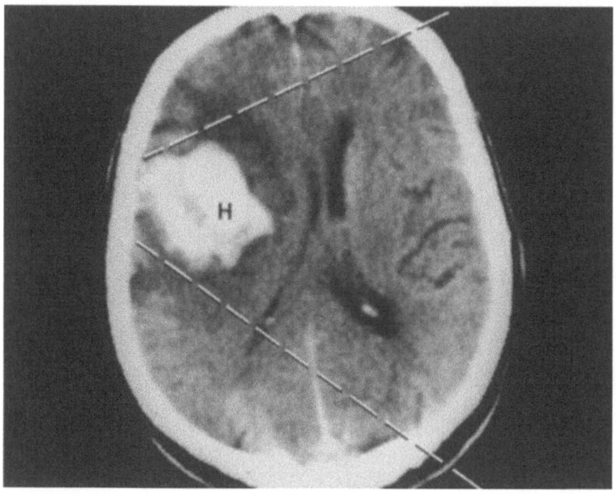

Fig. 426. Horizontal CT

C Cavity after evacuation of hematoma
H Hematoma
R Residual hematoma

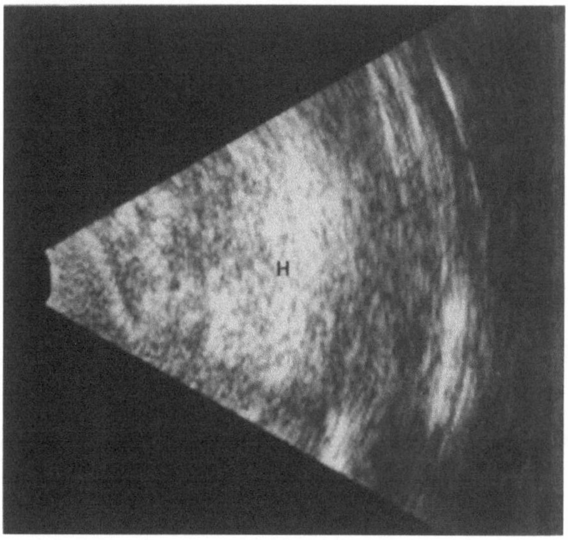

Fig. 427. Horizontal US. DRF 100, IOP probe, 5 MHz

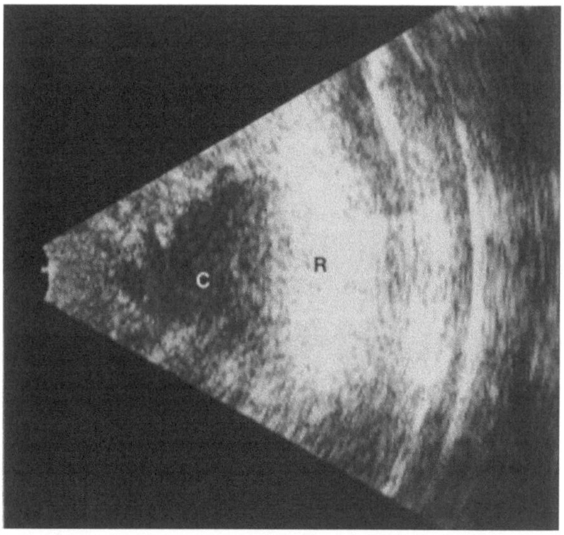

Fig. 428. Horizontal US. DRF 100, IOP probe, 5 MHz

CASE 96 (Figs. 429-431)

Temporooccipital hematoma in a 77-year-old woman. US-guided endoscopic evacuation (consecutive technique) was done through a burrhole over the lesion.

Fig. 430 shows the hyperechoic clot before evacuation. Fig. 431 shows an intraoperative control image revealing partial evacuation of the hematoma.

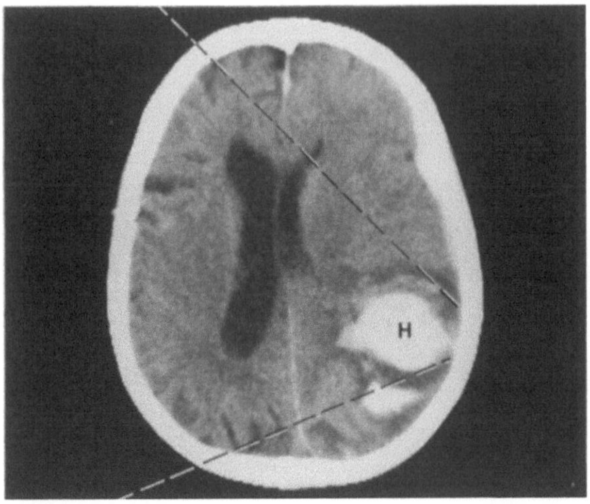

Fig. 429. Horizontal CT

C Cavity after evacuation of hematoma
H Hematoma
R Residual hematoma

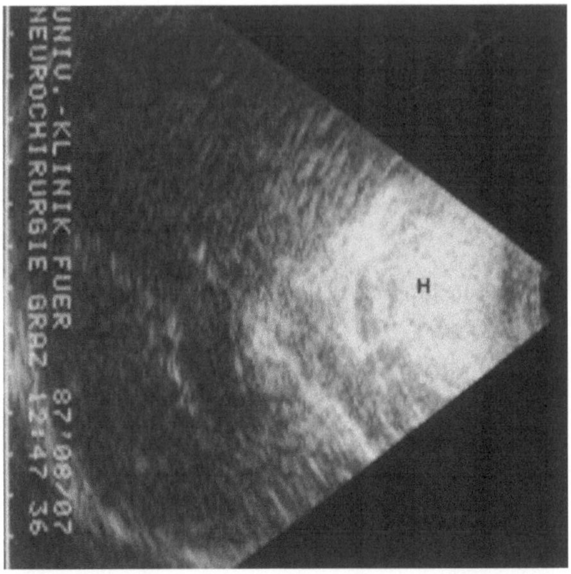

Fig. 430. Horizontal US. DRF 100, GPS probe, 5 MHz

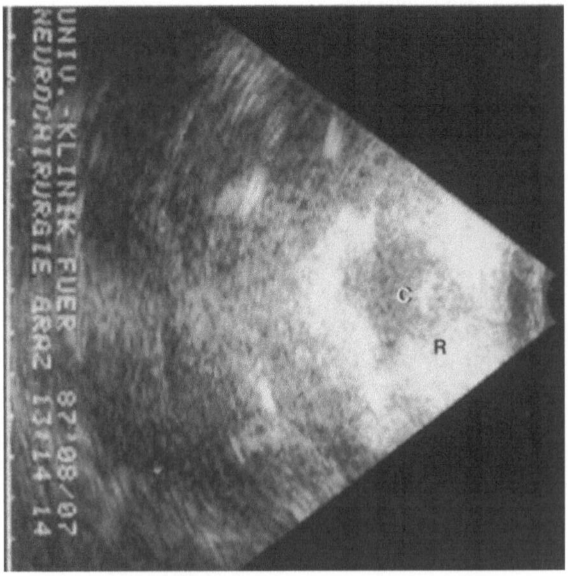

Fig. 431. Horizontal US. DRF 100, GPS probe, 5 MHz

Endoscopic Biopsy of Cystic Brain Tumors

CASE 97 (Figs. 432–441)

Anaplastic cystic astrocytoma in a 55-year-old woman. Since the patient was suffering only minor weakness of the left extremities, US-guided cyst drainage and endoscopic biopsy (consecutive technique) were carried out as a first step through a parietal burrhole.

The sequence of sagittal US images (Figs. 439–441) shows the hypoechoic cyst before (Fig. 439) and after (Fig. 441) evacuation. The channel of approach with the endoscope can be seen on the magnification (Fig. 440) of the US control and on the postoperative CT (Fig. 438), which also shows the shrunken cyst (cf. preoperative CT, Fig. 437).

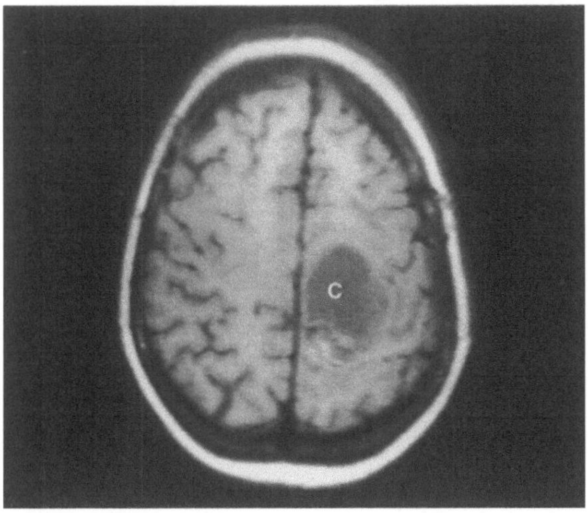

Fig. 432. Horizontal MRI

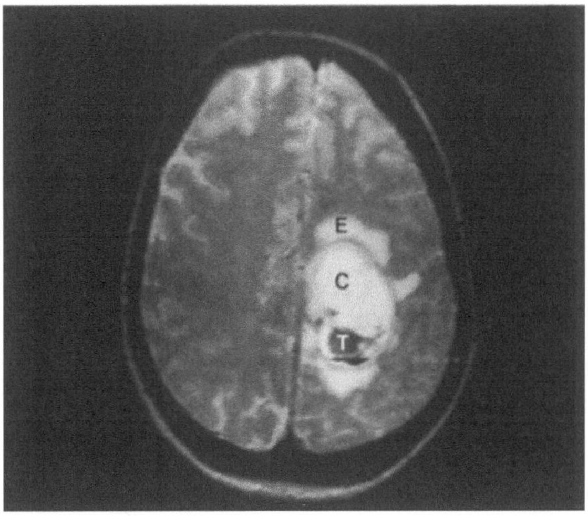

Fig. 433. Horizontal MRI

C Cystic part of tumor
E Edema
T Solid part of tumor

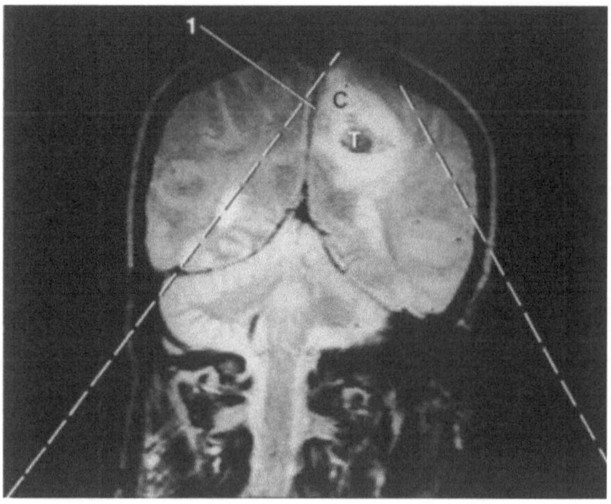

Fig. 434. Coronal MRI

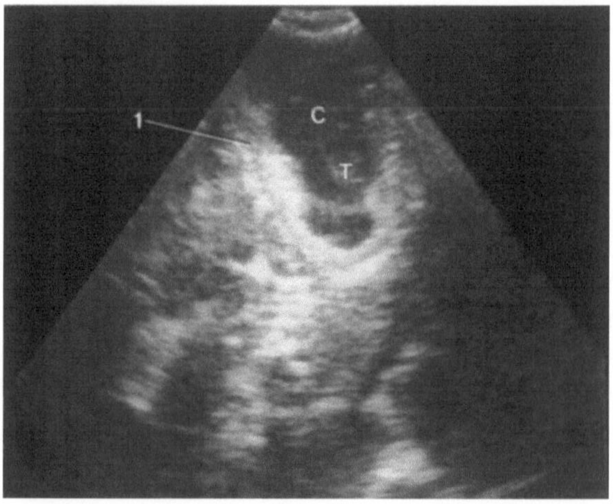

Fig. 435. Coronal US through right parietal burrhole. DRF 100, GPS probe, 5 MHz

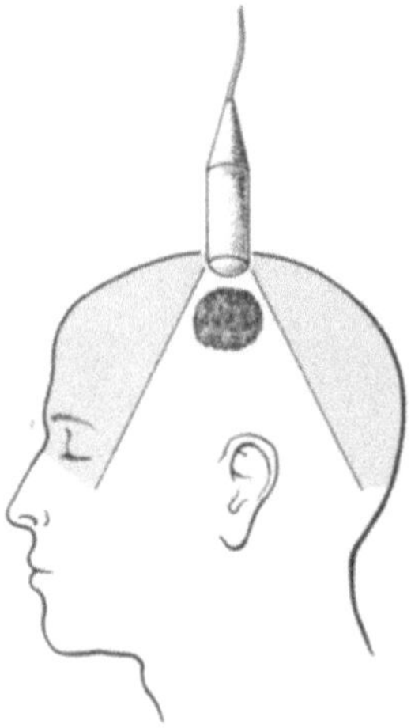

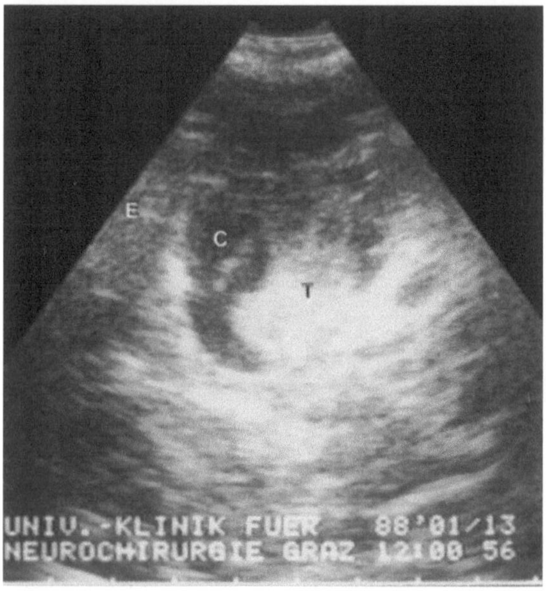

Fig. 436. Sagittal US. DRF 100, GPS probe, 5 MHz (see schema)

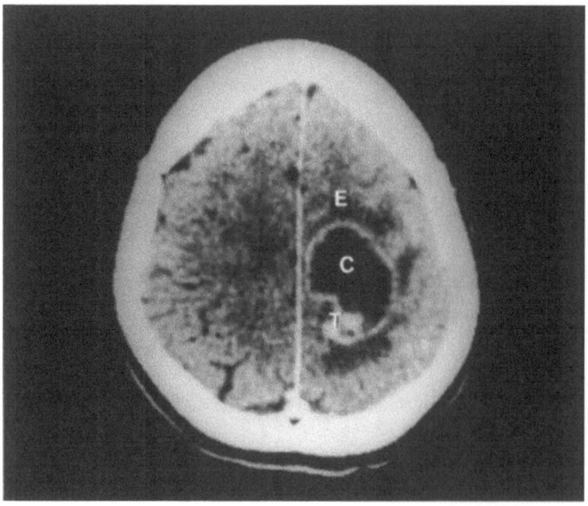

Fig. 437. Horizontal CT

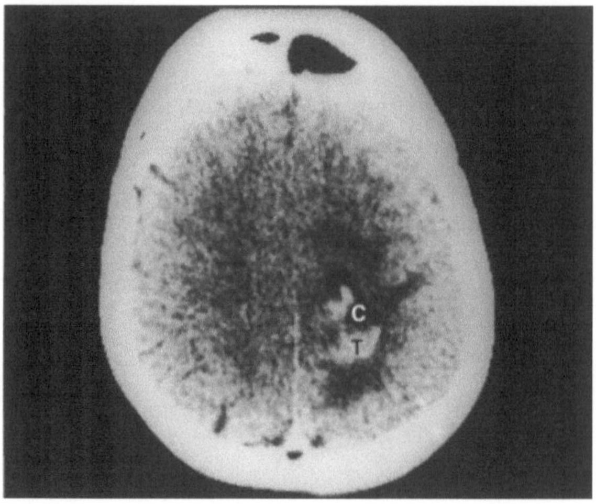

Fig. 438. Postoperative horizontal CT

1 Interhemispheric space
C Cystic part of tumor
E Edema
T Solid part of tumor
* Pathway of endoscope

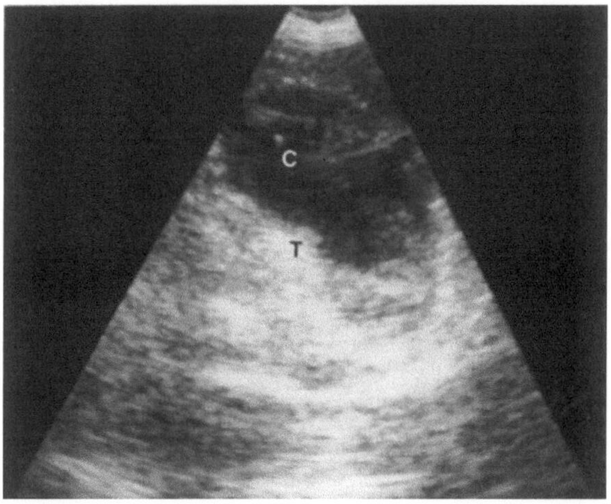

Fig. 439

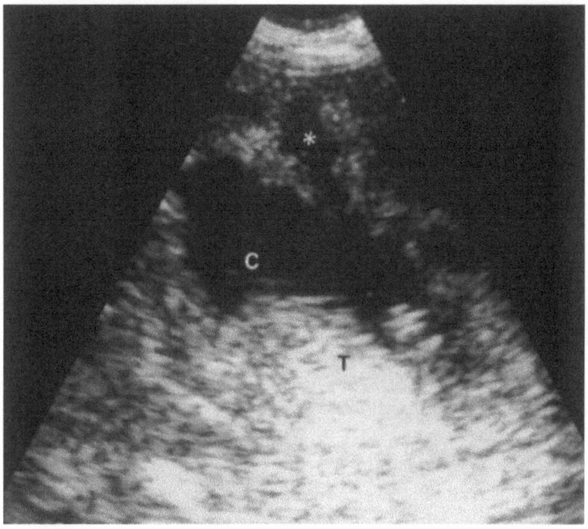

Fig. 440

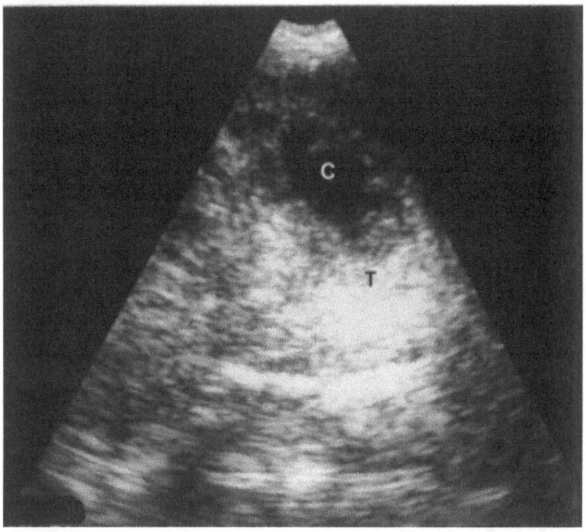

Fig. 441

Figs. 439-441. Sagittal US showing the relation between the cystic and solid parts of the tumor in slightly different planes. DRF 100, IOP probe, 5 MHz

CASE 98 (Figs. 442–444)

Cystic left frontal tumor in a 52-year-old man. US-guided drainage of the cyst and endoscopic biopsy (consecutive technique) of the cyst wall were performed through a left frontal burrhole. Histology revealed a metastasis from pulmonary carcinoma.

Fig. 444 shows the postoperative CT control with the shrunken cyst.

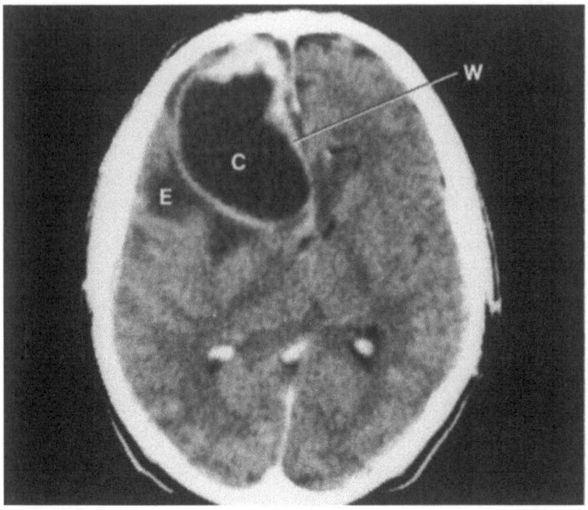

Fig. 442. Preoperative horizontal CT

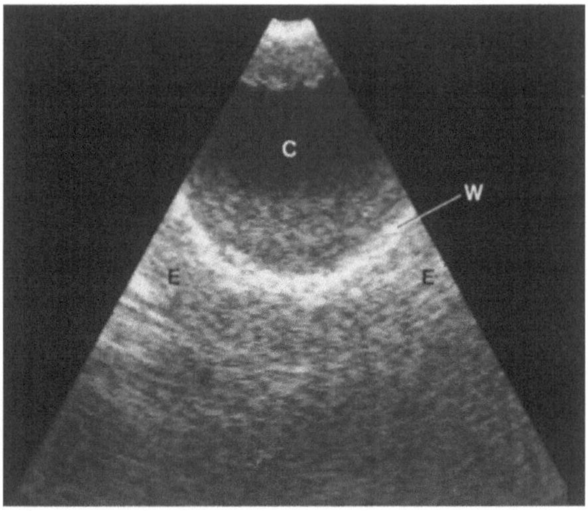

Fig. 443. Sagittal US. DRF 100, IOP probe, 5 MHz

C Cystic part of tumor
E Edema
W Cyst wall
* Catheter

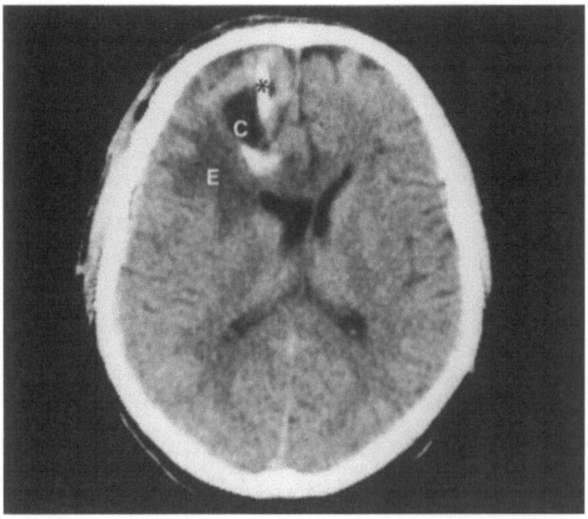

Fig. 444. Postoperative horizontal CT

CASE 99 (Figs. 445, 446)

A *left frontal cystic tumor* in a 54-year-old man operated upon by endoscopy (consecutive technique) via a left frontal burrhole.

MRI (Fig. 445) shows a huge cyst with a frontolateral solid part reaching into the cyst cavity. The parasagittal US (Fig. 446) section shows the hypoechoic cyst. The shape and thickness of the cyst wall cannot be clearly identified. From the left side, the solid tumor nodule looks into the cavity. On operation, the medial wall of the cyst turned out to have a maximal thickness of 1 mm and to have practically no contact with the surrounding brain tissue, so that it was floating as a membrane between the brain tissue on the medial side and the solid tumor nodule on the lateral side. The solid tumor nodule was resected through the endoscope. Histological investigation revealed a glioblastoma.

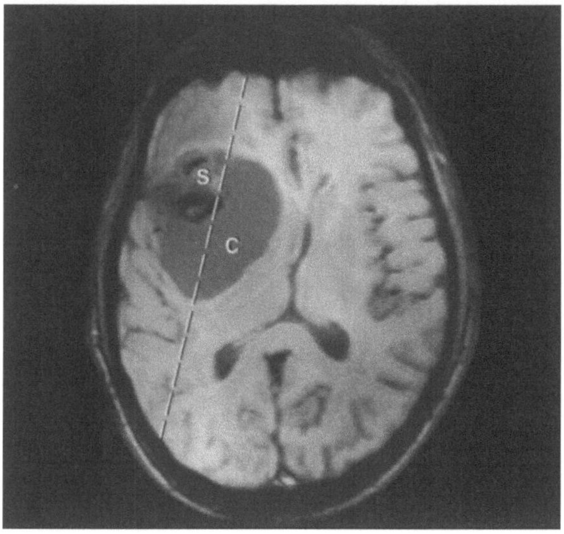

Fig. 445. Horizontal MRI. Stippled line = sector plane for Fig. 446; see also schema

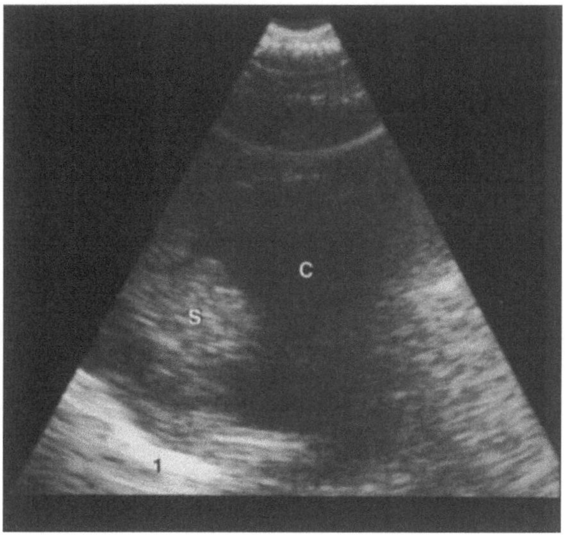

Fig. 446. Sagittal US. DRF 100, IOP probe, 5 MHz

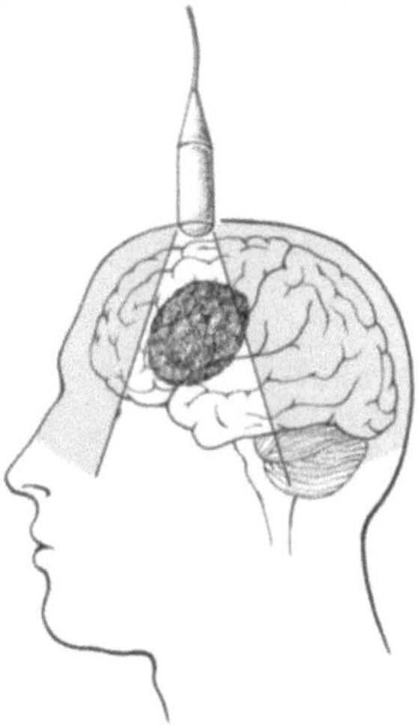

1 Frontal skull base
C Cystic part of tumor
S Solid part of tumor

CASE 100 (Figs. 447, 448)

Cystic anaplastic astrocytoma in a 53-year-old woman. Endoscopic biopsy (consecutive technique) and drainage of the cyst were carried out through a left parietooccipital burrhole under US guidance.

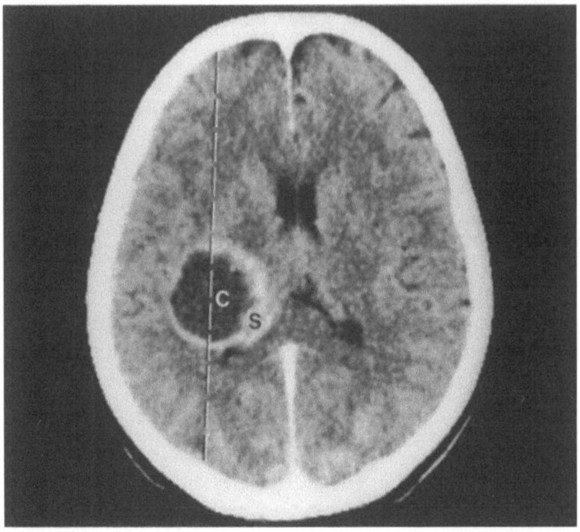

Fig. 447. Horizontal CT. Stippled line = sector plane for Fig. 448; see also schema

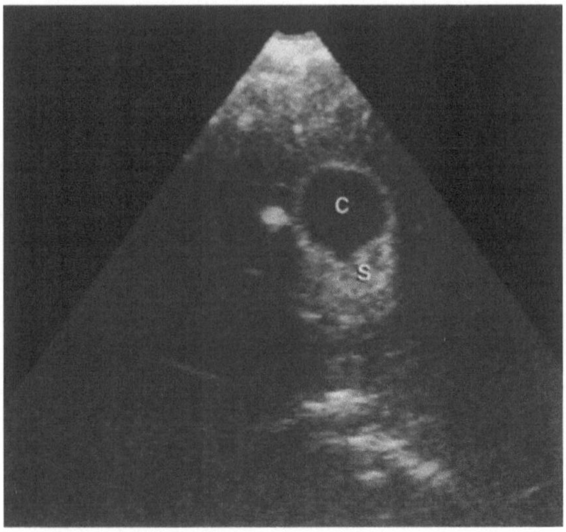

Fig. 448. Sagittal US. DRF 100, GPS probe, 5 MHz

C Cystic part of tumor
S Solid part of tumor

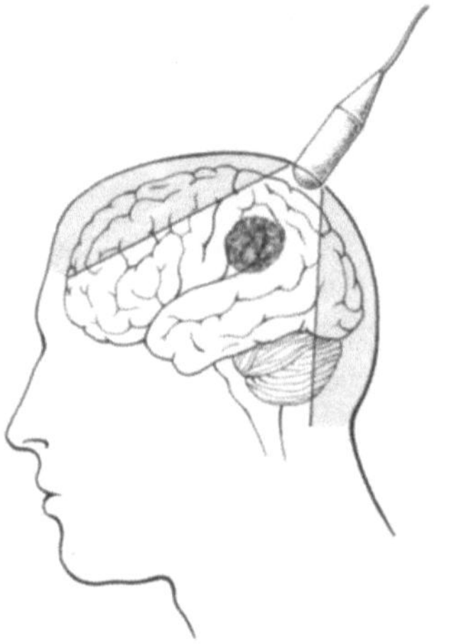

CASE 101 (Figs. 449-451)

Cystic glioma in the temporal region of a 46-year-old woman. US-guided drainage of the cyst and endoscopic biopsy (consecutive technique) were carried out through a left temporal burrhole. After transendoscopic tumor resection, a catheter was placed into the emptied cavity and connected to a subcutaneous Ommaya reservoir.

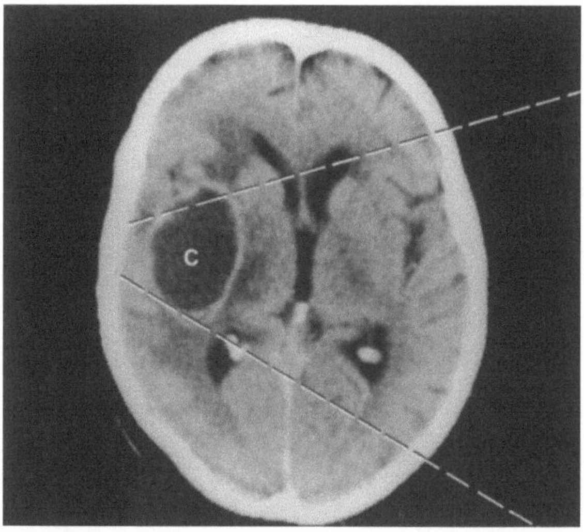

Fig. 449. Preoperative horizontal CT

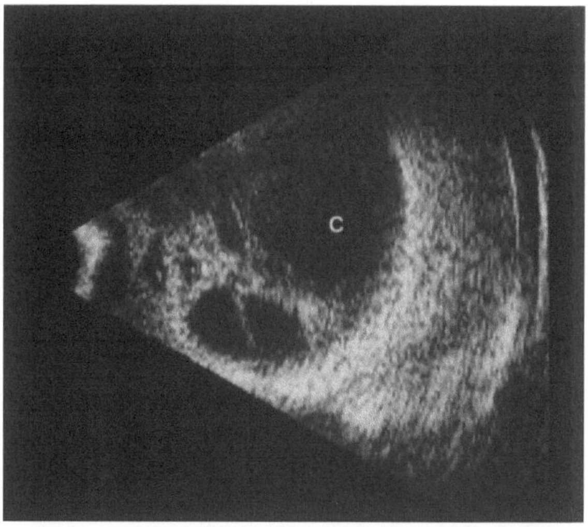

Fig. 450. Horizontal US. DRF 100, IOP probe, 7.5 MHz

C Cystic part of tumor
S Solid part of tumor
* Tip of catheter
↗ Subgaleal Ommaya reservoir

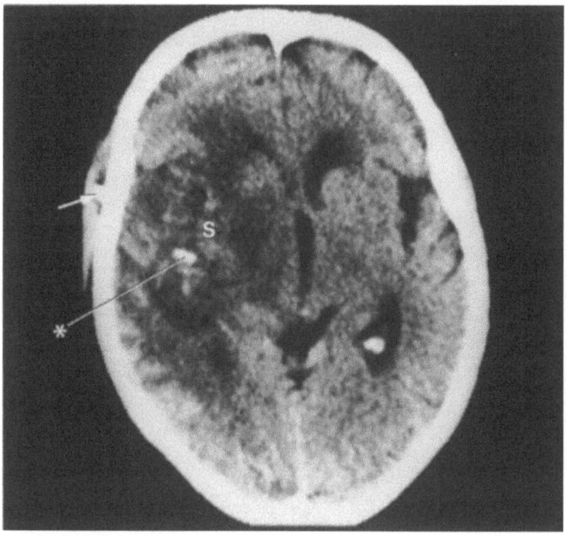

Fig. 451. Postoperative horizontal CT

US-Guided Biopsy of Brain Tumors

CASE 102 (Figs. 452-455)

US-guided puncture and biopsy of a deep-seated *left temporal cystic fibrillary astrocytoma* in a 14-year-old boy operated upon via left temporal craniotomy, using the simultaneous US-guided biopsy technique.

At the moment of the entry of the needle into the roof of the large cyst (↗, Fig. 453), the wall of the cyst is pushed inward. In Fig. 454, the needle's tip has entered the lumen of the cyst. The metal of the tip causes a shadow artifact (➧). As fluid is removed, the cyst shrinks, and the needle is retracted again (Fig. 455).

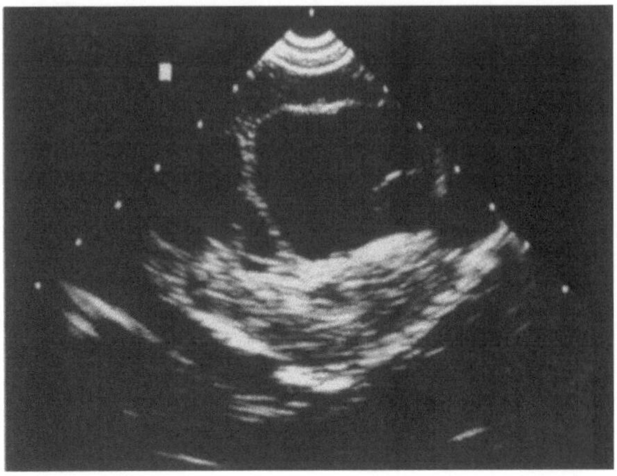

Fig. 452. Diagonal US during puncture of cystic astrocytoma. ATL, ADR, 3.5 MHz

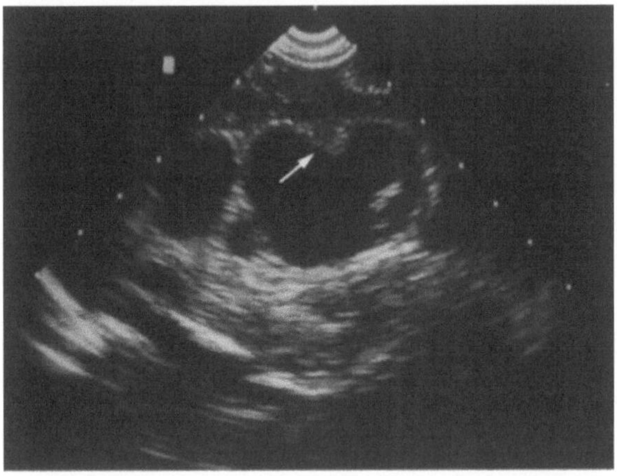

Fig. 453. Diagonal US during puncture of cystic astrocytoma. ATL, ADR, 3.5 MHz

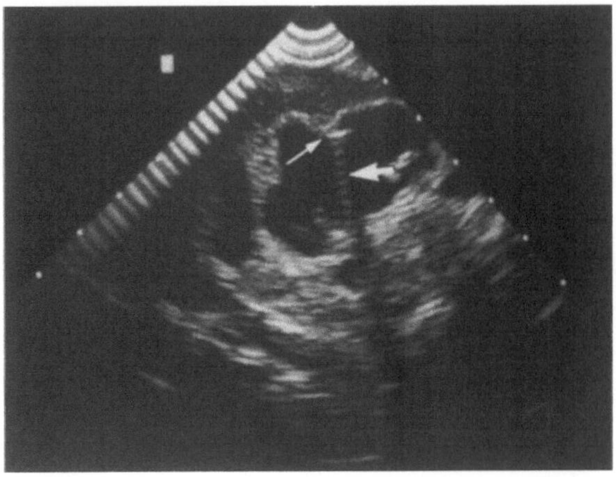

Fig. 454. Diagonal US during puncture of cystic astrocytoma. ATL, ADR, 3.5 MHz

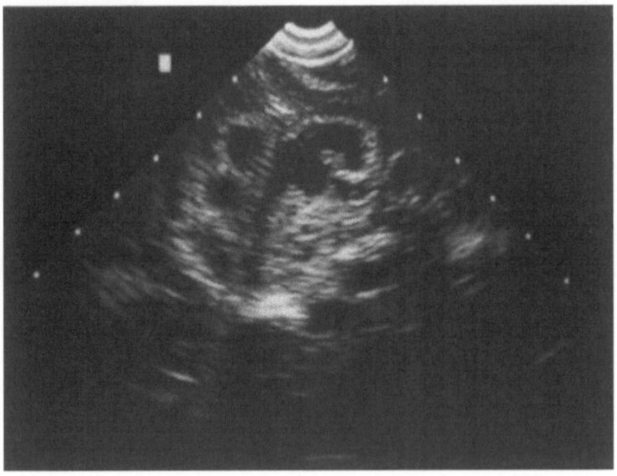

Fig. 455. Diagonal US during puncture of cystic astrocytoma. ATL, ADR, 3.5 Mhz

CASE 103 (Figs. 456–458)

US-guided biopsy (consecutive technique) via a right occipital burrhole: *glioblastoma* in a 36-year-old man.

The very slightly hyperechoic tumor can be recognized mainly because of the more markedly hyperechoic border. Fig. 457 shows the target point and the distance to target (distance between white cross and black cross). Fig. 458 shows a US control image taken 7 min after biopsy: the hyperechoic trace from surface to target point is due to minor oozing in the puncture channel.

C Border of tumor
F Falx
T Center of tumor

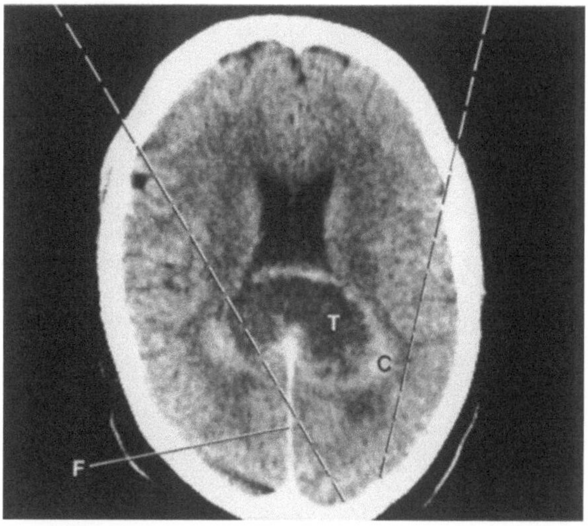

Fig. 456. Horizontal CT

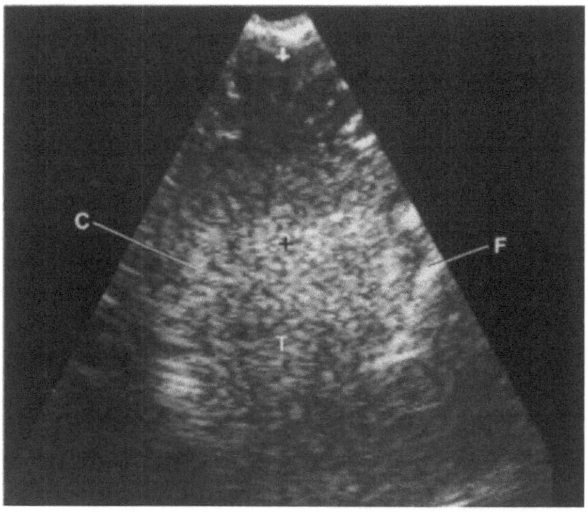

Fig. 457. Horizontal US. DRF 100, IOP probe, 5 MHz

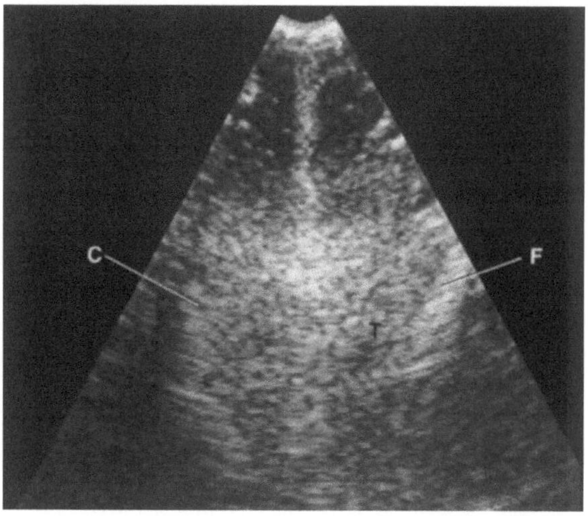

Fig. 458. Horizontal US. DRF 100, IOP probe, 5 MHz

CASE 104 (Figs. 459–461)

Thalamic oligoastrocytoma in a 7-year-old girl. US-guided endoscopic inspection of the ventricular tumor surface and biopsy (consecutive technique) were performed through a right frontal burrhole.

For other examples of US-guided endoscopic biopsy, see pp. 159–165.

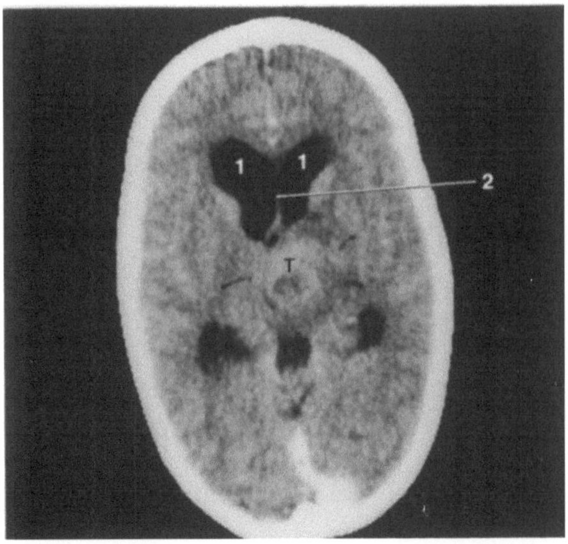

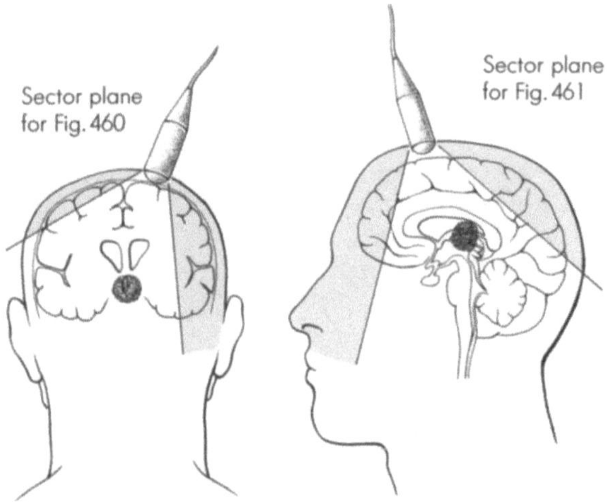

Fig. 459. Horizontal CT

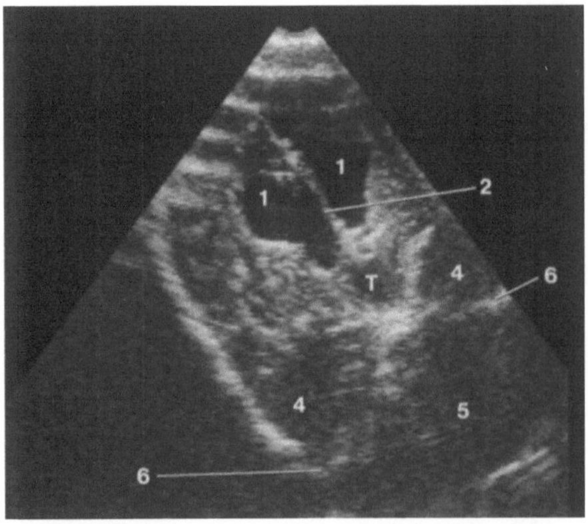

Fig. 460. Coronal US. DRF 100, GPS probe, 5 MHz

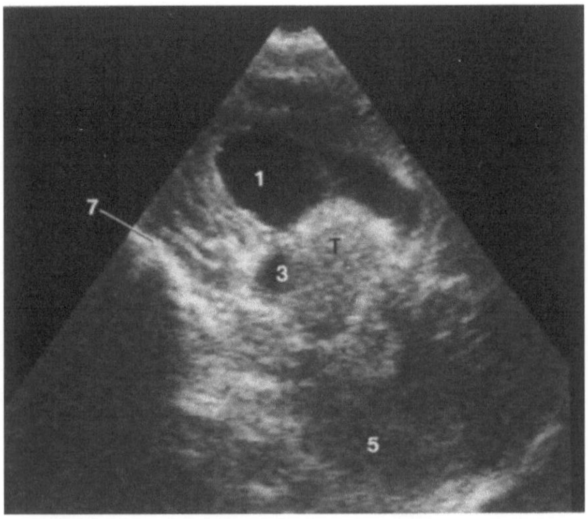

Fig. 461. Sagittal US. DRF 100, GPS probe, 5 MHz

1 Lateral ventricle
2 Septum pellucidum
3 Third ventricle
4 Middle cranial fossa
5 Posterior cranial fossa
6 Pyramidal edge
7 Frontal skull base
T Tumor

US-Guided Drainage of Brain Abscesses

CASE 105 (Figs. 462-466)

Abscess in the right operculum frontale of a 40-year-old man. The abscess, which had occurred after removal of a malignant meningioma and reoperation including removal of the bone flap, was punctured percutaneously under US guidance (simultaneous technique).

Figs. 464-466 show the shrinkage and collapse of the capsule during aspiration of the content through the introduced needle. On these US images, the capsule of the abscess is markedly hyperechoic, while the surrounding edema is slightly hyperechoic. The center of the abscess, hypodense on CT, displays higher echo intensity than does the brain tissue, apart from the edematous area. Toward the capsule can be seen a markedly hypoechoic ring which disappears during drainage.

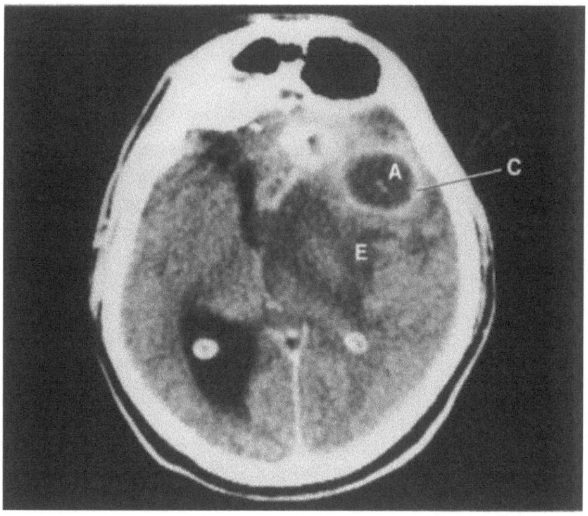

Fig. 462. Horizontal CT

A Abscess
C Capsule
E Edema
N Needle

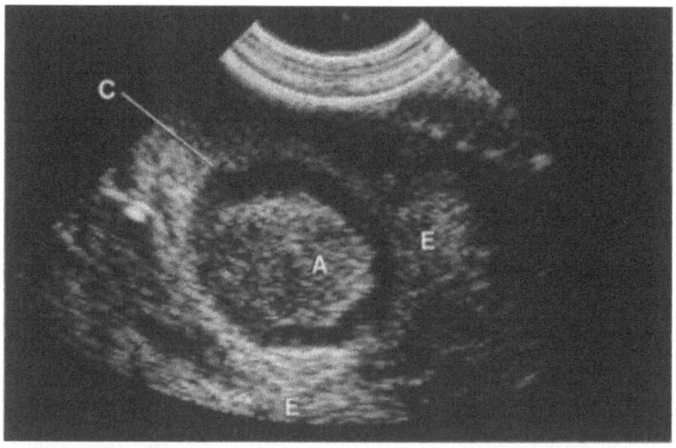

Fig. 463. Highly magnified US. NS, 5 MHz

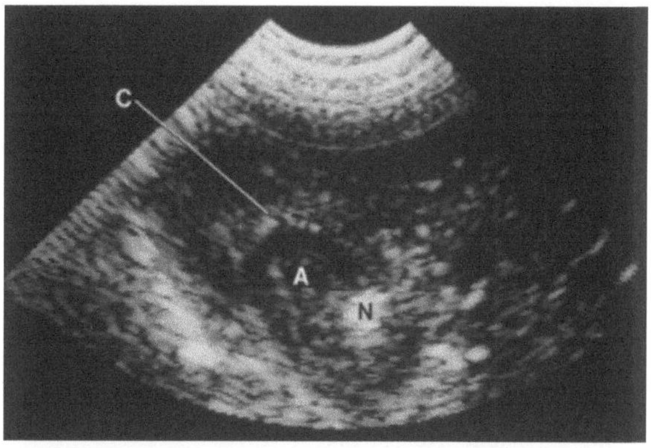

Fig. 464. Highly magnified US. NS, 5 MHz

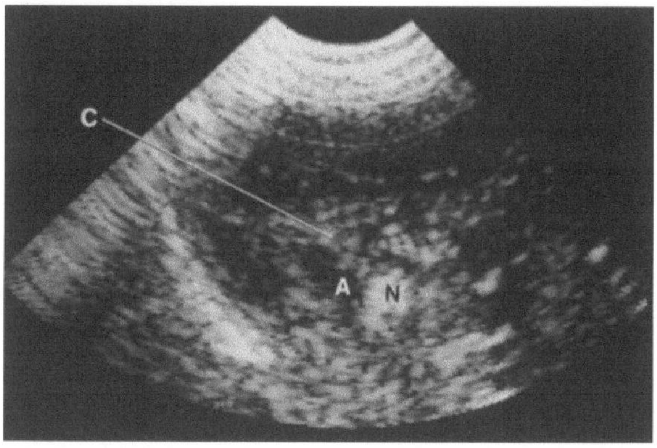

Fig. 465. Highly magnified US. NS, 5 MHz

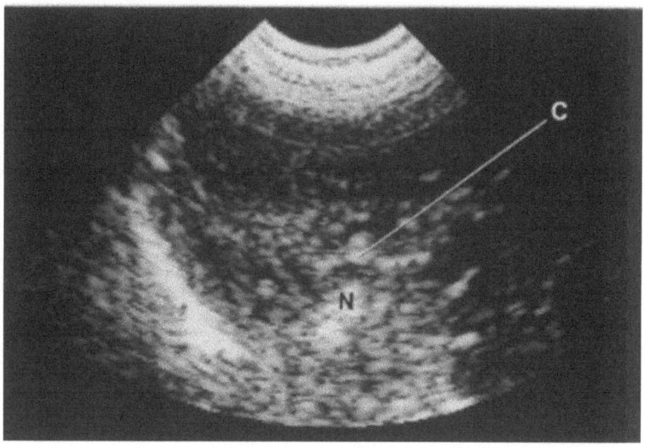

Fig. 466. Highly magnified US. NS, 5 MHz

References

1a. Auer LM, Holzer P, Ascher PW, Heppner F (1988) Endoscopic Neurosurgery. Acta Neurochir 90: 1-14

1b. Avecilla LS (1979) The physics and instrumentation of diagnostic ultrasound: a review, part I. Medical Ultrasound 3: 11-15

2. Baker ML, Dalrymple GV (1978) Biological effects of diagnostic ultrasound: a review. Radiology 126: 479-483

3. Bejar R, Cohen RW, Ekpoudia I, James HE, Gluck L (1985) Real time ultrasound diagnosis of hemorrhagic pathological conditions in the posterior fossa of preterm infants. Neurosurgery 16: 281-289

4. Berger MS (1985) Ultrasound guided stereotactic biopsy using the Diasonics neuro-biopsy device for deep seated intracranial lesions. Presented at the Annual Meeting of the American Association of Neurological Surgeons, Atlanta, Georgia, April 21-25

5. Brown FD, Rachlin JR, Rubin JM, Fessler RG, Smith LJ, Schaible KL (1984) Ultrasound-guided stereotaxis. Neurosurgery 15: 162-164

6. Chandler WF, Knake JE (1983) Intraoperative use of ultrasound in neurosurgery. Clin Neurosurg 31: 550-563

7. Chandler WF, Knake JE, McGillicuddy JE, Lillehei KO, Silver TM (1982) Intraoperative use of real time ultrasonography in neurosurgery. J Neurosurg 57: 157-163

8. Corrales M, Del Villar S, Hevia R, Saez M (1983) Sonography of the posterior fossa. AJNR 4: 665-667

9. Curie J, Curie P (1880) Sur l'electricite polaire dans cristaux hemiedres a face inclinees. Compt Rend Seances Acad Sci 91: 383

10. Dohrmann GJ, Rubin JM (1981) Use of ultrasound in neurosurgical operations: a preliminary report. Surg Neurol 16: 362-366

11. Dohrmann GJ, Rubin JM (1985) Dynamic intraoperative imaging and instrumentation of brain and spinal cord using ultrasound. Neurol Clin 3: 425-437

12. Dussik KT (1942) Über die Möglichkeit hochfrequente mechanische Schwingungen als diagnostisches Hilfsmittel zu verwerten. Z Neurol Psychiatr 174: 153-168

13. Duthel R, Portafaix M (1986) Biopsies echoguidees des tumeurs cerebrales. Neurochirurgie 32: 547-552

14. Enzmann DR, Britt RH, Lyons B, Buxton TL, Wilson DA (1981) Experimental study of high-resolution ultrasound imaging of hemorrhage, bone fragments and foreign bodies in head trauma. J Neurosurg 54: 304-309

15. Enzmann DR, Britt RH, Lyons BE, Buxton JL, Wilson DA (1981) Natural history of experimental intracerebral hemorrhage: sonography, computed tomography and neuropathology. AJNR 2: 517-526

16. Enzmann DR, Britt RH, Lyons B, Caroll B, Wilson DA, Buxton J (1982) High resolution ultrasound evaluation of experimental brain abscess evolution: comparison with CT and neuropathology. Radiology 142: 95-102

17. Enzmann DR, Lyons BE, Caroll B, Placone RC, Rasor J, Britt RH, Buxton J, Wilson D (1982) Experimental brain abscess: enhanced sonography and pathological correlation. AJNR 3: 41-45

18. Enzmann DR, Murphy Irwin K, Marshall WH, Silverberg GD, Britt RH, Hanbery JW (1984) Intraoperative sonography through a burrhole guide for brain biopsy. AJNR 5: 243-246

19. Enzmann DR, Murphy Irwin K, Ine M, Silverberg GM, Hanbery JW (1984) Case report. Intraoperative and outpatient echoencephalography through a burrhole. Neuroradiology 26: 57-59

20. Enzmann DR, Wheat R, Marshall WH, Bird R, Murphy-Irwin K, Karbon K, Hanbery J, Silverberg GD, Britt RH, Shuer L (1985) Tumors of the central nervous system studied by computed tomography and ultrasound. Radiology 154: 393-399

21. French LA, Wild JJ, Neal D (1950) Detection of cerebral tumors by ultrasonic pulses. Pilot studies on postmortem material. Cancer 3: 705-708

22. Gilsbach JM, Hassler WE (1984) Intraoperative Doppler and real-time sonography in neurosurgery. Neurosurg Rev 7: 199-208

23. Gooding GAW, Boggan JE, Bank WO, Beglin B, Edwards MSB (1981) Sonography of the adult brain through surgical defects. AJNR 2: 449-452

24. Gooding GAW, Edwards MSB, Rabkin AE, Powers SK (1983) Intraoperative real-time ultrasound in the localization of intracranial neoplasms. Radiology 146: 459-462

25. Gooding GAW, Boggan JE, Weinstein PR (1984) Characterization of intracranial neoplasms by CT and intraoperative sonography. AJNR 5: 517-520

26. Gooding GAW, Boggan JE, Powers SK, Martin NA, Weinstein PR (1984) Neurosurgical sonography: intraoperative and postoperative imaging of the brain. AJNR 5: 521-525

27. Grode ML, Komaiko MS (1983) The role of intraoperative ultrasound in neurosurgery. Neurosurgery 12: 624-628

28. Havlice JF, Taenzer JC (1979) Medical ultrasonic imaging: an overview of principles and instrumentation. Proceedings of the IEEE 67 (4): 620-640

29. Helzer MV, Herold S (1983) Nachweis eines Hirntumorrezidivs durch Ultraschall. RO FO 138: 753-755

30. Hyodo A, Mizukami M, Tazawa T, Togashi I (1983) Intraoperative use of real time ultrasonography applied to aneurysm surgery. Neurosurgery 13: 642-645

31. Jurine N, Allard D, Portafaix M (1986) L'echographie cerebrale transfontanellaire. Neurochirurgie 32: 537-546

32. Knake JE, Silver TM, Chandler WF (1982) Intraoperative cranial sonography for neurosurgical procedures. Semin Ultrasound 3: 200-308

33. Knake JE, Chandler WF, McGillicuddy JE, Silver TM, Gabrielsen TO (1982) Intraoperative sonography for brain tumor localization and ventricular shunt placement. AJNR 3: 425-430
34. Knake JE, Chandler WF, McGillicuddy JE, Silver TM, Gabrielsen TO (1982) Intraoperative sonography for brain tumor localization and ventricular shunt placement. AJR 139: 733-738
35. Knake JE, Chandler WF, Gabrielsen TO, Latack JT, Gebarski SS (1984) Intraoperative sonographic delineation of low grade brain neoplasms defined poorly by computed tomography. Radiology 151: 735-739
36. Laing FC (1983) Commonly encountered artifacts in clinical ultrasound. Semin Ultrasound 4: 27-43
37. Lange SC, Howe JF, Shuman WP, Rogers JV (1982) Intraoperative ultrasound detection of metastatic tumors in the central cortex. Neurosurgery 11: 219-222
38. Latchaw RE, Gold LHA, More JS Jr, Payne JT (1977) The nonspecificity of absorption coefficients in the differentiation of solid tumors and cystic lesions. Radiology 125: 141-144
39. Leksell L (1958) Echoencephalography: midline echo from the pineal body as an index of pineal displacement. Acta Chir Scand 115: 255-259
40. Levene MI, Williams JL, Fawer C-L (1985) Ultrasound of the infant brain. Developmental Medicine No. 92, Spastics International Medical Publications, London
41. Liebeskind D, Bases R, Elequin F, Neubort S, Leifer R, Goldberg R, Koenigsberg M (1979) Diagnostic ultrasound: effects on the DNA and growth patterns of animal cells. Radiology 131: 177-184
42. Liebeskind D, Koenigsberg M, Koss L, Raventos C (1981) Morphological changes in the surface characteristics of cultured cells after exposure to diagnostic ultrasound. Radiology 138: 419-423
43. Machado HR, Pariente D, Hirsch E, Sauvegrain J, Hirsch JF (1986) L'echographie peroperatoire en neurochirurgie pediatrique (Experience sur une serie de 40 interventions) Neurochirurgie 32: 287-295
44. Martin AO (1984) Can ultrasound cause genetic damage? J Clin Ultrasound 12: 11-20
45. Masuzawa H, Kamitani H, Sato J et al. (1981) Intraoperative application of sector scanning electronic ultrasound in neurosurgery. Neurol Med Chir 21: 277-285
46. Merritt CRB, Covlon R, Connolly E (1983) Intraoperative neurosurgical ultrasound: transdural and transfontanellar applications. Radiology 148: 513-517
47. Norman D, Stevens EA, Wing SD, Levin V, Newton TH (1978) Quantitative aspects of contrast enhancement in cranial computed tomography. Radiology 129: 683-688
48. Oldendorf WH (1980) Ultrasound. In: Oldendorf WH (ed) The quest for an image of brain. Raven Press, New York, pp. 49-59
49. Olislagers-De Slegte RGM, Smeets RWMC, Valk J, Crezee F (1984) Ultrasound in follow up of the postoperative brain. Neuroradiology 26: 267-272
50. Pigadas A, Thompson JR, Grube GL (1981) Normal infant brain anatomy: correlated real-time sonograms and brain specimens. AJNR 2: 339-344
51. Portafaix M, Motuo-Fosto MJ (1986) Surveillance echographique postoperatoire. Neurochirurgie 32: 568-571
52. Reizine D, George B, Rey A, Roux FX, Riche MC, Merland JJ (1984) L'echographie peroperatoire en neurochirurgie. Ann Radiol (Paris) 27: 401-404
53. Rogers JV, Shuman WP, Hirsch JH, Lange SC, Howe JF, Burchiel K (1984) Intraoperative neurosonography: application and technique. AJNR 5: 755-760
54. Roux FX, Ben Simon JL, Rey A, George B, Melki JP, Reizine D, Cophignon J (1983) Utilisation de l'ultrasonographie en temps reel en neurochirurgie. Neurochirurgie 29: 31-35
55. Roux FX, Constans JP, Cioloca C, Meder JF, Sermet A (1986) Ultrasonographie en temps reel en neurochirurgie. Ponction d'une cavite hypoechogene intracraniene. Neurochirurgie 32: 553-558
56. Rubin JM, Dohrmann GJ (1982) Use of ultrasonically guided probes and catheters in neurosurgery. Surg Neurol 18: 143-148
57. Rubin JM, Dohrmann GJ (1983) Intraoperative neurosurgical ultrasound in the localisation and characterisation of intracranial masses. Radiology 148: 519-524
58. Rubin JM, Mirfakhraee M, Duda EE, Dohrmann GJ, Brown F (1980) Intraoperative ultrasound examination of the brain. Radiology 137: 831-832
59. Rubin JM, Dohrmann GJ, Greenberg M, Duda EE, Beezold C (1982) Intraoperative sonography of meningeomas. AJNR 3: 305-308
60. Shkolnik A, McLone DG (1981) Intraoperative real time ultrasonic guidance of ventricular shunt placement in infants. Radiology 141: 515-517
61. Shkolnik A, Tomita T, Raimondi AJ, Hahn YS, McLone DG (1983) Work in progress. Intraoperative neurosurgical ultrasound: localization of brain tumors in infants and children. Radiology 148: 525-527
62. Sjolander U, Lindgren PG, Hugosson R (1983) Ultrasound sector scanning for the localization and biopsy of intracerebral lesions. J Neurosurg 58: 7-10
63. Slegte RGM de, Valk J, Broere G, Waal F de (1986) Further experience with ultrasound examinations in the postoperative brain. Acta Neurochir 81: 106-112
64. Sommer FG, Filly RA, Minton MJ (1979) Acoustic shadowing due to refractive and reflective effects. Am J Roentgenol 132: 973-977
65. Tsutsumi Y, Andoh Y, Inove N (1982) Ultrasound guided biopsy for deep-seated brain tumors. J Neurosurg 57: 164-167
66. Tsutsumi Y, Andoh Y, Matsutani M, Sai A (1985) New technique for removable implantation of radionuclides in central nervous system neoplasm by ultrasonic guidance. Surg Neurol 23: 520-524
67. Voorhies RM, Engel I, Gamache FW, Patterson RH, Fraser RAR, Lavyne MH, Schneider M (1983) Intraoperative localization of subcortical brain tumors: further experience with B-mode real time sector scanning. Neurosurgery 12: 189-194

Subject Index

abscess 97, 169
acoustic impedance 4
acoustic lens 3, 4
acoustic neurinoma 83, 84
anaplastic oligoastrocytoma 26
anaplastic oligodendroglioma 44
aneurysm 108, 110, 112, 114, 116
  giant 116
  internal carotid artery 110, 112
  ophthalamic artery 114
  pericallosal artery 116
  thrombosed giant 116
annular array 5
anterior cranial fossa 55
aqueduct stenosis 100
arachnoid cyst 96
Archimedes screw 154
arteriovenous malformation 108, 118, 120
arteriovenous malformation trigonal 118
artifact 6
astrocytoma
  anaplastic 29, 32, 33, 34, 35, 159, 164
  fibrillary 166
  grade 2 28, 80, 136
  grade 3 31
  pilocytic 25
  polycystic 30
attenuation 6
axial resolution 6
AVM nidus 118, 121

basal cistern 110
basal ganglia 100
biological effect 7
biopsy 154, 166, 167
brain abscess 97, 98, 169
brainstem 14, 59
burrhole evacuation 154

caudate nucleus 34, 48, 81
cavernous hemangioma 94
cavum vergae 81
ceramic crystal 3
cerebellar hemisphere 90, 137
cerebellar lobuli 137
cerebellum 20, 30, 121
choroid plexus 12, 77
cisterna magna 44, 77
clivus 20, 53, 55, 61, 85, 89, 121
collateral fissure 27
columnae fornicis 81
contrecoup lesion 107
coronal view 18
corpus callosum 17, 46, 53, 111, 136
craniopharyngioma 78

crura cerebri 40, 95, 111
crystal 3, 4, 5
cuneus 61
cyst 163
  drainage 159, 162
cystic glioma 165, 166
cystic metastasis 66, 70
cystic tumor 159, 162, 163, 164, 165, 166

drainage 155, 159, 162
dura 10
dysgerminoma 95

echo 3
echointensity 5
echotomogram 4
edema 24, 47, 55, 65
electromagnetic wave 3
endoscopic biopsy 155, 159, 162, 164, 165, 168
endoscopic evacuation 155, 156, 157, 158
endoscopy 163, 168
ependymoma 45, 82

foramen magnum 35, 44
foramen of Monro 28, 107
fourth ventricle 14, 20, 58, 62, 85, 109, 111, 121
frontal fontanelle 144, 145
frontal skull base 67

ganglioglioma 46
gelfoam 149
glioblastoma 36, 37, 38, 39, 40, 41, 163
glioma 24
gray scale 4
gyrus, cingulate 17, 46, 136
gyrus, inferior temporal 27
gyrus, parahippocampal 27
gyrus, postcentral 132
gyrus, precentral 132
gyrus rectus 109, 111, 113

hemangioblastoma 87, 88, 89
hematoma
  basal ganglionic 125, 126
  cavity 156, 157, 158
  cerebellar 91
  of choroid plexus 127
  chronic intracerebral 128, 130
  chronic subdural 90
  intracerebral 122, 156, 158
  intraventricular 127
  residual 157, 158
  traumatic 123
hemorrhage hypertensive 125, 127
hippocampus 20

horizontal view 12
hydrocephalus 99, 145
  occlusive 100, 106
  posthemorrhagic 104, 144
  posttraumatic 107
hypoechoic 5
  cyst 163

interface 4
interhemispheric fissure 14
interhemispheric space 12
internal acoustic meatus 83, 85
interpeduncular cistern 58, 109, 111
interpeduncular fossa 113
intraoperative control 147

landmarks for orientation 11
lateral resolution 6
lesser sphenoid wing 31

medulla oblongata 30
medulloblastoma 79
megahertz 6
meningioma 47
  cavernous sinus 59, 60
  cerebellopontine angle 86
  convexity 48, 50, 52
  falx 139, 142
  frontal 54
  lateral sphenoid wing 57
  of Meckel's cavity 58, 59
  medial sphenoid wing 56
  olfactory groove 55
  parasagittal 50, 52
  en plaque 60
  pyramidal 58
  temporoparietal 48
  tentorial 61, 62, 64
metastasis 65, 148, 150, 151
  from colon carcinoma 137
  from hypernephroma 75
  from melanoma 74
  from osteosarcoma 70
  from pulmonary carcinoma 66, 72, 76, 132, 133, 134, 162
  from renal cell carcinoma 135, 138
  from unknown origin 69
midbrain 109, 113
middle cranial fossa 55

needle aspiration 154, 169
needle biopsy 155, 166, 167
nidus of arteriovenous malformation 118, 121

oligoastrocytoma 168
oligodendroglioma 42, 44
Ommaya reservoir 165
operculum frontale 60
oscillating crystal 5

paracentral lobule 136
parasagittal view 16
pars centralis 40
periarteriitis nodosa 99
petrous bone 20, 85
phased array 5
piezo electric effect 3
pineal body 88
pineal region astrocytoma 30
pineal region meningioma 62
pineal region tumor 106
placement of burrhole 155
pons 14, 20, 58, 77, 85, 89, 109, 121
porencephaly 102
posterior cranial fossa 55
posterior fossa 20, 83
probe 4, 8, 9
puncture 166
puncturing channel 167
putamen 35
pyramid 58, 59

quadrigeminal cistern 17, 40, 77
quadrigeminal plate 62, 77
quartz 3

real time 3, 4
real time ultrasound echotomography 3
reflection 4
refraction 4
rolandic fissure 132
rotating crystal 5

sagittal sinus 140, 143
sagittal view 16
sector plane 11
sella turcica 53, 55, 67
septum pellucidum 4, 19, 40, 127, 168
shunt catheter 101, 107
shunt implantation 144
sphenoid body 31
sphenoid bone 77
sphenoid wing 35, 58, 67
splenium of corpus callosum 17, 88, 140
stereotactic techniques 152
subarachnoid hemorrhage 108, 109
sulcus, cingulate 17, 46, 135, 136
sulcus, paracentral 135, 136
superior frontal lobule 135
superior sagittal sinus 101
Sylvian cistern 111
Sylvian fissure 104

tentorial notch 62
tentorium 20, 30, 35, 44, 58, 61
thalamus 55, 77, 103, 104
third ventricle 19, 48, 58, 81, 107, 111, 168
tissue echo 4
transducer 5
trigonum 20, 77, 149
tumor 24
  cavity 150, 151

ultrasound beam 4
ultrasound frequency 6
ultrasound guided stereotaxy 152
ultrasound probe 4, 8, 9, 11
ultrasound waves 3
uncus 28, 95

ventricular bleeding 101
ventricular catheter 101, 107, 144, 145
ventricular tumor 78
vermis 14, 62, 77, 88

M. Samii, Hannover;
W. Draf, Fulda

Surgery of the Skull Base

An Interdisciplinary Approach

With a Chapter on Anatomy by J. Lang

1989. 512 pp. 289 figs. in 840 sep. illus. Hardcover
ISBN 3-540-18448-1

Contents: Surgery of the Anterior Skull Base: Surgery of Malformations of the Anterior Skull Base. - Surgery for Trauma to the Anterior Skull Base. - Surgery for Inflammatory Complications in the Region of the Anterior Skull Base. - Surgery of Space-Occupying Lesions of the Anterior Skull Base. - Surgery of Tumors of the Orbit and Adjacent Skull Base. - Special Operative Techniques. Surgery of the Middle Skull Base: Surgery of Traumatic Lesions of the Middle Skull Base. - Surgery of Inflammatory Disorders of the Middle Skull Base. Surgery of Space-Occupying Lesions of the Middle Skull Base. Surgery of the Posterior Skull Base: Surgery of the Internal Auditory Canal and Cerebellopontine Angle. - Surgery of Tumors of the Lateral Posterior Skull Base and Petrous Bone. - On the Problem of Paralytic Dysphagia Caused by Posterior Skull Base Tumors. Surgery of the Clivus: Introductory Remarks. - General Operative Techniques. Surgery of the Craniocervical Junction: Introductory Remarks. - Operative Technique. Surgery of the Facial Nerve and Skull Base: Introductory Remarks. - General Operative Technqiues. - Special Operative Techniques.

This is the first text to consider the skull base as a whole and from an interdisciplinary point of view. It analyzes the wide spectrum of pathological entities which can affect this crossroad region, including anomalies, traumatology, tumors and infectious processes.
The book considers general as well as specific surgical aspects and offers a wealth of excellent drawings and pictures to complement the text.
The reader will find himself equipped with a complete textbook on skull base surgery that emphasizes clinical applications and reflects valuable relevant experience from the fields of both ENT and neurosurgery.

Springer-Verlag
Berlin Heidelberg
New York London Paris
Tokyo Hong Kong

Springer

E. Kazner, S. Wende,
T. Grumme,
O. Stochdorph, R. Felix,
C. Claussen (Eds.)

Computed Tomography and Magnetic Resonance Tomography of Intracranial Tumors

A Clinical Perspective

2nd fully revised and expanded edition. 1989.
XIV, 685 pp. 738 figs. in 2993 sep. illus. Hardcover
ISBN 3-540-50576-8

This internationally recognized standard work on cerebral computer tomography has been completely revised and expanded to include magnetic resonance imaging. It systematically presents the clinical diagnosis and differential diagnosis of virtually all cerebral tumors. Cranial base and orbital lesions are also included. The authors' vast experience with CT and MRI in almost 10,000 cases of verified space-occupying lesions and orbital diseases lays a solid foundation for this second edition. The comprehensive illustrations include not just the typical, but also the rare tumors and atypical sites. The new WHO classification was used for the tumor categorization. The section on differential diagnosis offers complete coverage of all non-neoplastic, space-occupying intracranial lesions: inflammatory diseases, AIDS related diseases, acute demyelinization, granulomas, cysts, parasites, hemorrhages, vascular anomalies and brain infarctions.

Springer-Verlag
Berlin Heidelberg
New York London Paris
Tokyo Hong Kong

Springer

MIX
Papier aus verantwortungsvollen Quellen
Paper from responsible sources
FSC® C105338

If you have any concerns about our products,
you can contact us on
ProductSafety@springernature.com

In case Publisher is established outside the EU,
the EU authorized representative is:
Springer Nature Customer Service Center GmbH
Europaplatz 3, 69115 Heidelberg, Germany

Printed by Libri Plureos GmbH
in Hamburg, Germany